AF689520

Neocortical Modularity and the Cell Minicolumn

NEOCORTICAL MODULARITY AND THE CELL MINICOLUMN

MANUEL F. CASANOVA
EDITOR

Nova Biomedical Books
New York

Copyright © 2005 by Nova Science Publishers, Inc.

All rights reserved. No part of this book may be reproduced, stored in a retrieval system or transmitted in any form or by any means: electronic, electrostatic, magnetic, tape, mechanical photocopying, recording or otherwise without the written permission of the Publisher.

For permission to use material from this book please contact us:
Telephone 631-231-7269; Fax 631-231-8175
Web Site: http://www.novapublishers.com

NOTICE TO THE READER

The Publisher has taken reasonable care in the preparation of this book, but makes no expressed or implied warranty of any kind and assumes no responsibility for any errors or omissions. No liability is assumed for incidental or consequential damages in connection with or arising out of information contained in this book. The Publisher shall not be liable for any special, consequential, or exemplary damages resulting, in whole or in part, from the readers' use of, or reliance upon, this material.

This publication is designed to provide accurate and authoritative information with regard to the subject matter covered herein. It is sold with the clear understanding that the Publisher is not engaged in rendering legal or any other professional services. If legal or any other expert assistance is required, the services of a competent person should be sought. FROM A DECLARATION OF PARTICIPANTS JOINTLY ADOPTED BY A COMMITTEE OF THE AMERICAN BAR ASSOCIATION AND A COMMITTEE OF PUBLISHERS.

Library of Congress Cataloging-in-Publication Data
Neocortical modularity and the cell minicolumn / Manuel F. Casanova, editor.
p. cm.
Includes index.
ISBN 1-59454-301-1 (hardcover)
1. Neocortex. 2. Neurons. I. Casanova, Manuel F.
QP383.12.N465 2005
612.8'043--dc22 2005002276

Published by Nova Science Publishers, Inc. ✣ New York

CONTENTS

ACKNOWLEDGEMENTS

Many people have generously contributed of their time and energy to help us in editing this book. I am especially indebted to those academicians whose comments and insights helped chisel the biographical chapter on Vernon Mountcastle: Carlos Acuna, Robert Dykes, Kenneth Johnson, Hans Kornhuber, James Lynch, Edward Perl, and Gian Poggio. I am also grateful of the efforts from Nova Science Publishers for their editorial assistance.

Manuel F. Casanova, MD
Gottfried and Gisela Kolb Endowed Chair in Psychiatry
University of Louisville

INTRODUCTION

> Vernon Mountcastle, regarding his success in neurosciences: "For certainly much of what I have accomplished has been by the good fortune of being in a great institution and having first class colleagues...I think the answer is that given a certain level of competence, one has to be totally dedicated—and lucky!" (personal communication, 2004).

Many years ago the chess grandmaster Jose Raul Capablanca wrote an introductory textbook for his game. Contrary to previous authors who belabored the opening of the game, he emphasized the ending from the very first chapter. This approach received mixed reviews, as in this stage of the game, the outcome had usually been already decided. Mr. Capablanca, however, defended his approach. He explained that the endgame was purified to such an extent that only the essential elements remained, making piece–piece interactions more easily understood by the novice. Like Capablanca, neuropathologists approach their craft by learning the properties of the basic units before tackling more complicated tissue reactions. In effect, there is a covert understanding that observations on the morphology of cells provide a window to physiology in both health and disease.

Nature in its wisdom has simplified the job of the neuropathologist by limiting the number of ways a neuron may react to injury. Neurons are the most highly specialized cells of the body. Specialization, however, carries with it some dubious distinctions. As a jack–of–all–trades, the neuron ends up master of none. It may be said that a neuron has been so intensively "inbred" that it has lost some of its natural resistance to disease. Neurons therefore need help from outside sources to cope effectively with environmental exigencies. Among neurons' coping mechanisms are the blood brain barrier and the capacity of astrocytes to dispose of certain toxins. Furthermore, a neuron can only process information efficiently by deleting a large number of otherwise extraneous activities. Only primitive cells (e.g., tumor cells) exhibit such a variety of processes that confuses their internal logic and makes them react erratically.

In the case of the brain, many different lesions manifest the same patterns of cellular and tissue disruption. Hypoxia, hypoglycemia, infections, and trauma often produce homogenization (so called ischemic changes) of neurons. These cells stain more darkly, obscuring their individual elements. As a primary attempt to adapt to a particular stressor, the cell will repress its more highly differentiated functions, those that usually require a major amount of energy expenditure. The incapacitated cell becomes smaller (atrophic), somewhat triangular and shriveled. The neuropil, or the background of the gray matter, is pale staining. These changes, following dissimilar injuries, bear a temporal profile. After the first few hours of an insult, properly fixed neurons will exhibit microvacuolation of their somas. Homogenization of the cellular constituents is evident during the first day while an increase in microglia and early neuronophagia occurs after 48 hours. The end result is atrophy, cell loss, and gliosis. None of these changes characterize the pathology of mental illnesses.

Our everyday view of the world may not necessarily be the most comprehensive one. In this regard neuropathologists should temper opinions based on a limited representation of reality. Microscopy freezes in time a two-dimensional representation of a minute histological process. One must acquire knowledge of the physiology of the lesion before reaching a multidimensional diagnosis. In the case of mental disorders, the modular organization of the cortex may offer some clues to underlying etiology. It is tissue, rather than individual cells, that provides for the phenomena of perceptual binding and gamma frequencies. It is the continuous reentry of excitation into neuronal networks that provides for selective attention. The basis for language and its semantic content resides in the conjoint activation of topographically diverse brain regions. We may conclude that although molecular biologists placed the neuron on the rack and forced it to reveal its secrets, they learned very little about mental disorders.

Researchers may still wait to apply their molecular trade to single gene-dependent neuropsychiatric disorders. However, in clinical practice conditions such as Huntington's disease, familial Alzheimer's, and Zellweger's syndrome are few and far between. Still these conditions are not completely determined at the DNA level. Placing mice carrying the Huntington's gene in an enriched environment delays the onset of symptomatology. In similar fashion physical and mental exercise appears to protect against the ravaging effects of Alzheimer's disease. Possibly the most inheritable mental disorder is autism, with 92 % of monozygotic twins having a condition within the DSM spectrum of related disorders. Studies on the inheritance of autism suggest the involvement of three to ten genes. It has been proposed that mutations surpassing a threshold number of genes could cause classical autism, while a smaller number provides less significant deficits, e.g., social shyness or delays in language acquisition. It is mind-boggling the number of permutations (extreme coincidences) scientists quote to explain a condition as being completely determined by genes. There is something unsavory and inchoate about attempts to understand the brain/mind relationship based on complex statistical relationships between genes. These mathematical manipulations are subsumed under the euphemism of "genetic complexity," a clear evolutionary step from its predecessor the "Oh GOD" principle (One Gene, One Disease) and its parodies (one gene, one enzyme and one molecule, one postdoc). Genetic complexity views psychiatric illnesses as chimeras of molecular events. However, most neuropsychiatric conditions fall within the psychobiosocial framework of which genetics is only one aspect. Adolf Meyer would have stressed that mental conditions involve the whole person along with his/her environment.

Researchers should learn from the difficulty in targeting genes to create animal models with specific phenotypes. Generally, it is impossible to assess the impact of specific gene deletions on the phenotype/behavior of the animal. One of my favorite observations is the fact that within aligned regions, the genomes of chimpanzees and humans are almost identical. However, phenotypic and behavioral differences between these species are quite obvious. In surmising the recent surge of research in molecular biology and the corresponding scarcity of results, a geneticist may say that you need to break a few eggshells to make an omelet. Thus far we have been walking on egg shells and lost sight of the omelet.

Token physicalism is the view that each and every mental event is the result of a physical event, usually at the cellular or molecular level. It assumes that for every mental state there exists a set of physical causes that taken together produce that effect or even necessitate the same. The impracticability of such a view has only recently been realized. Take for example the paradigm shift in our perception of neuropharmacological interventions. With newer drugs only a small fraction of a given receptor occupancy correlates with maximum clinical response. The initial strategy of drug design based on targeting specific receptors has therefore yielded drugs that affect various combinations of adrenergic, dopaminergic, serotonergic, and histaminergic receptors. Thus, the systemic approach that escapes the molecular level of resolution has proven to be more successful in neuropharmacology. The relevance of a molecular event to the clinical applications of a specific disease may be of use in conditions due to bacteria and viruses. Thus far this medical model has failed to explain psychiatric disorders.

I have never heard a psychiatric patient complain of abnormalities in his/her dopamine receptor or second messenger system. I have never heard of a psychiatrist treating a patient based on the insertion of double-stranded DNA into a plasmid. Outside of psychiatry, even the 20 or so clinical trials of gene therapy in cystic fibrosis have found no or little effect of the inserted gene. The vectors used in these experiments have produced more side effects than benefits. However, both the failures and side effects may all be related to genetic engineering problems that may be overcome in the future. The problem is whether we have learned enough from these trials and at what expense.

Higher levels of resolution simplify the analysis of molecular interactions but fail to reflect the complexity ingrained in psychiatric symptoms. An intermediate level of resolution lying between the realm of cells and organs (Figure 1) may more suitably explain complex and disturbing behaviors. Unfortunately, neuroscience textbooks cover only half of the field, emphasizing manifestations within a reductionistic scale. Different chapters offer a collage of molecular events, scattered attention to neuronal nets, and hardly a mention of either mini- or macrocolumns. The attention paid to the neuron at the expense of modular arrangements is an atavism tantamount to chronological snobbery. This lack of acknowledgment is more perplexing when considering the range of complexity exhibited by the arrangement between and within cortical modules. In effect, modular abnormalities could explain a cornucopia of pathologies capable of dwarfing the limited response of the single neuron. It is by looking outside of the neuron that we may answer the pathological riddle of mental disorders.

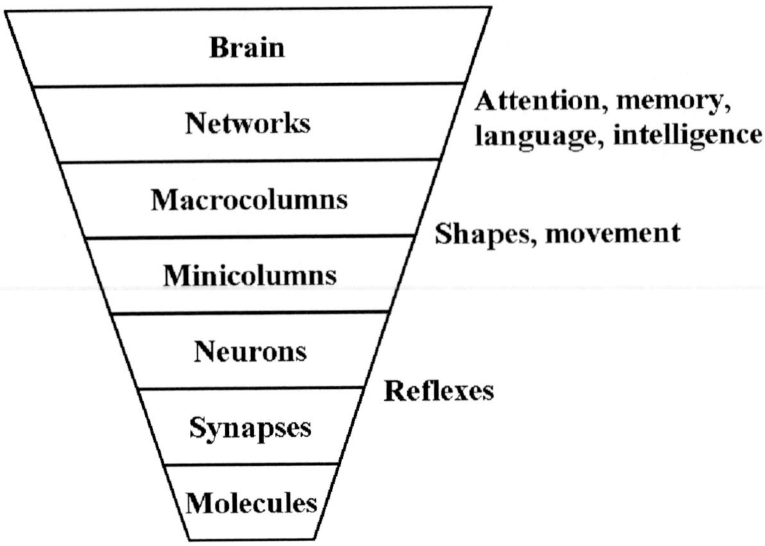

Figure 1.

It has been my intent in editing this book to focus on the lowest hierarchical element within the modular organization of the brain: the cell minicolumn. The minicolumn is a self-contained ecosystem of neurons and their connections that repeats itself throughout the extent of the neocortex. Although a few neuroanatomists at the turn of the century called attention to the vertical arrangement of the cortex, Vernon Mountcastle provided physiological proof in the 1950's for its existence and its role in perception. I feel an affinity for Dr. Mountcastle. We constantly deal in our writings with similar problems but from different perspectives. Initially, reading Mountcastle was akin to performing mental gymnastics. You do not read Mountcastle in a hurry. You have to be prepared to frequently reread a paragraph. Over time, however, my understanding of Mountcastle's work has flourished into reverence. My appreciation of minicolumns is now a mosaic of facts that makes sense of most neuroscience. A deaf person can't appreciate the beauty of Beethoven's symphonies anymore than minicolumnar illiterates can understand neuroscience.

Mountcastle is an outsized character that marched to his own beat. Never the person he "ought" to be, he was never boxed into preconceived ideas. This character trait was of immense help throughout his research career: Having no shoulders to stand on, he set his own goals and built upon his strengths. He aspired to an objective truth, the Holy Grail of neurosciences. In his search he overcame narrowness of scientific vision and became an heir to Socrates. While others went for easily accessible and exploitable prizes, Mountcastle claimed no glory, no acclaim. Personally he treated others by the categorical imperative: with respect and dignity as ends in themselves. He is a unique individual: We can't exchange Mountcastle for someone else and have an equal. At 85 years of age he presently pursues research with the same enthusiasm of his younger days. Therefore, I have devoted this book to Mountcastle, his life and scientific work.

In: Neocortical Modularity and the Cell Minicolumn
Editor: Manuel F. Casanova, pp. 1-13
ISBN 1-59454-301
© 2005 Nova Science Publishers, Inc.

Chapter I

VERNON B. MOUNTCASTLE: A LIFE THAT TRANSFORMED THE NEUROSCIENCES

Manuel F. Casanova*
University of Louisville, Louisville, KY

> "I discovered in the heavens many things that had not been seen before our own age. The novelty of these things, as well as some consequences which followed from them in contradiction to the physical notions commonly held among academic philosophers, stirred up against me no small number of professors—as if I had placed these things in the sky with my own hands in order to upset Nature and overturn the sciences."
> *Galileo Galilei, Letter to Grand Duchess Cristina, 1615* [1].

NEUROSCIENCE AT MID-TWENTIETH CENTURY

In the mid-20th century, neuroscientists intensified efforts to assemble the workings of the brain with its social and humanistic functions. They also broadened their inquiry: by including nonhuman species, they made new discoveries about the nerve impulses in peripheral tracts—cranial and spinal areas. By mid-century, probes had extended deep into the brain, made possible by invention of the stereotaxic apparatus.

Ramón y Cajal had applied morphological techniques to the cerebral cortex—the highest and most elaborate part of the brain. His work revealed precisely the interconnections between groups of individual nerve cells. Extending Cajal's insights, Vernon B. Mountcastle along with David Hubel and Torsten Wiesel used modern cell physiological techniques, studying not only how the nervous system is put together but how it works. They showed how links between neurons filter and transform sensory information on the way to and within

* Corresponding author: Manuel F. Casanova, MD, Gottfried and Gisela Kolb Endowed Chair in Psychiatry, University of Louisville, Department of Psychiatry, 500 South Preston St., A Bldg., Rm. 217; Louisville, KY 40292. Tel: (502)852-4077; Fax: (502)852-4078; E-mail: M0CASA02@louisville.edu

the cortex, that the cortex is grouped into functional sections or modules, and that experience can change this organization.

The Breadth of Mountcastle's Contributions

Mountcastle focused his particular research interests on the central neural mechanisms in perception, intentionality—or decision-making, and the higher functions of the brain. He has contributed to understanding brain function in four major areas: the organization of sensory systems and cerebral cortex, the neural mechanisms of information processing in sensory systems—the way the body registers sensations like touch and pain felt in shallow and deep surface areas, the ways in which neural events in sensory systems of primates—experiences recorded on the brain—affect the way they interpret sensations, and the cortical mechanisms of perception.

MOUNTCASTLE'S PERSONAL HISTORY

Vernon B. Mountcastle, Jr., was born in 1918 in Shelbyville, Kentucky, into a family of farmers from a long line of Virginians. His father was a railroad contractor and his mother a one-time teacher. The family soon moved back to Virginia. There, Mountcastle recalls, his mother treated him and his siblings as students, asking them to repeat their school lessons to her. In the process Vernon learned to read and write by the age of four. He attended primary and secondary schools in Roanoke, Virginia, from 1925–1935. He recalls growing up with "a marvelous group of twelve boys" within a few blocks of his home. "Their homes were all open," he recalls, forming "one great big family, producing empathy between people. It was an extraordinary time to grow up." Mountcastle goes back several times a year, joking, "You mustn't tell anyone you're a Virginian because people will be embarrassed that they're not."

In 1935 he enrolled in Roanoke College in Salem, Virginia, during the depths of the Depression. It was, he recalls, "a wonderful college with wonderful teachers and only 5–7 people" in his classes. He earned his B.S. in Chemistry with Honors in 1938. Influenced by a chemistry professor with a Ph.D. from Johns Hopkins, Mountcastle then applied to the Johns Hopkins Medical School, which accepted him. He doesn't recall reasons for his interest in medicine: his family had no doctors, no professional people. Moreover, he had never been out of the state, and his mother objected to his "going to school with Yankees."

At Johns Hopkins, then struggling through the Depression, the teachers accepted the students—only 75 of them—as fellows. His introductory class in anatomy was taught by "great teachers" such as Marion Hines and Sarah Tower. They were productive experimentalists, who taught from that viewpoint. Mountcastle recalls that while attending neuroanatomy several times a week, the teachers sat by students and taught them neuroanatomy by examining serial sections of the human brain. Arnold Rich in Pathology was "one of the best brains Johns Hopkins ever had." Warfield Longcope, the Director of Medicine, was a "great influence," providing the most intensive learning experience of his life, which came during the Medicine Quarter in the third year of medical school. It was total immersion: 24 patients, 5 students, 1 assistant resident, 2 interns, and a visiting physician—Maxwell Wintrobe.

Mountcastle has half-jokingly termed Johns Hopkins "a conceited place" whose internal mystique plays an important role in the development of young people. To "become something good," they must live up to it. He recalls Philip Bard's greatness in neurophysiology, his belief that teaching should be "personal." He also recalls the heavy influence of Dr. Alfred Blalock, who arrived when Mountcastle was a junior. "I had the most fantastic experience," Mountcastle recalls.

> "I felt that I was welcomed into a society of scholars. For example, we never got any grades. I learned later that there was a very detailed grading of everything. But you were never told. And that produced a fantastic atmosphere. You never felt that you were competing with another student; you were competing with the subject."

Mountcastle earned his M.D. in 1942 and interned in Surgery at the Johns Hopkins Hospital, July 1942–1943. He then served in the U.S. Naval Amphibious Forces for three years, with two major campaigns in the European Theater: Anzio, Italy, and Normandy, France. After the war ended, he married Nancy Clayton Pierpont in September, 1945. Three children followed: Vernon B. Mountcastle III in 1947; Anne Clayton Mountcastle (Bainbridge) in 1948; and George Earle Pierpont Mountcastle in 1949 (deceased in 1969). He now has six grandchildren.

After the war, in July, 1946, Mountcastle's future was "up for grabs." Since Johns Hopkins' School of Medicine emphasized clinical medicine and surgery, Mountcastle never considered going into neuroscience. He returned to Johns Hopkins, hoping to work with the surgeon Dr. Walter Dandy, a "distant figure." At that time, he recalls, Dandy had "magic." It was said, "God whispers in his ear." Dandy was a glamorous figure at the apogee of his career when he died in 1946. In Mountcastle's opinion he was "a bit behind the times" and less advanced than such figures as Penfield. However, he had developed ways of doing surgery very well and possessed great manual dexterity. Along with Frank Ford, an "exceptional teacher," he created an interest Mountcastle never lost. Dr. Blalock suggested Vernon pursue a residency with Dr. Woodall at Duke, who suggested, in turn, he spend a year with Bard. "If Bard will have you around for a year, you can have my residency." Mountcastle recalls his subsequent discussion with Bard:

> Bard: Regarding motion sickness, do you know of any psychosocial implications?
> Mountcastle: No.
> Bard: You can come.

Mountcastle accepted a year's appointment as a postdoctoral fellow working under Bard, waiting for a job to open in physiology. He recalls that in the late 1940s, Bard relied on his own great skill and experience in simply observing behavior. This was just when others (e.g., Harlow, Pribram) were developing objective methods for measuring changes in behavior, which Bard never took up. While Bard worked on the motor system, his discoveries were anatomical not physiological. Mountcastle stayed as a postdoc with Bard, being paid as he worked without needing to publish. After working only six months, he became aware that both Bard and the dean knew he was there: both thought Mountcastle was "better than *I* thought I was," he recalls. Rather than trying to teach his students anything directly, Bard gave his students confidence they could discover things; they responded by trying to live up to his belief in them.

Modern research on the role of the cerebral cortex in somatic sensation had begun in the Johns Hopkins Department of Physiology in the 1930s, with the work of Phillip Bard and Clinton Woolsey. Phillip Bard was 34 years old and an Assistant Professor in the Harvard Medical School Department of Physiology when he was called to chair the Department of Physiology at Johns Hopkins. Soon after arriving, he teamed up with Clinton Woolsey and Wade Marshall. Using gross electrophysiological recording techniques developed by Marshall and a strategy developed by Woolsey, these three young men discovered that the body surface of monkeys was systematically represented on the surface of the brain [2]. This was soon confirmed in humans by the Canadian neurosurgeon, Wilder Penfield. His work proved that not only monkeys but each of us has within our brain a naked representation of our own body, the closest thing to our true self-image [3].

Penfield's remarkable discovery raised a number of issues. Somatic sensation is not unitary; rather, it is comprised of several distinct sensations called *submodalities*. We can, for example, readily distinguish pressure on deep tissue from a light touch on the skin. However, the maps for these deep and surface submodalities appeared to fit together. Clearly, with the relatively gross techniques used by Marshall, Woolsey and Bard—techniques that averaged the responses from thousands of nerve cells—some critical dimension in the map was overlooked.

The particular question of submodality perception was tackled in 1948 by Mountcastle, Bard's most gifted student. Mountcastle did his first microelectrode experiment in 1949 and published his first paper in 1954. Otherwise, he had worked in electrophysiological experiments from 1946 on with gross electrode recording methods. He has written, "How we apprehend objects and events in the world around us and how they are represented in our brains are continuing themes in man's endeavor to understand himself"—and might have added, in his own research. He understood that we experience the outside world through our five senses: touch-pressure (and the related skin or somatic sensations), sight, hearing, taste, and smell. After the appropriate receptors analyze each sensation, lower relay stages code it. Based on our experiences with similar sensations, the cerebral cortex creates a meaningful image of it. Mountcastle had soon realized the value of cellular techniques that became available in the late 1940s. These procedures might help him detect new dimensions in the map of the somatic sensory system that eluded the gross recording techniques used by Bard and his colleagues.

This task required a number of major technical innovations, including new microelectrodes to precisely quantify natural stimuli—innovations to which Mountcastle contributed importantly. Other tools developed in the 1960s contributed to Mountcastle's insights. Mountcastle's laboratory was one of the first privileged to use one of the first 12 LINC computers developed at MIT's Lincoln Laboratory. Incredibly basic by today's standards, it represented (according to former postdoc James Lynch) a great advance over the large racks of relays that investigators had previously used to control experimental paradigms and the cumbersome photographic techniques used to record single-neuron data. In addition, to successfully isolate the relatively small neurons found in association cortex for lengthy periods, Mountcastle, in conjunction with John Chubbuck at the Johns Hopkins Applied Physics Laboratory, was developing a microdrive that used a special stepping motor to control the movement of the microelectrode far more smoothly and precisely than any previous microdrive design made possible. In addition, the microdrive's hermetically sealed chamber minimized the arterial pulsations of the brain.

Dr. Hideo Sakata recalls that Mountcastle "stuck to quantitative analysis as far as possible," (personal communication, June 9, 2003). Yet the detailed protocols of previous experiments were "full of descriptions of observations that could not be expressed in numbers." Mountcastle once told Sakata, "Quantitative study is important but it is more valuable to find a qualitative difference."

With these tools in hand—tools that formed the basis of modern cortical physiology—Mountcastle addressed the question of submodality specificity. He found that gross recordings at the cellular level missed a segregation of submodalities within all areas of the somatic sensory system. First, he found that single nerve cells respond specifically either to superficial touch stimuli or to deep pressure stimuli, but almost never to both. Second, he found that cells responding to one submodality were located together and segregated from cells responding to other submodalities.

Mountcastle found the most fascinating example of segregation in the cortex. His early research led to one of the central ideas in the functioning of the brain—the organization of the cerebral cortex into computational modules consisting of vertical columns of nerve cells, now called minicolumns or microcolumns. Within them can be seen layers. That is, neurons are arranged vertically like strings of pearls, with several hundred million of these columns bundled together. Within sensory cortex each column is submodality-specific, e.g., all the cells in a column receive information from a particular point on the skin and from a particular class of receptors, either superficial or deep.

Thus, each region of the skin projects to a particular area of the cortex, and the separate receptor classes are distributed in adjacent columns. The cortex uses the distribution of neurons in columns to handle different functions for the same small region of the body map. Each column is an integrating unit, or logical module, comprising thousands of neurons. It forms the initial stage in the cortex for elaborating sensory experience into consciousness. Mountcastle's technique involved opening the skulls of anesthetized cats and making microelectrode penetrations through the depth of the cortex. He then tested the responses of neurons related to the skin by moving hairs or manipulating the skin, deep tissues, and joints of the experimental animals—a process he called a "combined experiment."

Mountcastle described the experimental design used to investigate the neural coding problem in his 1968 study [2] of the neural mechanisms of the perception of vibratory stimuli. The general form of the design, which is used universally, is the following:

Identify a form of behavior that is well matched to the neural mechanisms of interest.

Design psychophysical experiments to obtain a quantitative characterization of that behavior over a wide range of stimulus conditions.

Use exactly the same experimental conditions in neurophysiological experiments to obtain a complete characterization of the neural activity that underlines the observed behavior.

"Inquire which quantitative aspects of the neural response tally with psychophysical measurements" [3]—i.e., advance all the plausible hypotheses and eliminate them one by one until a single hypothesis remains or another experiment is required to further reduce the possibilities.

At the time Mountcastle had not read Lorente de Nó's "Cerebral cortex, architecture, intracortical connections, motor programs" first published in nineteen thirty-eight. Lorente had earlier referred to the "vertical cylinders of cells" and was perhaps the first to assign them a basic physiological role:

> "All the elements of the cortex are represented in it, and therefore it may be called an elementary unit, in which, theoretically, the whole process of transmission of impulses from the afferent fiber to the efferent axon may be accomplished" [4].

The "bombshell" insight that neurons were arranged the same from top to bottom of the cortex came to Mountcastle independently from looking at the data exhaustively. Most important about his experimental technique, he had discovered that one could carry out his tests simultaneously in a waking primate.

Although two colleagues worked with him on his experiment, they refused to put their names on an article on columnar structure. Thus, he got full credit—and blame—for authoring the breakthrough article, "Modality and topographic properties of single neurons of cat's somatic sensory cortex" (1957). One of his postdocs during this period, Kenneth Johnson, recalls Tom Powell, his collaborator of the late 1950s, telling him that Vernon was ridiculed mercilessly over the columnar hypothesis by almost all neuroanatomists. It is clear, however, that such responses were driven by strong emotion from personal feelings about Mountcastle's personality and previous interactions with him. Thus, while attending a meeting of the American Federation of Biological Societies in 1967 or 1968 after a student had given a 10-minute oral presentation, Mountcastle stood up and destroyed the entire basis of the presentation. The student's professor tried to come to his defense but fared no better. The talk was seriously flawed. The questions could have been couched more diplomatically. Nevertheless, some researchers never forgot their utter public embarrassment. Instead of taking the positive side of the criticism and growing from the experience, they muttered at his back their own shortcomings and lack of insight. Anyone siding with Mountcastle was debased as being eccentric. "Minicolumns are figments of the old-man's imagination," was said.

Edward O. Wilson remarked in his book *The Diversity of Life* on the problems of getting ideas accepted by fellow scientists:

> "First rule of the history of science: when a big new, persuasive idea is proposed, an army of critics soon gathers and tries to tear it down. Such a reaction is unavoidable because, aggressive yet abiding by the rules of civil discourse, this is simply how scientists work. It is further true that faced with adversity proponents will harden their

> resolve and struggle to make the case more convincing. Being human, most scientists conform to the psychological Principle of Certainty, which says that when there is evidence for and against a belief, the result is not a lessening but a heightening of convictions on both sides...Rule number two: the new idea will, like mother earth, take some serious hits. If good it will survive, probably in modified form." [6]

Similarly, in his own vindication, Mountcastle quotes Zeki:

> "When confronted with a difficult problem which goes against their way of thinking, scientists often begin by shutting their eyes firmly to the evidence and pretending that it does not exist. The next stage consists of accepting the evidence but pretending that it is not important or that it can be adequately explained by the known facts. The third and final stage consists of admitting the evidence and its significance, but pretending that it has all been said before" [7].

Despite mounting criticism Mountcastle proceeded to use the method of single neuron analysis to explore the dynamic neuronal operations in the somatic afferent system, seeing how they relate to somatic sensory performance. He discovered that he could do this by direct, simultaneous application of the methods and concepts of psychophysics and neurophysiology. He applied them together with new methods for studying the higher functions of the brain in awake, performing, nonhuman primates. James Lynch recalls a major discovery never observed before: neuronal activity was not only related to somatosensory stimuli but was strongly modulated by whether or not the monkey was *interested* in a given stimulus at a given moment.

This general method is now a widely used, highly productive method in CNS sensory physiology. Mountcastle's series of investigations led to the emergence of a general principle: the relation of the observer, monkey or human, to events in the external world varies along quantitative continua. They are set by the transducing properties of the receptors and first-order fibers engaged by the stimuli—that is, conversion of a signal from one form to another. Subsequently, the relation of performance to central neural events varies along a linear continuum. Research has since confirmed this generalization for a number of somesthetic submodalities.

By the mid-1950s, Mountcastle had begun contributing chapters to texts edited by others. Then, in 1962, with *Interhemispheric Relations and Cerebral Dominance* (JHU Press), he began editing volumes to which he contributed numerous chapters. His handbook writing has continued after retirement from active laboratory research. Looking back, Mountcastle has credited writing textbook chapters on neurophysiology with helping his research. If one writes on a field, he has to understand it. Because handbooks involve a compendium of knowledge for other investigators, he needed to work hard on them. He enjoyed that, he has said, and learned a lot. He particularly recalls a "most interesting" experience with Fred Plum, whom he has praised as "really a scholar," while writing a *Handbook of Physiology*, Vol. V, on The Higher Functions of the Nervous System [5]. He enjoyed encompassing a subject, learning to "know as much as you can about it."

Mountcastle found editing a journal less stimulating but "someone has to do it." Referring to the straightforward rigor required by the job, he has said an editor "must bite the bullet to say what the truth about a subject is." As a result of his efforts as an editor, and the distinguished editors who followed him (John Brookhart and Edward Evarts), the *Journal of Neurophysiology* now may be the most distinguished journal in the field.

Also, in the 1950s bright young people began gathering around him. He considered his postdocs more as mature, accomplished investigators than as students, training more than 50 of them in the course of his career. At least half of them had a degree of experience, and half of them became professors (32 of the 50 at last count). Gian Poggio, who joined Mountcastle in 1957 and remained at Johns Hopkins, comments on his willingness "to help with constructive criticisms, and to share his vast and deep knowledge of brain functions." Hans Helmut Kornhuber (personal communication; June 2, 2003) worked with Mountcastle in 1965, becoming Professor and Head of the Department of Neurology of Ulm University in 1966. He praises his mentor's "exactness, reliability, a real researcher, nobility."

Kenneth Johnson, who worked with him between 1965 and 1970, says, "Everyone who has known Vernon well has trouble describing him succinctly." He remarks on Mountcastle's "seriousness of purpose," his enormous productivity, his willingness to tackle new, uncharted territory, his ability to assemble the diverse literature on a new subject and combine it with experiments to produce order and new insights: "his more fundamental contribution in [Johnson's] view is the intellectual and empirical standard that he set for the field in his papers of the 1950s, '60s, and '70s. No conclusion was based on anecdotal observation," (personal communication; June 17, 2003).

Robert Dykes worked with him during the same period—the later 1960s, saying, "His example was a rigorous model of an extremely careful analytical approach to all aspects of science, from the way he analyzes published data to the meticulousness with which he prepares his recording electrodes.... He sets extremely high standards for himself and expects the same of others around him," (personal communication, June 9, 2003).

Carlos Acuña, who spent a year with him in 1970, sums up Mountcastle's contributions:

> "Through carefully designed combined behavioral and electrophysiological experiments, Mountcastle has established a well documented correlation between psychophysics and neural activity. In doing this, he paved the way to the study of brain mechanisms in higher functions. In fact, many people around the world are using the conceptual and experimental approaches he designed in the '70s. Although this approach can be traced to Jasper and other researchers, it was Mountcastle who refined it and took it to a new level of excellence," (personal communication; June 10, 2003).

Sociologists have considered why gifted scientists often train other exceptional scientists: they can teach their junior colleagues the importance of working on really significant problems. They also offer resources and visibility, and make important channels of communication available to their students. At the same time, they must rein in their own ambition and unreservedly encourage the creativity of their gifted young colleagues. Along with this goes building around them an exciting environment filled with gifted peers. This must be an environment where important science is routinely done, because it is consciously structured around one or more absolutely central ideas.

In this regard, Mountcastle has claimed he's "had fun all his life." He has pointed to the importance of playing with ideas, letting them bounce around. He also mentions a habit of mind, accepting willingly and gratefully the criticisms of one's colleagues—how they react to what you're saying. Thus, exceptional scientists combine a remarkable intuition of what is important in their field with an almost childlike enjoyment of the day-to-day experimental and intellectual activity of science. They enjoy day-to-day science as a satisfying end in itself, an ever-changing intellectual adventure.

Eric Kandel has placed Mountcastle's discoveries in a larger social context, commenting on the way small groups in a university shape social contexts to make them conducive to creativity. The special nature of his contribution, along with that of David Hubel and Torsten Wiesel, who built upon Mountcastle's discoveries, was fostered by the particular collegial environment to which they belonged. They, in turn, restructured their environment anew, so as to foster creative activity in their younger colleagues. Kandel has singled out the Department of Physiology at Johns Hopkins and the Department of Neurobiology at Harvard as laudable aspects of academic life. They were most conducive for the establishment of a powerful intellectual environment that was resistant to both external and administrative pressure. This environment is at once sensitive to a historical perspective while at the same time encouraging the emergence of novel and important ideas, Kandel has said.

Midway through his second decade at Johns Hopkins, Mountcastle assumed administrative responsibilities. Having achieved the rank of professor in 1959, he succeeded Bard as director of the Department of Physiology in 1964, a position he held for 17 years. He also took on the editorship of Bard's distinguished *Textbook of Physiology*. At the time, he recounts, great trust existed between the clinical departments. He would be happy, he said, if the future of physiology were put in the hands of the basic science and clinical departments, who had great concern for the welfare of researchers and wanted them to succeed. He enjoyed the opportunity to create new things, he has said, such as the creation of departments of clinical neurology (headed by Guy McGhann), of neuroengineering (directed by Richard Johns) and neuroscience (directed by Solomon Snyder). He also helped gain support for two endowed chairs in Neurology and for the Bard Lectureship.

In the late 1960s Mountcastle's research focus evolved. As Kenneth Johnson puts it:

> "He had discovered the columnar organization of the brain about a decade earlier but he referred to that as a static property of the brain. He was much more interested in what he called its dynamic properties—how it works. The combination of psychophysics and neurophysiology was essentially a study of neural coding—how the brain represents, processes, and deciphers information," (personal communication; June 17, 2003).

Mountcastle quickly decided to search for more precise correlations between elementary neuronal processes and complex perceptual phenomena outside the post central somatic cortex. He grappled with a challenging problem: neurons of the primary somatic cortex responded in a stereotyped fashion to mechanical stimulation applied to the glabrous skin of the hand, whether or not the monkey detected such stimulation. This lack of correlation led him to study the parietal cortex, which human neurological observations indicated was a possible site for such a correlation.

He was one of the first to demonstrate the presence within the parietal lobes of neuronal mechanisms related to the perception of the animal's extrapersonal space, and the coordinated movement of his eyes and hands within that space. Thanks to a very fine series of experiments, Mountcastle elaborated the idea of a congruent development of a "neural apparatus for the integration and governance of those operations."

Mountcastle realized that in order to understand the highly discriminative capacities of sensory systems, he needed to go beyond a simple static analysis of the connections between the peripheral apparatus and its central projection. He focused on describing the dynamic aspects of the sensory system, laying stress on the role played by afferent inhibition in the discrimination of place and quality. In doing so, Mountcastle distinguished importantly between two components in the somatic afferent system, the "lemniscal" component and the "extra-lemniscal" component. A remarkable specificity for place and an equally precise specificity for quality characterize the lemniscal component of the somatic afferent system, which conveys distinct reports about discriminative aspects of the somatic sensation. By contrast, the extra-lemniscal component carries information concerning pain and temperature, as well as some diffuse tactile information.

The lemniscal system includes the superficial cutaneous receptors and the "deep" receptors subserving joint position and rotation. It projects, through already identified relays, onto the post-central gyrus of the cerebral cortex where a map-like representation of the body is found. The neurons of the cortex, which receive signals from both types of receptors, are grouped into separate columns of cells vertically oriented across the cortical layers. Each cell of such a vertical column is related to nearly the same small region of the body, and all are activated by stimuli of the same quality. The columns are therefore the elementary units which compose the cortical map. As Mountcastle has said: "The overall representational pattern within the post-central gyrus is thus composed of an intricately fitted mosaic of vertical units." Robert Dykes, a Mountcastle postdoc between 1966 and 1971, has commented,

> "Although it is harder to grasp as a single concept, Dr Mountcastle was a pioneer in the description of the relationships between neural function and perception. His elegant experiments showed, in a number of different ways that there was a precise and generally quantitative relationship between neural activity and a particular sensory experience, whether the neural response was found in the peripheral nerve or in the cerebral cortex." (personal communication, June 9, 2003)

An incident and a mystery in Mountcastle's life seem intertwined. "The greatest shock in his life was the unfortunate death of one of his sons [George Earle]" in 1969 at the age of 20, a former postdoc H.H. Kornhuber has commented. By that time Mountcastle had fully established himself as a researcher, administrator, and authority on neurophysiology. The mystery was Mountcastle's failure to receive the Nobel Prize, first, in 1981, when Hubel and Wiesel each received a quarter of the Prize for their discoveries concerning information processing in the visual system. Given the close relationship of Hubel and Wiesel's work to his own, many have questioned Mountcastle's omission.

When questioned in 1981 by others puzzled that the Nobel Prize had passed Mountcastle, a former postdoc detected a deep reservoir of resentment toward him by peers and colleagues, particularly in his age group and including contacts in Sweden. It became clear to him that Mountcastle's high professional standards and public criticism of scientists had alienated many who did not forget what they perceived as public tongue lashings or pointed criticisms of their work (*vide supra*). At least to some extent, this observer blamed the resistance and rejection of Mountcastle's work on his tendency to bluntly comment on the work of others publicly and privately. Parallels between Mountcastle and Galileo suggest themselves: both men were trailblazers, both resented by contemporaries for their discoveries, and both strikingly unable to suffer fools gladly. James Lynch (personal communication; October 23, 2003) has encapsulated Mountcastle's persona as "the epitome of the classic Virginia gentleman—always polite and soft-spoken, but with a will of steel."

The death of Mountcastle's son shortly thereafter has been described by a former postdoc as a "pivotal event in his life," making him "more accepting of the failings and foibles of others." When the immediate shock passed, those around him found him much more approachable than he had been before. With the death of his son, some found his personal interactions with others more nuanced, making him more approachable, writes the same source.

Vernon Mountcastle's research over the last third of his experimental career from the mid-1970s on constituted the first major neurophysiological study of higher function—i.e., function in cerebral cortex beyond the purely sensory and motor areas. These include the analysis of the flow of information from skin to the cerebral cortex; a correlation between cellular responses and perception; and more recently, a study of the mechanisms underlying attention and the control of purposeful movements. Posterior parietal lesions in humans have no effect on basic sensory discriminative capacity, but they have a profound effect on attention, perception, and action in extrapersonal space on the opposite side of the lesion—a syndrome called contralateral neglect. Mountcastle published his first paper in this series in 1975 and summed up the entire experimental series in 1995. In his typical way, Mountcastle applied quantitative methods to thousands of neurons and turned what had been unknown into something that was known. He opened the field for all to follow. The effects of attention on neuronal responses in parietal cortex and the function of parietal cortex as a sensorimotor interface is now a major research field. Most important, this research led the way to neurophysiological studies of all higher brain function.

In 1981 Mountcastle was named University Professor of Neuroscience and from 1980 to 1989 director of the Philip Bard Laboratories of Neurophysiology, a subdivision of the Department of Neuroscience He was also partly instrumental in establishing the Johns Hopkins Mind-Brain Institute, located on the arts and sciences campus. He retired from active laboratory work in 1992 and has since engaged in writing monographs. His first one, *Perceptual Neuroscience* was published in 1998 by Harvard University Press. Still active at 85, he has just finished a second monograph, *The Primate Hand as Perceptual Organ,* scheduled to appear in late 2004 or early 2005.

In the 1970s Mountcastle moved to a seven-acre country place in northern Virginia, with a swimming pool and 12 Arabian horses. He lists his indoor hobbies as reading English literature and history, though he considers himself more an outdoors man devoted to tennis and horse riding. He likes living where he can ride freely, acknowledging his wife "was the better rider." He experienced his greatest sense of freedom riding a horse while snow lay on the ground, a feeling "close to paradise." Regretfully, he gave up riding horses at age 84: "old bones do not heal readily!" He always enjoyed playing tennis with younger people, feeling one must first become a good tennis player to become a good researcher: "In tennis, one can work out all your angers and frustrations without harming anyone."

Those students fortunate enough to study as postdocs under Mountcastle's direction often mention the warmth and generosity he displayed toward them. Dr. Sakata considers him "the dearest friend and teacher for me, almost like my father in neuroscience, always encouraging me, caring about my research and appreciating my new findings."

Robert Dykes has emphasized Mountcastle's role as a role model: "He has had a decidedly positive effect upon my career by setting an example of very high academic and scientific standards. Having him as an example of a good scientist gave me confidence as a young scientist to take the time and to do things a bit differently than others."

At the turn of the century, Mountcastle sees neuroscience in its glory but facing major problems. Molecular neuroscience as a method has attracted all the bright young people, he thinks, and created a new fund of knowledge. It is also much easier than studying systems, which has a terrific future, he believes, but an endeavor which is having difficulty attracting the best people. The true amalgamation of that area is basic neurophysiology. The most successful kind of lab in the future will focus on perception, Mountcastle predicts.

He has published monographs, textbooks, and more than 100 papers and has received a number of honorary awards, among them six honorary degrees. Mountcastle's awards include, but are not limited to, the Lashley Prize from the American Philosophical Society, the Schmitt Prize and Medal from the Massachusetts Institute of Technology, the Horowitz Prize from Columbia University, the Lasker Award, the National Medal of Science, the McGovern Medal and Prize from the American Association for the Advancement of Science, the Sherrington Gold Medal, the Helmholtz Medal, the Zotterman Prize, the Australia Prize, and the Cajal Award.

REFERENCES

[1] Sobel S. *Galileo's Daughter*. New York, NY: Penguin Books; 2000.

[2] Talbot WH, Darian-Smith I, Kornhuber HH, Mountcastle VB. The sense of flutter-vibration: comparison of the human capacity with the response patterns of mechanoreceptive afferents from the monkey's hand. *Journal of Neurophysiology*. 1968;31:301-334.

[3] Mountcastle VB, Poggio GF, Werner G. The relation of thalamic cell response to peripheral stimuli varied over an intensive continuum. *Journal of Neurophysiology*. 1963;26:807-834. Cited by: Mountcastle VB. *Perceptual Neuroscience: The Cerebral Cortex*. Cambridge, MA: Harvard University Press; 1998.

[4] Lorente de Nó R. Cerebral Cortex Architecture, intracranial connections, motor projections. In: Fulton JF, ed. *Physiology of the Nervous System*. Oxford, UK: Oxford University Press; 1938.

[5] Mountcastle VB. The higher functions of the nervous system (volume V). In: Mountcastle VB, Geiger SR, eds; Plum F, volume ed. *Handbook of Physiology:A Critical, Comprehensive Presentation of Physiological Knowledge and Concepts, Section I: The Nervous System*. Bethesda, MD: American Physiological Society; 1987.

[6] Wilson EO. *The Diversity of Life.* New York, NY: W.W. Norton; 1993.
[7] Zeki S. *A Vision of the Brain.* Oxford: Blackwell; 1993:87. Quoted by: Mountcastle VB. *Perceptual Neuroscience: The Cerebral Cortex.* Cambridge, MA: Harvard; 1998.

ACKNOWLEDGEMENTS

The author wishes to acknowledge the following helpful documents and contributions:

American Association of Neurological Surgeons. *Vernon B. Mountcastle, M.D.* [videotape]. Rolling Meadows, IL: AANS; 1993. Leaders in Neuroscience Series.

Eccles JC. Nobel Nomination: Scientific Contributions of Vernon B. Mountcastle. January, 1986.

Imbert M. International Prize of the Fyssen Foundation. 1983.

Johnson KO. Nomination of Vernon Mountcastle for the Bristol-Myers Squibb Award. February, 2001.

Kandel E. Introductory Comments: 1978 Louisa Gross Horwitz Award to Mountcastle, Hubel and Wiesel.

Venere E. Vernon Mountcastle: head honcho. *The Gazette: The Newspaper of the Johns Hopkins University*. April 20, 1998;27(31). Available at: <http://www.jhu.edu/~gazette/aprjun98/apr2098/20mount.html>.

In: Neocortical Modularity and the Cell Minicolumn
Editor: Manuel F. Casanova, pp. 15-32
ISBN 1-59454-301
© 2005 Nova Science Publishers, Inc.

Chapter II

Vernon B. Mountcastle: Scientific Achievements

Juan Trippe II and Manuel F. Casanova*
University of Louisville, Louisville, KY

Introduction

Well into the Twentieth Century, theories of the brain had been dominated by the concept of cortical localization. Discrete and autonomous cognitive attributes were to be assigned to discrete and autonomous cytoarchitectonic areas of the cortex. All attributes would function in a hierarchy of control: phylogenetically more recent areas superordinate to older areas, and more cephalad brain structures controlling subcortical nuclei and brainstem. These ideas were grounded in the nineteenth century neurology of Broca and Jackson according to which local function could be inferred from area-specific deficits. As neurohistologic methods were refined at the turn of the last century by Golgi, Nissl, Waldeyer, Ramón y Cajal, and others, neuroanatomists were able to identify more-or-less discrete regions of cortical cytoarchitecture on the basis of cell morphology, cell count and density in the various laminae. The Vogts systematically mapped distinctive cytoarchitectonic areas throughout the cortex and sought to assign specific and discrete functions to each area. Brodmann's division of the cortex into about fifty cytoarchitectonically distinct areas remains the canonical basis for brain mapping to the present day. Their findings seemed to confirm the approach of mapping function to area.

At the turn of the twentieth century, events of the age would conspire to undermine the principle of cortical localization. Gordon Holmes, a British Army neurologist, and W.T. Lister meticulously catalogued and analyzed deficits incurred as the result of head trauma

* Corresponding author: Manuel F. Casanova, MD, Gottfried and Gisela Kolb Endowed Chair in Psychiatry, University of Louisville, Department of Psychiatry, 500 South Preston St., A Bldg., Rm. 217; Louisville, KY 40292. Tel: (502)852-4077; Fax: (502)852-4078; E-mail: M0CASA02@louisville.edu

during World War I, and were thus able to roughly map retinotopic projections onto occipital cortex [1]. In the same way, Holmes was able to deduce the principle of somatotopic mapping onto parietal cortex and describe deficits of attention and spatial perception in soldiers with damage to the posterior parietal cortex. These observations supported the idea that a specific function—perception via a specific modality—is distributed topographically within a relatively large region of cortex and that complex perceptual functions such as spatial localization of an object similarly could not be localized to a specific discrete area.

World War I also resulted in improvement in electrical circuit components for radio and other purposes. Over fifty years after Caton first described electrical activity in the brain, electroencephalic techniques became available which allowed for mapping the electrical activity of the cortex with vastly greater resolution than had hitherto been possible. These techniques, pioneered by Berger, Adrian, and others [2], became widely adopted. Global or widely distributed patterns of activity could be correlated with specific behavioral states, in particular states of relative global arousal such as sleep. The sought-for correlations between specific behaviors and corresponding areas of local electrical activity could not be found, however.

More detailed cortical mapping would become possible with the advent of measurement of electrical activity directly from peripheral nerves and the cortical surface. Gerard, Marshall, and Saul [3] were the first to apply macroelectrodes to the surface of somatic sensory cortex in order to measure the slow-wave potential evoked by activation of peripheral somatosensory receptors. However, it was at Johns Hopkins from the mid-nineteen-thirties onward that Philip Bard, the young and dynamic Physiology Department Chairman, directed a research program which fully explored the possibilities afforded by this technique. Clinton Woolsey, an extremely gifted and ambitious research fellow recruited out of the surgery program, together with Marshall and Bard, systematically mapped the somatotopic representation of a monkey's body onto the surface of cortex [4] and, following Adrian in Britain, subsequently detailed a *second* somatotopic map on an adjoining parietal region [5]. All at Hopkins were in their thirties at the time this ground-breaking work was being conducted. Meanwhile, at McGill in Montreal, Wilder Penfield experimented with electrode stimulation of the cortical surface in patients conscious during surgery. The practice was implemented in order to assess the potential extent of functional deficit following excision of brain tissue. At the same time, it allowed Penfield to construct cortical sensorimotor maps in the human which corresponded well with those created by the Hopkins group for the monkey.

Despite their successes, it was recognized that evoked potential techniques lacked sufficient resolution to truly investigate the physiological basis of perception in detail. Such investigations into the functional activity of cortical microstructures and subcortical nuclei would require a technique that would revolutionize neurophysiology. The technique, recording the electrical activity of single neurons with an extracellular microelectrode, continues today to transform our understanding of the brain.

The development of the single-unit recording approach continued throughout the nineteen-forties. Working at the University of Chicago, Gilbert Ling improved the precision and reliability of the microelectrode recording technique, which supported its widespread adoption [6]. Studies during this period were conducted in a variety of invertebrate and vertebrate species by Hartline, Barlow, Adrian and others [7]. Herbert Jasper, working with

Penfield in Montreal at the time, used the technique in nonhuman species to investigate auditory brainstem nuclei, and in thalamic nuclei involved in behavioral arousal [8]. Moving to Hopkins from Australia following the end of World War II, Stephen Kuffler [9] employed microelectrodes to investigate the receptive fields of retinal ganglion cells in the cat and made his now-famous observations of their center-surround properties. Mountcastle and colleagues [10]–[13] refined use of the technique in their studies of the somatosensory receptive-field properties of the thalamus in the cat, rabbit, and monkey and further used it to investigate cortex in the early and mid-fifties. The development and improvement of equipment and techniques used in these studies further facilitated progress, notably the Horsley-Clarke head-holder and the Davies isolation chamber, which dampened vibrations from vascular pulsations and physiologic tremor and without which precise microelectrode recording would have been impossible. Furthermore, neurohistologic techniques reconstructing the microelectrode's path of penetration in the cortex and allowing for precise location and identification of neurons analyzed in test animals were perfected by Mountcastle's colleague, Jerzy Rose.

Mountcastle's Discovery of Cortical Columns

All of these developments set the stage for what is truly the landmark result of single-unit recording studies in living cortex: Vernon Mountcastle's discovery of functional cortical columns in the somatosensory cortex of cats and monkeys [14]–[16]. Recordings were made from twenty-three hundred neurons over the course of these investigations. The latency and spiking frequency of large numbers of these were carefully quantified. The spiking response of each neuron was analyzed in terms of its receptive field and modality, i.e. the nature of the external energy stimulus transduced by its afferent receptors. It must be remembered that there was no prior expectation that the studies would reveal columnar organization of information processing. Rather, it was by dint of careful observation and quantification of each response that the receptive fields of cells in the successive laminae penetrated were determined to overlap to a great degree, with all responses specific to a given modality and only to afferents from the contralateral side of the body. This was recognized early on and great care was taken to guide subsequent penetrations perpendicular to the cortical surface. A critical confirmation of the columnar hypothesis came with two early experiments in which slanting penetrations were made at an angle of 45 degrees to the tangential plane, demonstrating a change in modality as the microelectrode passed through adjoining regions from layer to layer [15].

The picture of somatic sensory cortex emerging from these investigations encompassed a number of important findings. First, neuronal populations within each column responded to one specific submodality and dermatomal locale. Columns extending from layers II through VI were disposed topographically along the mediolateral axis and according to submodality along the anteroposterior axis, with three distinct submodalities identified. Cells activated by deformation of hairs demonstrated rapid adaptation of spiking activity, while those cells responding to constant pressure on the skin surface showed slow adaptation, or spiking activity sustained according to length of time pressure was applied. The third submodality of cell response observed was that of joint motion and position. Within proprioceptive columns, cells in adjacent areas were identified exhibiting reciprocal activation to alternating flexion and extension of joints in their receptive field. Because tonic activity was suppressed in a cell as the opposing cell was activated, Mountcastle inferred the mechanism of reciprocal lateral inhibition. For all submodalities, spiking frequency correlated with stimulus intensity. It was also observed that cells in all layers of a column responded with approximately the same latency, at least for early responses. This common latency served as another dimension for functionally identifying a given column. Finally, a pattern of surround inhibition in the receptive fields of somatic sensory cortical neurons was identified whereby stimulation in areas peripheral to a central excitatory region actually inhibited cell activity.

These investigations of columnar physiology served to undermine the dogma linking functions with specific cytoarchitectonic areas. Neuroanatomists earlier in the Twentieth Century had described the organization of cortex in terms of neurons bundled into structures oriented perpendicular to the cortical surface, notably von Economo [17] in his description of auditory cortex. Lorente de Nó [18] was the first to posit a vertical flow of information into and out of the cortex through radially-oriented chains of interneurons extending through the full thickness of cortex with relative limitation of information flow horizontally into surrounding cortical areas.

Even into the Fifties, such was the hold on thinking in neurophysiology of the idea that a given function must be integrated over the entire surface of a cytoarchitectonic area presumed to subserve that function that Mountcastle felt compelled to cite the experiments of Roger Sperry [19] with subpial cortical dicing in support of his own findings. Sperry isolated numerous μm-scale segments of the visual cortex in monkeys and cats with transections through cortical gray matter but sparing the underlying white-matter afferent connections of each segment. These animals' capacities for visual discrimination remained largely intact, suggesting that at least in striate cortex these μm-scale segments are capable of high-level information abstraction with relatively little contribution required from horizontal interaction of neighboring segments.

The work of Mountcastle with single unit recording, and the subsequent studies of Hubel and Wiesel in striate and extrastriate cortex confirming the ubiquity of columnar organization, fostered an explosion of work in the perceptual physiology of the cortex and were the source of several important principles which emerged early on. Namely, investigations of static physiologic properties such as surround inhibition and partially overlapping receptive fields support formulation of testable assertions both about underlying neuroanatomy and about perceptual information processing. With the results of these and subsequent studies, questions about perception could be phrased in the language of information theory, in terms of thresholds, triggers, parsing, and feature detection.

Characterizing the Elements of Perception

Mountcastle understood early on the limitations of investigations of the static features of single neurons in anesthetized animals. During the Sixties he sought to study dynamic properties of afferent and cortical neuronal populations interacting with each other and with homotypic cortex in order ultimately to understand the relation of perception to decision-making and action. In keeping with his systematic and visionary approach to research, Mountcastle sought initially to quantitatively characterize the signal-transduction properties of all the somatic sensory receptor types. He appreciated that in order to understand the interactions of these primary afferents generating higher-order perceptual processes, it would be necessary to quantify signal-processing in elemental afferents using psychometric functions—i.e. relating stimulus intensity to probability of detection and discriminative response. A decade earlier, Stevens [20] had formulated the generic relation between a stimulus and its perceived intensity as being that of a power function. Mountcastle [21] found that, for the specific case of somatic sensation in glabrous skin, this relation was in fact linear—i.e. the exponent was unity. He also noted that the relation of afferent spiking frequency to stimulus intensity was also linear and that spiking frequency therefore corresponded directly to perceived intensity. In relating detection thresholds to frequency of sine-wave mechanical stimuli, a biphasic function curve was generated, suggesting that two distinct populations of afferents underlie the sense of flutter-vibration. He characterized the psychophysical properties of mechanoreceptors found in the glabrous skin of the palm in monkeys, showing that, in response to a sinusoidal flutter/vibration stimulus, rapidly-adapting Pacinian corpuscles responded optimally to vibration in the bandwidth of 50 Hz to 300 Hz, allowing for exquisite discrimination of the deflection of individual hairs. Meissner's corpuscles were also rapidly-adapting, but responding to lower frequencies in the range of 10 Hz to 100 Hz, and finally deeper-situated Merkel disks were slow-adapting, giving a sustained response to lower frequency flutter stimuli.

Combining Neurophysiology and Psychophysics

This work, conducted during the mid Nineteen-Sixties, laid the foundation for what has become the paradigmatic method for examining the neural basis of behavior: the combined psychophysical-neurophysiological experiment. This technique, pioneered in classical conditioning studies in the late Fifties by Herbert Jasper [22], and by Edward Evarts [23] working in motor cortex in the early Sixties, applied the single unit recording method in awake, behaving monkeys that were conditioned to emit behaviors manifesting perceptual detection and discrimination in response to carefully quantified stimuli. In time the method would be extended by Mountcastle and others to encompass conditioning regimes shaping complex behaviors manifesting not only perceptual discrimination but also potentially activity modulated by attention and including the coordination of complex perceptual and motor programs [24].

The combined experiment methodology, as employed by Mountcastle, incorporated three elements: First, psychophysical experiments were devised in which nonhuman primate test subjects were operantly conditioned to emit behaviors manifesting detection and perceptual discrimination, shifts in attention or other perceptual phenomena in response to a given stimulus continuum. It was necessary that these regimes be amenable to the use of statistical methods of decision theory and designed in such a way that subjects could respond to the full range of stimuli necessary to elucidate neuronal operations. Second, single unit recording studies would be conducted simultaneously with psychophysical experiments adapted to the neuronal activity being investigated—i.e., to "inquire which quantitative aspects of the neuronal response tally with psychophysical measurements." [25] Recordings from a sequence of such neurons would be obtained with the idea of retrospectively re-constructing the population activity of neurons underlying perceptual operations. Third, it was necessary to develop the theoretical constructs with which to make generalizations about neuronal population activity from these series of single unit recordings and to relate that activity to the simultaneously obtained results of psychophysical testing [26,27].

The employment of flutter-vibration stimuli was the experimental paradigm chosen because variations in patterns of temporal activity could be investigated with populations of afferent and cortical neurons subserving a single receptive field serving as self-controls. The periodicity of the mechanical sine wave oscillatory stimulus predicted patterns of neural activity with first order periods corresponding to the period of the stimulus of mechanical oscillation. Changes in frequency and amplitude of the stimulus thus allowed for study of how temporal aspects of somatic sensory stimuli are translated into temporal spiking patterns in primary afferents and cortex. Combined experiments were conducted in primary afferents subserving glabrous skin in the monkey hand [28] and in monkey cortex [29]. Populations of both primary afferents and cortical neurons exhibiting distinctive patterns of activity were identified, each of which corresponded exclusively to input from either Meissner's or Pacinian corpuscles. These studies supported the hypothesis that the relation between external stimulus intensity and both magnitude of spiking activity and subjective estimate of intensity—i.e. the exponent value in Stevens's equation—is encoded peripherally at the stage of receptor transduction or in the primary afferent.

Psychophysical comparisons between human and monkey were made of the ability to detect and discriminate vibratory stimuli of varying frequencies [30,31]. From these it was shown that both human and monkey responses could be described with identical biphasic stimulus-response curves over the range of 5 Hz to 500 Hz, reflecting the activation of discrete populations of receptors: Meissner's corpuscles at lower frequencies (5 Hz to 50 Hz) and Pacinian corpuscles, with a different slope coefficient, at higher frequencies (50 Hz to 500 Hz). Echoing Weber's law, frequency discrimination was found to vary directly with increasing frequency; that is, larger periods of vibration corresponded to larger just-noticeable-differences (JNDs). Further, variability in frequency of response of cortical neurons was found to be reflected in the range of responses of observers.

As will be explored in the following pages, the combined experimental paradigm of recording neuronal activity in awake, behaving animals was revolutionary in leading to the birth of a major new field of inquiry: cognitive neural science. The method allowed for direct investigation of higher mental processes, so-called, which had hitherto fore been largely inaccessible, including those underlying attention, learning and memory, and decision-making. Several important principles have emerged from this approach as well as from electrophysiological studies employing slice preparations of metabolically active brain tissue, work with preparations of simple neuronal circuits in invertebrate and simple vertebrates, and more recent work employing sophisticated imaging technologies achieving resolutions approaching the cellular scale.

First, as has been well established, there is no "grandmother neuron" functioning as a central node for information processing relating to any given percept. In general, signal processing in the brain is mediated by patterns of activity in radially-oriented neuronal populations comprising in most instances from eighty to one hundred neurons. These populations do not simply sum inputs stochastically; rather, there is an ordered flow of information through well-defined input, output, and intermediate processing channels that constitute the elemental microcircuit, or minicolumn, of the neocortex.

Second, there is no grandmother minicolumn. Rather, the integrated activity of these minicolumns yields an actively processed, or constructed, representation of the perceived environment. The processing underlying these constructions encompasses differential activation of subsets of cortical minicolumns integrating input, either interspersed or superimposed, from thalamocortical sensory afferents; from intra-areal, transcortical, and transcallosal projections; and from modulatory projections of subcortical and brainstem structures. These connections provide the anatomic substrate for the dynamic activity that defines cortical macrocolumns.

To elaborate, there is no passively projected, congruent image of grandma represented anywhere in cortex. Rather, the components of perception are processed in a distributed network of patterns of minicolumnar activity. These are specialized to process information from afferents channeling information specific to various types of sensory receptors. These patterns are compounded into parallel cortical streams, each to some degree insulated from the rest and specialized for a specific functional aspect of the perceptual whole. There has been some preliminary success in functionally defining some of these patterns of activity in terms of operational transforms upon inputs to produce outputs. The following list of some candidate cortical functions is adapted from Mountcastle [32] (p 287)]:

Thresholding: a nonlinear relation between the level of presynaptic input and cortical neuronal discharge.

Amplification of inputs: e.g., a single impulse in a single myelinated fiber of a peripheral nerve in an attending human suffices to evoke a conscious perception.

The derivative function: cortical operations tend to accentuate and amplify transient inputs, adapt to constant ones.

Feature convergence: the creation of a neural representation of a complex feature or set of features by combining signals of two or more simpler ones.

The distribution function: some areas receive the neural signals of certain simpler features of sensory stimuli and distribute them separately to other cortical areas. Areas 3b and V1 in addition to having other functions, serve as distribution centers.

Coincidence detection by convergence of excitation, linking together two events that occur closely in time.

Synchronization and coherence of activity in the different nodes of distributed systems.

Pattern generation: creation of spatial and temporal patterns in output signals that are not present in inputs (e.g., induced rhythms).

Where instantiated in cortex, these functions are *emergent* properties. They are stable operations arising from the dynamic activity of distributed networks of minicolumns. That is, the properties of these operations cannot be predicted from the characteristics of the individual elements of the network—i.e. neurons, glia, and microcircuits—observed in isolation. The analysis of emergent phenomena in neural circuits had a notable precedent in the work of Hodgkin and Huxley [33], who investigated how action potentials arise from the dynamic properties of the squid giant axon membrane with respect to voltage-dependent conductance to sodium and potassium ions. They were able to derive empirically a set of equations that describe the nonlinear behavior of the action potential spike, the velocity of its propagation along the axon, and other properties. They did this by systematically varying the membrane potential of the axon and recording the effect on conductance to sodium and potassium ions without any knowledge of the properties of the individual ion channels themselves. The hope has been that, in similar fashion, the dynamic properties of distributed networks of minicolumns can be investigated without direct reference to the intrinsic operations of the minicolumn or the properties of the neurons that constitute it.

EXPLORATIONS OF THE PARIETAL LOBE

By 1970 Mountcastle and his colleagues had established a correlation between increasing stimulus amplitude for a mechanical oscillation at 10 Hz to 40 Hz, probability of correct detection in psychophysical measurements, and increased entrainment of neuronal spiking activity at the given frequency [34]. Recording in the postcentral somatic sensory cortex, they were unable to distinguish between patterns of neuronal discharge associated with correct detection and those associated with misses at the 50 % detection level. The question was thus posed: where was the locus of neural activity driving detection of the stimulus.

It was in this setting that Mountcastle and his colleagues initiated their first survey studies of posterior parietal cortex in alert, behaving monkeys. Their first forays were conducted without a clear experimental agenda, but, as Mountcastle put it: "What we observed in those exploratory experiments determined my experimental life for fifteen years: neurons that were active if and only if the animal 'had a mind' to deal with the stimulus in a behaviorally meaningful way!" [35] In their preliminary studies of area 5 and later area 7 of posterior parietal cortex, they observed neurons discharging only when the monkey reached for a reward, as opposed to a bland object stimulus in the environment; neurons which were active only in the grasping as opposed to the reaching phase of reward-object manipulation, and vice versa. Other neurons had broadly distributed, bilateral receptive fields responsive to cutaneous stimulation. Still others were responsive to only motivationally significant objects perceived in large sectors of the visual field. It soon became apparent that certain qualities were common to the receptive fields of most neuronal populations examined: namely, those of the perception and attention to motivationally significant objects found in immediate extrapersonal space, intentionality, and the shaping of motor and oculomotor schemas for manipulating such objects.

In preparing for these early studies of the posterior parietal cortex, Mountcastle reviewed the clinical literature concerning "parietal lobe syndrome," looking at the effect of various parietal lobe lesions in humans and non-human primates. Lesions of the parietal lobe do not affect primary sensory or motor function per se, but rather the "higher" functions of spatial and object perception, attention, and willed movement. Discrete lesions may create functional dissociations among these, and yet each function arises from dynamic activity in a widely distributed network in which lesioned parietal tissue may serve as only one component. Since such lesions affect activity throughout the network, the function of a given area cannot simply be said to be the reciprocal of the deficit caused by damage to that area. The hallmark deficit of parietal lobe syndrome is hemispheric neglect in which attention to the contralateral body and surrounding extrapersonal space is compromised, frequently with denial of such neglect. Thus, a patient will not recognize one side of his body as his and may actually complain of foreign body parts in his bed. Other patients demonstrate avolition, or difficulty in initiating guided movement in extrapersonal space. Inability to recognize familiar objects, or anosognosia, is another common deficit, as are deficits in distinguishing spatial relations among objects. Still other patients exhibit difficulty with visually guided reaching or grasping movements, termed optic ataxia. While the literature describing these clinical syndromes had some heuristic value in guiding early investigations in posterior parietal cortex, it nevertheless became apparent early on that qualitative methods involving the techniques available to clinical neurology were inadequate to the task. It would be necessary to devise well-controlled quantitative study protocols in which complex, conditional behavioral tasks were matched to the complex, conditional behavioral repertoires reflecting the activity of parietal homotypic cortex.

The first surveys of posterior parietal cortex were significant first for what they failed to reveal: in the cortical region putatively concerned with the construction of spatial representations, there has yet to be found any topographic mapping of visual space or body surface onto cortex. Instead the area is organized into discrete units or groupings of neurons, organized into macrocolumnar structures at a scale of a millimeter or less which demonstrate specific perceptual and motor response characteristics. Adjacent units may form ensembles whose individual functions are coordinated in the execution of complex sensorimotor schemas [36-39]. These survey studies identified five major classes of neurons found in functional groupings: reach/hand-manipulation, oculomotor, fixation, and visual neurons, as well as special neurons combining more than one of the response characteristics, often involving visual receptive fields with complex response properties. A relatively large proportion of the total number of neurons sampled was represented in each category, with a correspondingly large set of neurons not exhibiting any of the defined response characteristics.

Studies of reach-hand manipulation neurons, as well as fixation and oculomotor neurons were conducted with a behavioral paradigm involving detection alone or detection plus reach of the arm to manipulate a computer-controlled target moving along a circular track at arms length [38]. 11 % of neurons sampled in area 5 as well as 33 % of neurons sampled in area 7 exhibited reach-hand manipulation response characteristics. These neurons were not activated directly by sensory stimuli, but rather discharged at high rates when an animal executed a command function to obtain and manipulate a reward object located within arms reach. This function was conditional in that it would not be activated by motivationally bland objects or by objects located outside of immediate extrapersonal space. In addition, patterns of neuronal discharge were not directly correlated with particular patterns of joint or muscle movement suggesting that the command function was not a motor sequencing program but rather was intentionally oriented toward a particular goal object in the environment. Further, these patterns were independent of the source of the stimulus, whether visual or tactile; as well, they were independent of the time interval between stimulus cueing and execution of the reach-manipulation movement. Finally, arm reaching and hand manipulation were found to be dissociable with distinct populations of neurons discharging during each action. Thus, designated HM (hand manipulation) neurons would be largely inactive during the reach phase of visually-guided arm movements, yet become highly active as the monkey shaped its hand to grasp an object.

With the exception of the reach-hand manipulation cells described above, most neurons of area 7 of posterior parietal cortex appear to be responsive primarily to visual stimuli. Three distinct classes of visually responsive neurons have been identified in this area of cortex with a fourth special class combining attributes of the first three classes. Visual fixation neurons discharge at a high rate when the test subject attends to a motivationally significant object in the visual field. High rates of discharge continue with smooth-pursuit tracking movements of the reward object in visual space and continue without regard to the direction of movement of the object in the visual field. The activity of visual fixation neurons, like the activity of reach-hand manipulation neurons, is dependent on the rewarding nature of the object, the motivational state of the test subject, and the location of the object within arm's reach in extrapersonal space. High rates of discharge are maintained until the subject obtains the reward or until the object is made inaccessible to reaching and grasping.

Oculomotor neurons as a class comprise two different types of cells. Tracking neurons preferentially discharge as the eyes lock onto and pursue objects slowly moving through the visual field. These neurons exhibit a level of activity inverse to that of fixation neurons, as they are relatively silent during fixation of a reward target. Discrete populations of tracking neurons are preferentially sensitive for different directions of eye movement, but are relatively insensitive to tracking speed. Saccade neurons discharge preferentially immediately before and during rapid movement of the eyes across large arcs of the visual field in order to focus on an object in the field periphery. They are active during eye movements prompted by motivationally significant stimuli but are relatively inactive during spontaneous saccades. Saccade neurons are also preferentially active with respect to direction; cell populations discharge most readily during saccades directed contralaterally to the hemisphere in which they are located. Their discharge rate is relatively insensitive to the amplitude of the saccade. Both tracking neurons and saccade neurons are subject to an angle of gaze effect. For eye movements of identical amplitude and direction the neurons will tend to discharge at different rates as the eyes track through different regions of the field of vision.

Mountcastle and his colleagues then undertook to investigate the inferior parietal lobule, studying the visually responsive neurons located there that exhibited complex receptive field properties. Of the two classes of neurons identified, the class I PVN (parietal visual neurons) exhibited large, typically bilateral receptive fields often encompassing the entire field of vision (as opposed to class II neurons which had smaller receptive fields limited to the parafoveal region of the contralateral visual field). Discharge rates for class I neurons were greatest for target stimuli moving through the periphery of the visual field. These neurons were relatively insensitive to the rate of movement of the stimulus and adapted slowly to sustained stimulation.

Most notable was the effect of attentive fixation on the activity of class I PVNs. Whereas response was strongly suppressed to perifoveal stimulation, it was actively facilitated for moving stimuli in the periphery of the field. This pattern of activity of inferior parietal lobule neurons was in contrast to that seen in striate-temporal lobe pathways in which foveal or perifoveal stimulation elicited neural activity. The activity of class I PVNs has obvious adaptive value for the primate subject who can suppress response to an attended object and rapidly shift attention to moving stimuli in the visual periphery representing a potential threat. It was shown that the response vectors of individual parietal neurons could be summed to yield a population vector that accurately represents the direction of stimulus movement. Population vectors could be derived for the full distribution of meridional directional preferences in the visual field [40]. The response properties of these neurons are also well suited for representing the flow fields of movement in the visual field occurring as the subject moves through its environment. These properties allow for the appropriate discrimination of visual self-image from background and of movement of self versus movement of surrounding objects in extrapersonal space [41-43].

Cortical Columnarity as an Organizing Principle

Vernon Mountcastle's long and distinguished career in neuroscience has yielded many notable contributions to the field, including development of the combined psychophysical-single unit recording experiment which has been and remains the paradigm for research in neurophysiology. His later work laid the foundation for a broad and active research agenda, focused on the perceptual processes of the posterior parietal cortex, notably the work of Ungerleider and Mishkin establishing parallel paths of visual processing in extrastriate cortex [44]. Most fundamentally, it was his early discovery of the physiological basis of columnarity in somatic sensory cortex that has proven seminal in transforming our understanding of how the brain is organized. His work during the late Nineteen-Fifties demonstrated cortex that was organized into modular regions that were somatotopically and modality specific. These studies in somatic sensory cortex provided a foundation and reference for the subsequent vast literature documenting modular organization throughout other areas of heterotypic and homotypic cortex.

The landmark work of Hubel and Weisel [45,46] determined the columnar organization of striate cortex with respect to ocularity, retinotopic location, and orientation as a matrix-like arrangement of orientation hypercolumns and orthogonally arranged ocular dominance hypercolumns. The former are composed of a set of orientation slabs, or columns, each responsive to a segment of specific orientation in a full sequence comprising 180 degrees. The basic model has been confirmed and elaborated upon in numerous subsequent studies (see Peters [47] for review). Studies have extended understanding of columnar organization in extrastriate visual cortex with respect to responsiveness to orientation to moving stimuli in area MT of the macaque [48] and in inferotemporal cortex with respect to object shape and feature processing [49,50]. Columnar organization has been well documented in primary auditory cortex (see Wong [51] for review), motor cortex [52], and in prefrontal association cortex [53,54].

Mountcastle recognized that columnar properties arise from the interaction of architectonic features—afferent inflows and the radially-oriented cortical neuronal circuits subtended by them—together with dynamic intracortical operations. He identified columns displaying a specific electrophysiological response with the "elementary unit of organization in the somatic cortex made up of a vertical group of cells extending through all the cellular layers" [15]. At the same time, he emphasized that the columnar discharges represented "the first response of cortical cells to a peripheral stimulus," with observations suggesting "later and more complex discharge patterns" overlying the columnar pattern might emerge.

Numerous studies have since supported Mountcastle's findings and have elaborated understanding of the modular organization of somatosensory cortex. Favorov and Whitsel [55] conducted micromapping studies in cat and monkey demonstrating the minicolumnar basis of receptive field distribution. Vertical microelectrode penetrations through somatic sensory yielded superimposed receptive fields for the various cell layers encountered. With penetrations made slightly tangential to the vertical axis, abrupt changes in receptive field location occurred as the microelectrode tip traversed lateral intervals of 40 μm to 50 μm consistent with the diameter of minicolumns receiving afferents from discrete and juxtaposed receptive fields.

Additional evidence demonstrating the organization of minicolumns as elementary functional units of cortical macrocolumns was provided by a study [56] in which afferents innervating receptive fields on the glabrous surface of the monkey paw were severed and then allowed to regenerate. In intact animals, a microelectrode introduced at a small angle to the tangential plane passing through successive minicolumns would encounter adjacent and overlapping receptive fields blending into a continuum. Afferent fibers regenerating following median nerve transaction would re-innervate the glabrous surface in a random pattern. Receptive field locations would shift discontinuously as the microelectrode traversed intervals of 50 μm to 60 μm corresponding to the diameter of a minicolumn. Thus, discrete receptive fields were revealed for each minicolumn-size block of cortical tissue. Favorov and Diamond [57] subsequently mapped somatic sensory cortex in the cat using multiple, closely-spaced microelectrode penetrations to determine columnar patterning. Cortical columns were determined to be quasi-hexagonal in shape with a width of approximately 300 μm to 400 μm and encompassing 80–100 minicolumns.

Studies of cortical metabolism and blood flow have offered another approach in detailing minicolumnar composition of cortical columns. Correlated studies of electrophysiology and metabolic activity involving uptake of 2-deoxyglucose [58] demonstrate that a suitable somatosensory stimulus will activate a cortical column in contralateral somatic sensory cortex and, as well, will increase metabolic activity in a larger, encompassing segregate measuring approximately 500 μm by 1500 μm. Metabolic activity is not increased uniformly within the region but varies across the cortical surface in intervals of 18 μm to 30 μm [59] These observations reveal minicolumns as the physiological and metabolically active constitutive elements of cortical modules.

MODULAR ARCHITECTONICS

The revolution in neurophysiology led by Mountcastle, Hubel, and Wiesel fostered corresponding efforts in histology to find structural counterparts corresponding to the emerging picture of modular cortical function. The principle of modular architectonics had been anticipated by Lorente de Nó in his descriptions of the vertical orientation of neuronal cell assemblies in cortex, as well as those by Scheibel and Scheibel [60] of spatial ordering of dendritic and axonal processes in the brainstem. It was Szentagothai [61,62], however, who proposed the first explicit model of the modular organization of neuronal connectivity, for somatic sensory cortex. This model posited flow of information through an elemental circuit comprising thalamocortical afferents synapsing upon spiny stellate cells in layer IV, and whose tangential extent is defined in part by the field of synaptic connections formed by the axonal ramifications of those stellate cells with the dendritic arborizations of pyramidal cells found in layers II, III, and V. Szentagothai's cortical module was characterized additionally by corticocortical afferents and pyramidal cell collaterals whose axonal ramifications extending over the bases in layers VI and I with a width of 200 μm to 300 μm help define the extent of the module. It was further characterized by the presence of peripheral inhibitory interneurons, though firm knowledge at the time was limited to the large basket cells found principally in layer III. Szentagothai's characterization of columns defined by corticocortical afferents has been extended throughout sensory and motor cortex and subsequently into prefrontal association cortex where columnar interdigitation of contralateral and ipsilateral projections has been identified [63]. This model has since served as the basis for various modifications and refinements based on electrophysiology coordinated with microinjection labeling of individual cells. As a result, the morphology and columnar connectivity of the various classes of inhibitory interneurons has been established, including the role of double bouquet GABAergic interneurons in providing "curtains" of inhibitory activity around minicolumnar structures, 50 μm in diameter, partly defined by dendritic arborizations of bundles of vertically oriented pyramidal neurons.

It was Mountcastle and his colleagues [29] who first distinguished pyramidal cells from inhibitory interneurons on the basis of their physiological response properties. In single unit studies of somatic sensory cortex he identified different classes of cells exhibiting either regular or thin spike patterns, which he identified as corresponding to pyramidal cells and stellate inhibitory interneurons respectively. Intracellular studies in cortical slab preparations later confirmed the distinction between the two types of spiking waveforms. RS (regular spiking) waveforms were recorded from pyramidal neurons while FS (fast spiking) waveforms were associated with stellate inhibitory interneurons [64].

This class of interneuron exhibiting FS spiking characteristics comprises chandelier cells that provide inhibition within minicolumnar structures and basket cells located primarily in layer III whose collaterals provide inhibition over the range of hundreds of μm and which provide constraint of the dynamic physiological activity of macrocolumns [65] Recent investigations of RS and FS units in dorsolateral prefrontal cortex during an oculomotor delayed response task revealed that FS units showed similar isodirectional tuning as adjacent RS units during delay phase. It was shown that these FS units rather than providing nonspecific modulation of the activity of pyramidal neurons were providing direct isoorientation inhibition to associated pyramidal cells. These observations reveal the activity of inhibitory interneurons and pyramid cells as integrated into the function of local microcircuits subserving spatial working memory [66].

Mountcastle's Legacy

Vernon Mountcastle's reputation as one of the great original thinkers in neuroscience was established based upon the early work of his career: the large series of studies of somatosensory cortex employing innovative single unit recording techniques. These demonstrated the columnar organization of neocortex underlying the superimposition of related perceptual functions upon a common two-dimensional cortical somatotopic map. This principle of modular organization—Mountcastle's columnar hypothesis—has been confirmed in all areas of cortex and is established as a fundamental fact of the organization of the brain. Accepted as a commonplace today, the columnar hypothesis was met with disbelief, resistance, and even ridicule on the part of many neuroscientists when it was first proposed in the 1950s.

Having elucidated in terms of columnar organization what he referred to as the "static" properties of cortex, Mountcastle and his colleagues during the sixties and early seventies focused upon its dynamic properties. Neurophysiological and psychophysical experiments were coordinated in the same subject. This combined experimental approach made possible the understanding of information encoding and processing in single cells at the level of mechanoreceptor, afferent, and cortical neuron.

In order to investigate his original ideas, Mountcastle employed a comparably fundamental new approach to methodology. Experimental results were based not on qualitative comparisons or on anecdotal reports. Rather, conclusions were derived from the systematic analysis of recordings from large numbers of neurons. Single unit experiments required complex and exacting preparation and many consecutive hours for their execution. Study designs were based upon the quantification of stimulus-response relationships, pioneering the implementation of methods from information and statistical decision theory. This rigorous approach set the standard for all subsequent research in behavioral neurophysiology.

References

[1] Marshall LH, Magoun HW. *Discoveries in the Human Brain.* Totowa, NJ: Humana Press; 1998.

[2] Adrian ED, Yamigawa K. The origin of the Berger rhythm. *Brain.* 1935;58:323-351.

[3] Gerard R, Marshall W, Saul L. Electrical activity of the cat's brain. *Archives of Neurology and Psychiatry.* 1936;36:675-735.

[4] Marshall WH, Woolsey CN, Bard P. Observations on cortical somatic sensory mechanisms of cat and monkey. *Journal of Neurophysiology.* 1941;4:1-24.

[5] Woolsey CN, Marshall WH, Bard P. Representation of cutaneous tactile sensibility in the cerebral cortex of the monkey as indicated by evoked potentials. *Bulletin of the Johns Hopkins Hospital.* 1942;70:399-441.

[6] Harrison TS. Five scientists at Johns Hopkins in the modern evolution of neuroscience. *Journal of the History of the Neurosciences.* 2000;9:165-179.

[7] Finger S. *Origins of Neuroscience.* New York: Oxford; 1994:245-247

[8] Jasper HH. Diffuse projection systems: the integrative action of the thalamic reticular system. *Electroencephalography and Clinical Neurophysiology.* 1949;1:405-419.

[9] Kuffler SW. Discharge patterns and functional organization of the mammalian retina. *Journal of Neurophysiology.* 1953;16:37-68.

[10] Mountcastle VB, Henneman E. Pattern of tactile representation in thalamus of cat. *Journal of Neurophysiology.* 1949;12:85-100.

[11] Mountcastle VB, Henneman E. The representation of tactile sensibility in the thalamus of the monkey. *Journal of Comparative Neurology.* 1952;97:409-440.

[12] Rose JE, Mountcastle VB. The thalamic tactile region in rabbit and cat. *Journal of Comparative Neurology.* 1952;97:441-490.

[13] Rose JE, Mountcastle VB. Activity of single neurons in the thalamic tactile region of the cat in response to a transient peripheral stimulus. *Bulletin of the Johns Hopkins Hospital.*1954;94:238-282.

[14] Mountcastle VB, Berman AL, Davies PW. Topographic organization and modality representation in the first somatic area of cat's cerebral cortex by method of single unit analysis [abstract]. *American Journal of Physiology.* 1955;183:646.

[15] Mountcastle VB. Modality and topographic properties of single neurons of cat's somatic sensory cortex. *Journal of Neurophysiology.* 1957;20:408-434.

[16] Powell TPS, Mountcastle VB. Some aspects of the functional organization of the cortex of the postcentral gyrus of the monkey: a comparison of findings obtained in a single unit analysis with cytoarchitecture. *Bulletin of the Johns Hopkins Hospital.* 1959;105:133-162.

[17] von Economo CF. *The Cytoarchitectonics of the Human Cerebral Cortex.* Oxford, UK: Oxford University Press; 1929.

[18] Lorente de Nó R. Cerebral cortex: Architecture, intracortical connections, motor projections. In: Fulton JF, ed. *Physiology of the Nervous System.* Oxford, UK: Oxford University Press; 1938:291-339.

[19] Sperry RW, Miner N, Myers RE. Visual pattern perception following sub-pial slicing and tantalum wire implantations in the visual cortex. *Journal of Comparative and Physiological Psychology.* 1955;48:50-80.

[20] Stevens SS. On the brightness of lights and the loudness of sounds. *Science.* 1953;118:576.

[21] Mountcastle VB, Talbot WH, Kornhuber HH. The neural transformation of mechanical stimuli delivered to the monkeys hand. In: De Reuck AVS, Knight J, eds. *Ciba Foundation Symposium: Touch, Pain, and Itch.* London, UK: J & A Churchill; 1966:326-351.

[22] Jasper HH, Ricci G, Doane B. Microelectrode analysis of cortical cell discharge during avoidance conditioning in the monkey. *Electroencaphalography and Clinical Neurophysiology.* 1960;131:137-156.

[23] Evarts EV. Methods for recording activity of individual neurons in moving animals. In: Rushmer RF, ed. *Methods in Medical Research.* Vol. 2. Chicago: Yearbook; 1966:241-250.

[24] Stebbins WC, ed. *Animal Psychophysics: The Design and Conduct of Sensory Experiments.* New York: Plenum; 1970.

[25] Mountcastle VB, Poggio GF, Werner G. The relation of thalamic cell response to peripheral stimuli varied over an intensive continuum. *Journal of Neurophysiology.* 1963;26:807-834.

[26] Werner G, Mountcastle VB. The variability of central neural activity in a sensory system, and its implications for the central reflection of sensory events. *Journal of Neurophysiology.* 1963;26:958-977.

[27] Werner G, Mountcastle VB. Neural activity in mechano-receptive afferents: stimulus-response relations, Weber functions, and information transmission. *Journal of Neurophysiology.* 1965;28:359-397.

[28] Talbot WH, Darian-Smith I, Kornhuber HH, Mountcastle VB. The sense of flutter-vibration: comparison of the human capacity with the response patterns of mechanoreceptive afferents from the monkey's hand. *Journal of Neurophysiology.* 1968;31:301-334.

[29] Mountcastle VB, Talbot WH, Sakata H, Hyvarinen J. Cortical neuronal mechanisms in flutter-vibration studied in unanesthetized monkeys: neuronal periodicity and frequency discrimination. *Journal of Neurophysiology.* 1969;32:452-484.

[30] Mountcastle VB, LaMotte RH, Carli G. Detection thresholds for vibratory stimuli in humans and monkeys: comparison with threshold events in mechanoreceptive afferent nerve fibers innervating the monkey hand. *Journal of Neurophysiology.* 1972;35:122.

[31] LaMotte RH, Mountcastle VB. The capacities of humans and monkeys to discriminate between vibratory stimuli of different frequency and amplitude: a correlation between neural events and psychophysical measurements. *Journal of Neurophysiology.* 1975;38:539-559.

[32] Mountcastle VB. *Perceptual Neuroscience: The Cerebral Cortex.* Cambridge, MA: Harvard University Press; 1998.

[33] Hodgkin AL, Huxley AF. A quantitative description of membrane current and its application to conduction and excitation in nerve. *The Journal of Physiology.* 1952;117:500-544.

[34] Carli G, LaMotte RH, Mountcastle VB. A comparison of sensory behavior and the activity of postcentral neurons, observed simultaneously, elicited by oscillatory mechanical stimuli delivered to the contralateral hand in monkeys. Paper presented at: XXV International Congress of Physiological Sciences; 1971; Munich, Germany.

[35] Mountcastle VB. *The parietal system and some higher brain functions.* Cerebral Cortex. 1995;5:377-390.

[36] Lynch JC, Acuna C, Sakata H, Georgopoulos AP, Mountcastle VB. The parietal association cortex and immediate extrapersonal space. Paper presented at: Society for Neuroscience Annual Meeting; 1973; San Diego, CA.

[37] Lynch JC, Mountcastle VB, Talbot WH, Yin TCT. Parietal lobe mechanisms for directed visual attention. *Journal of Neurophysiology.* 1977;40:362-389.

[38] Mountcastle VB, Lynch JC, Georgopoulos AP, Sakata H, Acuna C. The posterior parietal association cortex of the monkey: command functions for operations within extrapersonal space. *Journal of Neurophysiology.* 1975;38:871-908.

[39] Mountcastle VB. The columnar organization of the neocortex. *Brain.* 1997;120:701-722.

[40] Steinmetz MA, Motter BC, Duffy CJ, Mountcastle VB. Functional properties of parietal visual neurons: radial organization of directionalities within the visual field. *Journal of Neuroscience.* 1987;7:177-191.

[41] Mountcastle VB, Andersen RA, Motter BC. The influence of attentive fixation upon the excitability of the light sensitive neurons of the posterior parietal cortex. *Journal of Neuroscience.* 1981;1:1218-1235.

[42] Mountcastle VB, Motter BC, Steinmetz MA, Duffy CJ. Looking and seeing: the visual functions of the parietal lobe. In: Edelman GM, Cowan WM, Gall WE, eds. *Dynamic Aspects of Neocortical Function.* New York, NY: John Wiley & Sons; 1984:159-193.

[43] Motter BC, Steinmetz MA, Duffy CJ, Mountcastle VB. The functional properties of parietal visual neurons: the mechanisms of directionality along a single axis. *Journal of Neuroscience.* 1987;7:154-176.

[44] Ungerleider LG, Mishkin M. Two cortical visual systems. In: Ingle DJ, Goodale MA, Mansfield RJW, eds. *Analysis of Visual Behavior.* Cambridge, MA: MIT Press; 1982:549-586.

[45] Hubel DH, Wiesel TN. Receptive fields of single neurons in the cat's striate cortex. *The Journal of Physiology.* 1962;148:574-591.

[46] Hubel DH, Wiesel TN. Receptive fields and functional architecture of monkey striate cortex. *The Journal of Physiology.* 1968;195:215-243.

[47] Peters A. The organization of the primary visual cortex in the macaque. In: Peters A, Rockland KS, eds. *Primary Visual Cortex in Primates.* Dordrecht, The Netherlands: Kluwer Academic; 1994:1-36. *Cerebral Cortex.* Vol. 10.

[48] Albright TD, Desimone R, Gross CG. Columnar organization of directionally selective cells in visual area MT of the macaque. *Journal of Neurophysiology.* 1984;51:16-31.

[49] Gross CG, Rocha-Miranda CE, Bender DB. Visual properties of neurons in the inferotemporal cortex of the macaque. *Journal of Neurophysiology.* 1972;35:96-111.

[50] Tanaka K. Inferotemporal cortex and object vision. *Annual Review of Neuroscience.* 1996;19:109-139.

[51] Wong D. Cellular organization of the cat's auditory cortex. In: Altschuler RA et al, eds. *The Neurobiology of Hearing.* New York: Raven; 1991:367-387.

[52] Meyer G. Forms and spatial arrangement of neurons in the primary motor cortex of man. *Journal of Comparative Neurology.* 1987;262:402-428.

[53] Goldman-Rakic PS. Modular organization of prefrontal cortex. *Trends in Neurosciences.* 1984;11:419-424.

[54] Kritzer MF, Goldman-Rakic PS. Intrinsic circuit organization of the major layers and sublayers of the dorsolateral prefrontal cortex in the rhesus monkey. *Journal of Comparative Neurology.* 1995;359:131-143.

[55] Favorov OV, Whitsel BL. Spatial organization of the peripheral input to area 1 cell columns, I: the detection of "segregates." *Brain Research Review.* 1988;13:25-42.

[56] Kaas JH, Nelson RJ, Sur M, Merzenich MM. Organization of somatosensory cortex of primates. In: Schmitt FO, Worden WG, Adelman G, Denis SG, eds. *Organization of Cerebral Cortex in Primates.* Cambridge, MA: MIT Press; 1981:237-261.

[57] Favorov OV, Diamond ME. Demonstration of discrete place-defined columns—segregates—in the cat SI. *Journal of Comparative Neurology.* 1990;298:97-112.

[58] Juliano SL, Whitsel BL. A combined 2-deoxyglucose and neurophysiological study of primate somatosensory cortex. *Journal of Comparative Neurology.* 1987;263:514-525.

[59] Tommerdahl M, Favorov O, Whitsel BL, Nakhle B, and Gonchar YA. Minicolumnar activation patterns in cat and monkey S1 cortex. *Cerebral Cortex.* 1993;3:399-411.

[60] Scheibel ME, Scheibel AB. Structural substrates for integrative patterns in the brain stem reticular core. In: Jasper HH, Proctor LP, Knighton RS, Noskay WC, Costello RT, eds. *Reticular Formation of the Brain.* Boston, MA: Little, Brown; 1958:31-68.

[61] Szentagothai, J. Architecture of the cerebral cortex. In: Jasper HH, Ward AA, Pope A, eds. *Basic Mechanisms of the Epilepsies.* Boston, MA: Little, Brown; 1969:13-28.

[62] Szentagothai, J. The module concept in cerebral cortical architecture. *Brain Research.* 1975;95:475-496.

[63] Goldman-Rakic PS, Schwartz ML. Interdigitation of contralateral and ipsilateral columnar projections to frontal association cortex in primates. *Science.* 1982;216:755-757.

[64] McCormick DA, Conners BW, Lighthall JW, Prince DA. Comparative electrophysiology of pyramidal and sparsely spiny stellate neurons of the neocortex. *Journal of Neurophysiology.* 1985;54:782-806.

[65] Jones EG. GABAergic neurons and their role in cortical plasticity in primates. *Cerebral Cortex.* 1993;3:361-372.

[66] Rao SG, Williams GV, Goldman-Rakic PS. Isodirectional tuning of adjacent interneurons and pyramidal cells during working memory: evidence for microcolumnar organization in PFC. *Journal of Neurophysiology.* 1999;81:1903-1916.

In: Neocortical Modularity and the Cell Minicolumn
Editor: Manuel F. Casanova, pp. 33-55 ISBN 1-59454-301
© 2005 Nova Science Publishers, Inc.

Chapter III

An Apologia for a Paradigm Shift in the Neurosciences

Manuel F. Casanova [*]
University of Louisville, Louisville, KY

John Dewey [1] on defining reflective thinking:

"Active, persistent, and careful consideration of a belief or supposed form of knowledge in the light of the grounds which support it and the further conclusions to which it tends."

Edward Glaser [2] on defining critical thinking:

"An attitude of being disposed to consider in a thoughtful way the problems and subjects that come within the range of one's experience. ... Critical thinking calls for a persistent effort to examine any belief or supposed form of knowledge in the light of the evidence that supports it and the further conclusions to which it tends."

Introduction

The neuronal doctrine states the principle that "the nerve cell is the anatomical, physiological, metabolic, and genetic unit of the nervous system" [3,4]. Throughout the last century the neuronal doctrine has acquired different connotations. Initially, researchers expounded the indisputable concept of the neuron as a particulate cell of the nervous system. This was nothing more than the application of Matthias Schleiden and Theodor Schwann's cell theory to the nervous system. A later school of researchers has been intensely

[*] Corresponding author: Manuel F. Casanova, MD, Gottfried and Gisela Kolb Endowed Chair in Psychiatry, University of Louisville, Department of Psychiatry, 500 South Preston St., A Bldg., Rm. 217, Louisville, KY 40292. Tel: (502)852-4077; Fax: (502)852-4078; E-mail: M0CASA02@louisville.edu

ideological. These scientists postulate that the neuron is the framework of neurosciences including, among others, neuropathology, learning, and theory of mind. This mode of thinking has transformed the neuron into an axis around which most of neurosciences revolve. In the hands of these neo-scientists, the neuronal doctrine has become the M-theory of neurosciences. "M" is said to stand for either metatheory (a theory about theories), mother of all theories, or meme theory. The term meme refers to the basic building blocks of our mind and culture [5]. Within this theoretical framework the truth of the premise guarantees the truth of the conclusion. In philosophy this type of postulate is known as begging the question. Good common sense should prompt us to ask how or why this is so. Can understanding the reasoning behind the neuronal doctrine or asking questions from a neuronal perspective provide the proper analytical context for those problems faced by neurologists, psychiatrists, and neuroscientists? Are terms such as neurology, neuroscience, and neuroanatomy appropriate, or are they examples of misguided intentionality? Since science is more than a belief system, it seems opportune to reassess the underlying tenets of the neuronal doctrine from the standpoint of a plausible alternative, i.e., the cell minicolumn.

This chapter extends the premise that existing research has not adequately validated the tenets for the neuronal doctrine. In other words, this chapter is primarily argumentative. Taken in this context the thrust of this narrative differs from that found in other scientific writings focusing on deductive sequences and the scientific method. That is, the main aim of this chapter is not whether other neuroscientists might or might not agree with my statements. The finality of the argument is for a problem not to be ignored. I wish to instill in the reader my own sense of risk taking and to consider the possibility of working outside of conventional reward structures. This chapter is therefore a biased appraisal of the literature that makes argumentative claims and intentionally leaves out reservations. I have taken this approach deliberately not only to attract criticism and learn from it but also in hope of capturing the readers' attention in a more engaging fashion. After reading this chapter, a constructive interpretation of its reasoning should lead readers to consider whether a paradigm shift in neurosciences is warranted [6]. Interested readers may benefit from reading texts espousing an alternative viewpoint [7,8].

Neuronal Pathology

Current medical nosology ascribes diagnostic importance to the presence of pathological findings, that is, abnormalities at the cellular and tissue levels. The evaluation of cells can be divided into those dealing with the nucleus and those pertaining to the cytoplasm. Put simplistically, nuclear characteristics regulate the metabolic or growth activity of a cell. By contrast, morphological characteristics of the cytoplasm regulate the functional differentiation of the cell. Under normal circumstances (i.e., euplasia) these morphological characteristics of the nucleus and cytoplasm are uniform and observed in similar cell types within a given sample of tissue.

Most cells display a round nucleus. This shape reflects a natural state by which objects (e.g., soap bubbles, planets) maximize volume and minimize surface area. Variations in the shape of the nucleus by means of prolongations and sharp angulations significantly increase its surface area and can potentially alter the structure/composition of the nuclear membrane. The new state veers from that attained by the mature or fully differentiated cellular element. Nuclear pleomorphism is therefore a signpost of lack of differentiation or anaplasia.

The cytoplasm surrounds the nucleus as a lake envelops an island, allowing visualization of organelles by light microscopy. The cytoplasm determines the amount of functional differentiation of a cell. This is reflected by prolongations of the soma (i.e., axons and dendrites of neurons, cilia of ependymal cells, and end-feet of astrocytes) rather than by the analysis of any intrinsic organelle. These extensions provide morphological adaptations that allow the proper functioning of the cell within its immediate environment.

The normal, biological state of the cell and its corresponding morphology are fairly constant. Morphological changes at the cellular level occur in patterns revealed by rigorous observation. Taken together they comprise "syndromes" that classify the particular cell or tissue by type, degree of differentiation or de-differentiation, and functional activity. Deviations from these patterns suggest pathology. As a clear example, some stressors act through the regulation of energy metabolism, e.g., ischemia, anoxia, and hypoglycemia. An acute insult inactivates the Na/K ATPase pump, and water flows into both cytoplasm and nucleus. The normal RNA basophilia fades, and eosin becomes increasingly bound to denatured intracytoplasmic proteins. The nucleus swells and fills empty areas of chromatin with a glassy substance. Severe proteolysis then blurs the margins of the nuclear chromatin. Eventually, large masses of (hetero)chromatin become visible, yielding transcriptionally inactive segments of the genome. At the same time, the nucleoli contracts and often disappears. If water loss supervenes, the nucleus shrinks and its membrane infolds, creating a small pyknotic nucleus. Usually, karyorrhexis does not appear within the central nervous system except under unusual circumstances. Given the limited capacity of the neuron for repair and division, the final outcome of a severe brain lesion (one indicative of great membrane damage) will be cell death.

By observing the temporal profile of morphological changes in the nucleus and cytoplasm of cells, as well as any adjacent tissue reaction, the neuropathologist learns the severity and length of an insult. Some of the main nuclear descriptors include size, shape, chromatin pattern, nuclear membrane configuration, and number of nucleoli. From the above description one might easily surmise that some defining elements of pathology include, among others, cell shrinkage or swelling, molding and shape abnormalities of the nucleus, homogenization of the cyto- and nucleoplasm, eosinophilia, and cell loss. Although researchers have traced neurological disorders to these changes, many psychiatric conditions appear to lack them, e.g., schizophrenia, autism, and bipolar disorders. In study after study, psychiatrists have engaged in a Sisyphean struggle to uncover the organic nature of mental conditions. More than a century of these failed attempts prompts questions as to whether our trust in a neuronocentric viewpoint is well founded.

The Plurality of Neurons

Histology textbooks apply the term neuron to a cell whose presence, along with its connections, defines the brain as an organ. According to classical histology, tissue consists of cells of the same type functioning as a unit. Tissues are then assembled into organs that serve a specific purpose. This grouping is thought to have resulted from the need of multicellular organisms to exploit ecological niches not available to any of its component cells acting alone.

Dissecting organs provides definition of representative tissue structures (e.g., epithelial, muscle, connective), each one having specialized cell types. In this sense muscle tissue has myofibers, while different types of connective tissue may have fibroblasts, chondroblasts, or adipocytes. If the organ is the brain, by analogy to other organs, it should have a representative cellular unit. This histological criterion established the existence of the neuron as a first principle of neuroscience. In other words, the neuron's *raison d'être* was to provide rational expectations about the structure and function of the brain in its normal and pathological states: a foundation upon which to base causality. However, the neuron itself is an idealized structure that unifies the attributes of countless others into a unified whole. The word neuron is therefore a plastic concept that writers adjust to their topic, applying an abbreviated description to a rather complex and diverse grouping of cells. Countless types of neurons exist in the brain, each one varying from others in shape, size, location, neurotransmission, and overall function. Epigenetic circumstances determine which type of neuron among hundreds of choices a particular cell will become at maturity. The plurality of neuron types, both in terms of anatomy and function, argues against their designation as the representative element of the brain.

The concept of the neuron as an idealized cell rather than a concrete entity has been a core tenet of neuroanatomy. Researchers have expanded on the "generalized neuron concept" to identify or represent concepts that illustrate the anatomy and physiology of some cells within the nervous system [9,10]. According to Shepherd and Koch [8], one of the main aims of the well-known neuroscience book *The Synaptic Organization of the Brain* is "to provide the reader with a sense of the canonical structure and function of the key neurons in different regions so that they can be incorporated into more realistic simulations of the neural operations of those regions." The current convention endows the generalized/canonical neuron with the following components [11]:

- A receptive component for input to the neuron either from other neurons or for sensory signals,
- An impulse-initiating and impulse-propagating component which sends the impulse,
- A transmitter-releasing component.

One must note this conceptual model does not specify the size and shape of the cell body (nucleus included): "The membrane functions of the neuron and the trophic functions are separated in this model and it is immaterial where in the cell the same is located." [11] This approach fails to distinguish among the different anatomical components of a neuron. Thus, it defines dendrites and axons as special membrane components of the neurons regardless of their spatial relationship to the cell soma. In this regard, it cloaks the terms axon and dendrite with the same plasticity as the word neuron.

Despite the long history of the generalized neuron concept within neuroscience, its use limits understanding of the nervous system. The majority of information-processing cells within the nervous system fail to adhere to the traditional simplistic model. Thus, axons may bear receptive surfaces, and dendrites may generate all-or-nothing impulses. Moreover, many nervous system elements characterized as neurons fail to obey Ramón y Cajal's law of dynamic polarization. These notable exceptions denote differences in kind rather than degree among neurons; in other words, the term neuron encompasses a large variety of different cells. This mode of existence stands in contrast to other organs of the body where cells resemble each other anatomically and physiologically.

The generalized neuron concept spawned its physiological counterpart in Barlow's neuronal doctrine of perception. Barlow [12] postulated the existence of cardinal or grandmother neurons capable of encoding precepts. His five postulates were as follows:

1. To understand nervous function one needs to look at interactions at a cellular level, rather than either a more macroscopic or microscopic level, because behavior depends upon the organized pattern of these intercellular interactions.
2. The sensory system is organized to achieve as complete a representation of the sensory stimulus as possible with the minimum number of active neurons.
3. Trigger features of sensory neurons are matched to redundant patterns of stimulation by experience as well as by developmental processes.
4. Perception corresponds to the activity of a small selection from the very numerous high-level neurons, each of which corresponds to a pattern of external events of the order of complexity of the events symbolized by a word.
5. High impulse frequency in such neurons corresponds to high certainty that the trigger feature is present.

However, the number of possible precepts is very high, far outstripping the total number of neurons within the nervous system. If they exist, cardinal neurons would have to be present everywhere in significant numbers. Neurophysiological experiments have found neurons with higher-order properties in only a few places [13].

The Interdependence of Neurons

Within the vertebrate nervous system, even simple actions require multiple neurons to coordinate their efforts. "A reflex arc consisting of just two neurons is an abstraction, useful for discussion, which does not exist in nature. Even in systems such as the monosynaptic myotatic reflex in mammals, in which there is one set of afferent and one set of efferent neurons, many neurons are involved." [11]. "No matter how complicated a single neuron may be, it cannot play a role in the processing of information without interacting with other neurons" [8]. The limited involvement of only two elements of an information processing chain severely restricts the possible outputs. Other cells and functionalities must be implicated for operational characteristics to emerge. It is thus unsurprising that convergence and divergence commonly occurs within the nervous system, even within the so-called "two-neuron arc." Convergence enables spatial summation or facilitation while divergence extends the influence of single neurons to a large number of other neurons. By adding inhibition to simple circuits, for example, more complex organizations attain further information processing capabilities.

Consider the biceps reflex [14]. To flex the arm one must make a coordinated effort: contracting the biceps muscle and relaxing the triceps. Both contraction and relaxation of muscles is mediated by the neurotransmitter acetylcholine. The presence of acetylcholine produces muscle excitation. In the absence of inhibitory neurotransmitters acting upon the muscle end-plate, relaxation is achieved by limiting the release of acetylcholine, that is, by lessening excitation. Intervening cells termed intrinsic, local, or interneurons mediate relaxation of the triceps by inhibiting innervating motor neurons. Even simple reflexes function properly only when neurons intimately contact other neurons. This interdependence is as apparent in three dimensions (the nervous system) as in two dimensions (cell culture).

As neuroscientists have labored to find an *in vitro* model of the neuron, they have achieved great success in culturing neurons. They can now manipulate cell lines to induce morphological changes characteristic of differentiated neuronal cells such as synaptogenesis and myelination. Still, the density of cells at which such cultures are initiated is critical for their survival. This factor, called the seeding density, has been claimed to vary between 80 and 300 cells/mm^2 [15]. Neurons cannot be cultured in isolation from other cellular elements.

When tissue stemming from sources outside of the nervous system is dissociated into single cells and planted in a culture dish, a series of characteristic events ensue. First, cells undergo a cycle of rapid division or log phase growth. Then, only as they become confluent and establish contact with each other, the rate of division slows, and cells begin to express features of differentiation. Primary cultures from brain tissue behave differently, in that dispersion of postmitotic cells will extend processes and form synapses with one another. Under these conditions neurons rarely divide and then acquire a neuronal phenotype [16]. In this regard neurons do not act in isolation, but they continue to exist because they communicate with other neurons. This basic understanding of neuronal function bolsters the claim that disruption of cellular interactions is the main culprit for either abnormal or incomplete differentiation in neuronal cell cultures [17].

Neuronal cultures recapitulate the knowledge we have gained on brain development. During a certain time window of brain development, the survival of individual neurons depends on making connections with adequate target structures. Removal of the target structure leads to cell death of neurons normally connected to the same.

The previous discussion illustrates the way neurons, as particulate cells of the nervous system, undergo an infinite regression. That is, neurons exist as chains of information processing cells. Within them, any element functions only by interacting with a similar entity. However, defining the physiology of neurons in terms of other neurons is implausible. Its absurdity is exemplified in the famous story of an elderly woman confronting Bertrand Russell after a lecture on orbital mechanics [18]:

> "The Earth is not a ball revolving around the Sun," she said, "It is a crust of earth on the back of a giant turtle."
> Trying to pursue the argument by following the lady's train of thought, Russell asked, "And what does that turtle stand on?"
> To what the lady answered, "You are a very clever young man, but it's turtles, turtles all the way down."

Moreover, causal explanations, telling why a phenomenon exists, are weakened by embedding the term in question within its framework.

When Daniel Dennett [19] undertook the ambitious project of explaining consciousness, many of his critics said he had failed to "save the appearance or phenomena." His definition not only failed to mention consciousness, but it also strayed from what the consciousness phenomena "seemed-like" in the conception of his critics. Dennett responded by arguing that for a definition to be useful, the phenomena it explains can not rightly appear within the framework of the explanation [20]. A comprehensive physiological definition of neurons should include the transference of information among similar elements, i.e., interdependence among cells. Such a definition would argue against considering the neuron the anatomical and physiological unit of the brain. Without resorting to gap junctions, one can argue on a physiological basis for the correctness of the "syncitium" concept developed by Camillio Golgi, although anatomically the presence of synapses is well recognized.

The idea of an infinite regress was the great flaw in vitalistic theory, which based human life on a vital force, i.e., life pre-existing itself. Such an explanation does not settle an argument but rather postpones it one additional step. Daniel Dennet [21] has called an infinite regress "a loan on intelligence" that must somehow be repaid. Furthermore, the idea of an infinite regression leads to a paradox. Take a normal male adult brain weighing 1400 g, having a normal complement of neocortical neurons, and expressing normal cognitive abilities. Take one neuron away and ask yourself whether losing a single cell would impinge on that person's cognitive abilities. The answer should be "of course not." Take another neuron away and ask the same question. The answer would still be "of course not." It is highly improbable to find two brains, one belonging to a cognitively impaired patient and the other to a normal individual, whose only difference is one neuron. Continuing this line of reasoning may lead to a nervous system of only a hundred neurons. Would we still deny any possible cognitive impairment? If not, when did the change happen? This paradox illustrates the vagueness surrounding the limits of a neuron. It is difficult, if not impossible, to define an amount of neurons accounting for cognition or the totality of the brain.

To solve the little-by-little (*sorites*) paradox, one might posit the existence of an alternate unit of anatomy and function. Changes in its basic template, reproduced many times throughout the neocortex, would provide for salient phenotypic manifestations. Some neuronal conditions, such as thesaurosis, approach this process. However, these conditions seldom affect the totality of neurons. Even when doing so, changes may not be specific but systemic, e.g., affecting all cell types. The differential diagnosis of these neonatal metabolic conditions includes asphyxia, perinatal ventricular hemorrhage, meningoencephalitis, etc. [22] However, these catastrophic events are related more to brain death than to alterations of higher cortical functions. The unit or basic template for which we are looking should serve as the simplest information processing "module" that reproduces itself throughout the neocortex.

Clinical Applications of Modular Connectivity: Landau-Kleffner Syndrome and Alzheimer's Disease

Strange Behavior by Harold Klawans [23] recounts an interesting story about a thoroughly delightful and precocious child who accompanied her grandfather to his scheduled medical appointments. Although normally gregarious, attentive and talkative, over the span of several weeks she became silent and depressed. Her mother referred to some autistic traits: "She's in her own world." Further, the child did not respond to verbal communication, not even the bark of her dog. This failure suggested to Klawans the possibility of aphasia. Furthermore, some automatisms indicated epileptic phenomena. A referral to a specialist resulted in the diagnosis of Landau-Kleffner syndrome or acquired epileptic aphasia. This syndrome becomes noticeable between two and six years of age. There is no hereditary predisposition, and patients lack a clear precedent for the seizures [24]. In patients whose epilepsy becomes refractory to medical treatment, some improvement has been reported after multiple subpial transactions. In Klawans' story, surgical intervention spared the child further seizures, and she began speaking before leaving the hospital.

Subpial transaction is based on physiological evidence suggestive of a columnar organization within the neocortex. Several decades ago, Sperry and associates [4] sliced the visual cortex of monkeys and cats into micro-scale segments. The animals retained their capacity for visual discrimination, suggesting that within columns communication occurs predominantly along the vertical axis. Horizontal contacts among columns are fewer by comparison but may allow the kindling of seizure activity observed in the Landau-Kleffner syndrome. According to Calvin [25]:

> "On average, a cortical neuron contacts fewer than 10 percent of all neurons within a radius of 0.3 mm. But roughly 70 percent of the excitatory synapses on any superficial-layer pyramidal neuron are derived from pyramidal neurons less than 0.3 mm away, so these neurons may be said to have an unusually strong propensity to excite one another. To a neurophysiologist, that raises all sorts of red flags: it's a perfect setup for instability and wild oscillations, unless carefully regulated."

These long collaterals give rise to clusters of terminal branches, one in the vicinity of the parent soma, another below the soma in layer V, and two more at a distance of some 500 μm from the soma [26]. It has been noted that this "skip-spacing" distance of 500 μm is the same as the distance between macrocolumns [25]. Long collaterals of superficial pyramidal cells may therefore provide positive feedback among columns. In the normal state, positive feedback may play a role in Hebbian learning, e.g., the establishment of ocular dominance patterns from an initial random state in which all neurons in the visual cortex receive equal signals from the left and right eyes [27]. In the abnormal state a runaway effect on positive feedback could provide kindling for seizure activity.

Pathology of intercolumnar connectivity is not confined to the kindling phenomena. But it may also play a role in the pathogenesis of some neurodegenerative conditions such as Alzheimer's disease. Based on quantitative observations, medial temporal lobe structures such as the entorhinal cortex and/or subiculum appear to be either the first or the principal region affected by pathology in Alzheimer's disease. These structures serve as a "gateway" between the hippocampus and other areas of the cortex. Since tangles are selective for corticopetal neurons [28,29,30,31], regions receiving projections from the entorhinal/subicular regions would themselves exhibit pathology based on their corticocortical connectivity. Such a stepwise progression has been observed in Alzheimer's disease where tangles stereotypically begin in the entorhinal cortex and "spread" first to the posterior parahippocampal gyrus and then to the frontal and occipital cortices [32,33,34]. This model assumes bilateral neuropathological change. Individual differences explain little of the total variance, duration of illness being the most important variable [35]. In effect, a recent article has detailed minicolumnar abnormalities in Alzheimer's disease [36].

MODULES

> "The interconnections and hence the function of the brain are built first a self-organizing system and second by experience. The self-organization of the early central nervous system is something marvelous and beyond our current understanding."
>
> *D.W. Ross [37]*

Brodal [38] in his textbook *Neurological Anatomy in Relation to Clinical Medicine* made three observations:

1. There is an extremely high degree of order in the anatomical organization of the central nervous system.
2. The nervous system is composed of a multitude of minor units, each with its particular structural organization, specific as regards its finer intrinsic organization as well as with its connections with other units.
3. Investigation of the structure of the nervous system in all its detail is a prerequisite for progress in studies of its function.

A module (Latin *modus* or measure) is usually defined in terms of its structure (standard of measure) and its function (a self-contained, replicable component that may function as part of a larger whole). Implicit in this "black box" characterization of the module's structure and function is its adaptability to the frameworks of various systems and levels of organization. The research literature is full of references to modular organization. Variations on the theme appear in fields as diverse as cognitive science, computer science, psychology, biology, genetics, and philosophy. Yet the concept of the module is used more infrequently in neuroscience than it should be. The reasoning of this observation can lead us into the territory of those non-modular approaches that have attempted to describe cortical organization, e.g., Hebbian cell assemblies, neural networks, and essential nodes. Alternatively, this approach can reveal fundamental differences between theorists. For example, Calvin [39] prefers using the terms "minicolumn" and "macrocolumn" instead of "module." He believes that modules should be restricted to repeating units with an internally identical architecture. They should not apply, as the term is used in so many fields, to something that is merely repeated, segmented, or grouped. In opposition to Calvin's narrow definition of modules, Purves [40] uses the term module to mean iterated or patchy areas. This prompted Calvin to respond that "by so loose a definition, both a dried-up river bed and the fur of a marmalade cat are also modular" [39].

Natural and artificial systems tend towards complexity and are usually composed of sublevels (e.g., components, assemblies, or connections). To understand the sublevels is to understand the system and vice versa. Biologists favor a "nested" rather than a hierarchical design where modules are semi-independent from each other, a function of a limited number of information channels between them. This process compartmentalizes a large number of neurons into circuits connected to their environment by a relatively small number of axons. A modular arrangement in this sense would enhance survival of that organ and its function.

Other properties of modules include emergence and a tendency towards self-organization. Emergence results when novel properties are ascribed to the module but whose components are irreducible. An often-quoted example comes from the statement that consciousness is an emergent property of the brain. Similarly, a car is an emergent property of its interconnected parts. Emergence is intimately linked to a cascade effect where small perturbations can have enormous effects. The story goes:

> For the want of a nail, the shoe was lost;
> For the want of the shoe, the horse was lost;
> For the want of the horse, the rider was lost;
> For the want of a rider, the battle was lost;
> For the want of the battle, the kingdom was lost;
> All for the want of a nail.

In this sense slight perturbations can make the future of a system unpredictable, or chaotic.

As previously mentioned, self-organization is another property of a module/system. The term self-organization denotes the ability of a system to structure itself without apparent constraints from outside forces. Self-organization usually permits a change of state: diminishing from a large space into a persistent smaller one. The preferred position for the system within a restricted volume of space is called an attractor. This is counter to the idea ingrained in the second law of thermodynamics (entropy), stating that all systems tend towards disorder.

Let's examine some examples of self-organization. Water chaotically washing off the drain in your bathroom sink suddenly organizes into a swirling whirlpool. During growth the florets of a cone flower acquire attractive spirals. The chambered shell of the Nautilus (a mollusk) reveals a mathematically exact logarithmic spiral. When a homogeneous liquid, e.g., oil, is heated from below, energy may be dissipated in terms of molecular collisions. However, if the temperature differs enough between the top and bottom of the liquid, one can observe coordinated movement. This is called the Rayleigh-Benard instability. This movement, a convection roll, acquires a hexagonal pattern where liquid rises in the center and sinks at the perimeter. The resultant mosaic of hexagonal cells is an attempt at reducing the surface area of the fluid. In all of these examples, form is acquired independent of "genetic" factors. Rather, the resultant shape depends on the interaction between components of the system independent of the physical nature of those components.

Sometimes self-organization leads to basic similarities in structure. In general two figures are said to be similar if they are scaled versions of each other. The term self-similar is more specific and defines a fractal property whereas the overall shape of a figure is the same as a smaller portion of the same figure. In this regard self-organization leads to similarities in shape that differ somewhat from the fractal pattern in terms of their telescoping properties. A spiral whirlpool siphoning down the drain or the shell of a Nautilus both recreate the shape of the larger organism/system to which they belong.

Columns provide a possible example of self-organization within the nervous system. "If we go around wiretapping the individual neurons in the cerebral cortex, we discover that neurons with similar interests tend to be vertically arrayed there, forming cylinders known as cortical columns, which cut through most of the layers. It's almost like a club that self-organizes out of a crowd at a party, where people of similar interests tend to cluster together." [25]. Noticeably, both neocortical mini- and macrocolumns acquire a putative hexagonal arrangement in a telescoping pattern.

Self-organization is an important concept within neuroscience because it helps constrain those interpretations we may derive from certain experimental procedures. Take for example the way we study the function of genes in the developing brain. In this regard we create mutations in experimental animals that prevent the generation of their protein products. These animals, "knock-out" mice, can be bred in a laboratory setting and examined for the effects that the particular gene may have on the growth, development, and survival of the animal. However, within systems, properties are not mathematical aggregates. Perturbations in the initial state of a system can have major and often unpredictable effects. Furthermore, variations may be imposed by the amount of change (the total absence of a gene vs. its dysfunction) and by when it occurs in the life of the animal. As quoted in the introduction to this book, more often than not, it is impossible to assess the impact of specific gene deletions on the phenotype and/or behavior of an animal.

Self-organization and emergence are byproducts of the way we define systems. However, the importance of modular arrangements may lie within a natural selection model. In this model, systems reveal a bias for moving in a particular direction that maximizes any advantageous interaction with their environment. The modular organization of the brain presents another advantage over the neuronal concept: A map of the path taken by information as it passes through the different processing way stations shows only a few connections. At a first glance it would seem likely that information-processing chains in the brain might be 20 to 30 links long. However, energy expenditure and the possibility that information may degenerate every time signals are transferred makes information chains much shorter than expected. Half a dozen links is a good thing; waste is an alien concept in nature. In large chains or cascades, small differences in the initial transmission would produce enormous and possibly unpredictable effects. Imagine a drop of water falling on a mountain. Depending on small changes as to where it might fall, the water cycle may include an underwater river or the Pacific Ocean. In our everyday life we must avoid perturbations accrued to lengthy information processing sequences. Try thinking of your mother's face under different circumstances, e.g., your birthday, at your high school graduation, or on Mother's day. It is clearly important that we always identify each memory trace with the same person and do not merely summon up an approximation.

Given the large variety of components (different cells and their connections), organizing them into a pattern (module) overcomes the problem of "complexity of substance" [27]. The brain has some 10^{10} neurons, 10^3–10^4 connections per neuron, and about 50 different neurotransmitters. Self-organization patterns would permit reproducibility. This capability addresses the way one pattern emerges out of the possible randomness of different environmental circumstances. It is this reproducibility that allows neurologists to localize and diagnose disease processes within the brain with considerable accuracy despite the differences presented by the patients, e.g., race, age, and nutrition. Overcoming the complexity of substance also explains how a limited number of genes acting during development affect the intricate anatomical interactions of the brain. Lastly, arranging circuits within units in a confined space shortens neuronal processes and, other things remaining equal, shortens conduction times.

Looking Outside of the Neuron

Decades of controversy regarding the representation of cerebral functions have been favorably settled in the opinion of most neuroscientists. Researchers have demonstrated beyond any reasonable doubt that different convolutions of the brain provide our motor, sensory, auditory, and visual abilities. Still, a vast span of the cerebral cortex appears to be terra incognita, and higher operations such as judgment, attention, and thinking lack a corresponding territory. These higher functions are not impaired by lesions affecting groups of neurons or particular gyri. This is in clear contrast to subcortical nuclei where lesions cause disorders of cranial nerves, motor, sensory and autonomic function, while leaving "mentation" unaffected. Neurologists assume that higher functions somehow result from the "rich connectivity of all parts of the so-called cortical centers" [22]. According to Passingham [41], the neocortex and its connections account for 80 % of the volume of the brain. Many behaviors engendered by the cortex may therefore be classified as emergent properties. These emergent properties derive from the underlying organization of the nervous system rather than as a byproduct of any of its individual components. The sheer abundance of these emergent properties indicates that the modular organization of the nervous system is at a premium within the neocortex.

A feature of science known as reductionism attempts to explain complex systems in terms of smaller or more basic features of reality. For many decades, dissecting the brain into smaller components gave rise to the idea that brain cells were the basic anatomical unit of the brain. This attempt brings to mind a favorite passage from an older textbook of neuroanatomy:

> "There are two ways of coming to know a machine: one is that the master who made it should show us its artifice; the other is to dismantle it and examine its most minute parts separately and as a combined unit....But since the brain is a machine, we need not hope to discover its artifice by methods other than those that are used to find such for other machines. There remains to be done; therefore, only what would be done for all other machines. I mean the dismantling of all its components, piece by piece, and consideration of what they can do separately and as a whole." —Niels Stensen [14,42]

This is the same as trying to study a radio by throwing it to the floor and examining its pieces.

When applied to the cortex, reductionism questions what quantum of tissue typifies the holistic properties of the cortex (i.e., afferent, central processing, and efferent) and reiterates itself throughout the extent of this structure. What structure provides a canonical circuit for cortical organization? [8] This approach should distinguish intrinsic features of the brain from those that are relative to some extrinsic use. It would also provide a template unit capable of performing parallel processing of information [19,43]. This would not only allow real time processing of information but also account for the physiological and evolutionary constraints imposed by the necessary interconnectivities of the units [44].

MINICOLUMNS

The neuron is a differentiated element. During development it gradually becomes fixed, less flexible, and more prone to injury, therefore creating the appearance that it has added importance of its own. The visibility and prominence of the neuron suggests that the central nervous system revolves around it. Unsurprisingly, neuronal changes appear to either drive the whole or be the main cause of change. This neuronocentric view of the brain engendered a long-standing debate on the relationship of primate brain size (encephalization) and cognition. The question posed was whether 1 gram of human brain tissue equals 1 gram of great ape tissue. Jerison [45] argued that an increase in brain tissue was the most important determinant of human intelligence. Holloway [46] championed a contradictory stance, arguing that brain circuitry reorganization caused or provided human mental capacities. Although the debate ricocheted through the neuroscience community for several decades, it can best be summarized as "what varies between species is the way neurons are used to build the neuromeres—or, alternatively, the way neurons are used to construct neural circuits or networks within the system as a whole" [14]. It is therefore worth noting that certain elements of neocortical circuitry reiterate themselves to reflect a pattern, such as apical dendritic bundles, the myelinated bundles of pyramidal cells, double bouquet axon bundles, synaptic compartments, and the relationship of the previously mentioned elements to pyramidal cells. These elements occur in fixed interrelationships within the cell minicolumn, itself a reiterative element found in all neocortical areas [47,48].

The cell minicolumn consists of 60 to 100 neurons along with their afferent, efferent, and interneuronal connections. Together the elements provide for a canonical circuit to the neocortex. Input is feed-forwarded through a short chain of two or three neurons within the same column and then transmitted to other target areas. Anatomically, cells are arranged along a radial scaffolding most noticeable in thick Nissl-stained sections. The juxtaposition of cells becomes less prominent with aging, providing a thickness dimension that is easily missed in thin paraffin sections. The genesis of the cell minicolumn occurs early in gestation when symmetrical divisions of periventricular germinal cells create their total number. After E40, both in macaque monkeys and humans, a subsequent series of asymmetrical divisions determines the cellular constituency of the minicolumn [49]. This radial organization is thus preeminent to other organizations based on either synapses or layering. The addition of minicolumns accomplishes the growth of the human neocortex as compared across species. This helps explain why the human neocortex is 1000-fold larger than that of the mouse while only a two or three-fold difference separates their cortical widths. Numerous studies using C-2-deoxyglucose, intrinsic optical signaling (IOS), nerve regeneration, and evoked potentials have established the minicolumn as a physiological unit of the brain [47,48]. Other chapters within this book cover the structure of the minicolumn in depth.

Interestingly, one could base the anatomical and physiological validity of the cell minicolumn on the presence of secondary structures. Astrocytes with interlaminar processes may maintain the spatial definition of the cell minicolumn and help isolate them from neighboring minicolumns [50,51,52]. Moreover, the cortical microvasculature has a columnar organization. Arterioles penetrate the cortex at right angles to the pial surface. The radial orientation provides a columnar pattern of blood flow, NADH/NAD+ redox state, and glucose metabolism, which can be seen during hypoxia or ischemia [53]. These vessels are not randomly distributed but follow a set geometry variously described as hexagons [54] or microcircles [55]. Vessels may act as radiators to the minicolumn. Water has a high capacity, meaning that it takes a long time for it to warm up. That is why cities that are near large bodies of water tend to have a moderate climate; they don't get too hot or too cold. If the system partakes in a dissipative thermal mechanism, heat or energy may not be distributed uniformly throughout the module. Rather, it may be concentrated along the structural flow of information. Of importance to functional neuroimaging is the hypothesis of Lierse [56], namely that capillary density provides an index of oxidative metabolism. Within a given region of the brain, this principle may apply primarily to the minicolumn rather than to individual cellular entities. In addition, this pattern of vascularization may explain why moderate changes in temperature have profound effects on brain functions.

Recently, variations in the basic template of the cell minicolumn have been reported in autism, dyslexia, Asperger and Rett syndromes [57-63]. The reports are significant because they relate pathology within the modular framework of the neocortex and provide an unexplored dimension within neuropathology. It is clear that if the minicolumn is accepted as a distinct anatomical structure, different disease processes may affect it. By analogy, cirrhosis affects the lobule of the liver by creating broad septal tracts due to collagen deposition. The study of kidney pathology is similarly facilitated by dividing cells into those that affect its four anatomical components: glomeruli, tubules, interstitium, and blood vessels. Some components are more vulnerable to specific pathological processes: Glomerular conditions are immunologically mediated whereas tubular and interstitial disorders are usually caused by toxic or infectious agents [64]. In a similar vein, certain pathological conditions may preferentially affect minicolumns. Clinically, aberrations of those emergent properties stemming from the neocortex should be salient manifestations of minicolumnopathies.

Similarly, aging is the great equalizer in terms of minicolumnopathies. A case report in Asperger's disease has already reported that minicolumns appear to "normalize" with aging [58]. In the following section we discuss additional characteristics of minicolumnopathies.

PUTATIVE CHARACTERISTICS OF MINICOLUMNOPATHIES

Comorbidity

This is a natural consequence of minicolumnopathies as they involve numerous neurotransmitter agents. Overall, transmission of information occurs vertically within the neocortex primarily by excitation and inhibition. The vast majority of connections within the neocortex are intrinsic to the same, thus giving rise to massive excitatory and inhibitory feedback circuits [65]. Modulatory effects are provided by horizontal components that innervate different layers of the minicolumn, e.g., monoaminergic agents that bypass the thalamus. The result provides a Cartesian system for the action of neurotransmitters. This fact may help explain why amino acids (e.g., glutamate and GABA) are the major transmitters in the mammalian nervous system. On the other hand, modulatory transmitters stemming primarily from sources outside of the minicolumn (acetylcholine, norepinephrine, dopamine, histamine, and 5-hydroxytryptamine) account for transmission at only a small percentage of central synaptic sites. Modulatory agents influence the afferent, internal processing, and efferent components of the minicolumn depending on the layers innervated. According to Diamond [66] regardless of neocortical location, layers II and III serve as associational cortex, layer IV as sensory, and layers V and VI as motor cortex. The complexity of modulatory interactions suggests that attempts at finding a single neuropharmacological abnormality for minicolumnopathies may be misguided.

Gender Differences

Brain size varies according to gender. Studies have found that per given stature or body surface area, brain volume is approximately 100 grams larger in men than in women [67]. One study of children 5 to 17 years of age reported a 10% increase in brain size for boys compared to girls. The results suggest "the presence of early gender-associated differences in cerebral development and organization" [68]. Brain size differences reflect changes in the gray/white matter ratio, with a significantly higher ratio of gray matter in women than in men [69]. Larger brains, those with supernumerary minicolumns, require a corresponding disproportionate increase in white matter (corticocorticoid) connectivity. These findings suggest concomitant differences in the number of neurons and their connectivities. Unsurprisingly, cytoarchitectural studies have found significantly higher neuronal densities and total number estimates in males and a reciprocal increase in neuropil and neuronal processes in female cortex [70,71]. Therefore, variations in the modular organization of the brain might help explain gender-related changes in brain volume and gray/white matter ratios.

Complex Genetic and Epigenetic Influences

This characteristic would be manifested by a complex medical history, e.g., birth difficulties, febrile illness, RH incompatibility, and maternal influenza. In our laboratory, analysis of minicolumnar width across a control population shows a continuous variation suggestive of additive polygenetic and environmental influences (Casanova, unpublished findings, 2005). The expected curve for a condition defined by a small number of genes (e.g., hair color) would have provided a jagged continuum of heights [72]. The superimposition of variations stemming from multiple genetic loci and environmental influences (e.g., body height or, in this case, minicolumnar width) accounts for the smoothness of the curve [72]. This also suggests that symptoms may appear within a spectrum, raising the possibility that parents and other relatives would exhibit some but not all of the symptomatology.

Attempts at treatment may permit remission of pathological symptomatology along with any advantage (e.g., multitasking in ADHD or savant skills in autistic individuals) accrued to their minicolumnar phenotype. Computer modeling studies provide some evidence for this assertion. At least one of them is based on self-organizing feature maps and columnar feature development, i.e., objects with similar features activate neighboring columns. However, the uneven distribution of synaptic weights among neurons in a column allows for variability. Gustafsson [73] concludes that narrow columns facilitate discrimination whereas wider columns facilitate generalization.

Language Impairment and Alterations of Cerebral Dominance

These traits may be manifested by an unusually high proportion of left-handers. In addition, since modern psycholinguists believe that language reflects the way the mind works, thought disturbance may also be related. Evidence is based on morphometric studies on minicolumns located within the planum temporale (Brodmann area 22) [74]. The study examined the brains of normal humans, chimpanzees (*Pan troglodytes*), and rhesus monkeys (*Macaca mulatta*) for width of cell columns, the peripheral neuropil space, the spacing density of neurons within columns, and the Gray Level index per minicolumn. Only human brain tissue revealed robust asymmetry in two aspects of minicolumn morphology: wider columns and more neuropil space on the left side. This asymmetry was absent in chimpanzee and rhesus monkey.

Change in Prevalence through Different Generations

The development of human civilization has removed many of the natural environment's checks and balances on behavioral phenotypes. Our present society is therefore unique in having created a man-made environment that is technologically driven. Differences in minicolumnar widths, and their attendant alternative way of perceiving information, offer an evolutionary improvisation that may prove adaptive within our technologically driven society. "The point is that the perceived value of any given trait is greatly dependent on a continually changing social and economic context—indeed, in the end, a changing biological context as well" [75]. Some authors have denoted this characteristic as a "cohort effect" to explain the increased incidence of both bipolar and unipolar depression. "The cohort effect cannot be attributed to genetic alteration because it occurred over too short a period of time. Instead, it must reflect a cultural influence on expression of vulnerability to the disorders. This suggests that genetic vulnerability may be necessary but, without certain stress factors, insufficient for the expression of an illness" [76].

Frontal Lobe Syndrome

This may be manifested as a pseudodepression, indifference so extreme as to reduce the response to pain, an inability to initiate any behavior, and being at the mercy of incidental distractions ("field dependent behavior"). The frontal lobe is probably the most connected part of the brain. According to Goldberg [77], "The prefrontal cortex is directly interconnected with every distinct functional unit of the brain…this particular connectivity also puts the frontal lobes at particular risk for disease." This may be due to the fact that the dorsolateral prefrontal cortex in amphibians may serve as the precursor to the neocortex [78]. In mammals connections from the dorsolateral prefrontal cortex to other annexed regions may serve to unify their function. In addition, the frontal lobe acts as gateway for the flow of information of multiple neurotransmitter systems as they undergo their rostrocaudal trajectory throughout the brain. Abnormal interactions at this initial point may provide for a cascade effect that is only exacerbated by the rich connectivity of this structure.

Abnormalities on EEG, Especially its High (Gamma) Frequency

The generation of EEG signals is facilitated by the summation of electrical potentials from pyramidal cells [79]. Pyramidal cells within minicolumns are especially suited for this role for many reasons. 1) The apical dendrites of pyramidal cells extend in bundles through nearly all cortical layers. This anatomical arrangement guides the flow of current generated by postsynaptic potentials through the entire thickness of the cortex. 2) Cortical pyramidal cells are packed into functional vertical units facilitating summation of signals. Groups of cells working on the same stimulus correlate their output at around 40 Hz, resulting in oscillatory patterns at that frequency. This characteristic suggests that synchronization of different areas at their gamma frequency denotes relatedness. Because distant cell groups are likely to be active simultaneously, precise time-locking is essential for either the segregation or amalgamation of separate cell ensembles [61].

Abnormalities in Brain Size, Gyrification, and Gray/White Matter Ratios

(See also Gender Differences, above.) Minicolumns have emergent properties that are not reducible to their input or to their individual neuronal components [62]. These properties are based, in part, on feedforward and feedback connections between minicolumns. The fraction of white matter devoted to connectivity between these modular units is the short association fibers underlying the cortex [80]. Estimates of cortical interconnectivity for the human brain suggest that each module is connected to a thousand other modules [44]. In other words, if a fixed percentage of interconnections are maintained with an increasing number of minicolumns, then a large fraction of the increased brain size is spent in wiring these modular units. Overall the addition of minicolumns during encephalization has resulted in: 1) small changes in the cortical gray matter when expressed as a percentage of brain volume, 2) large increases in white matter volume, 3) vast expansion in the surface area of the cortex, and 4) little change (or even diminution) in subcortical structures.

The Presence of Heterotopias

Heterotopias refer to abnormal clusters of gray matter. Microscopically, they are comprised of neurons and glial tissue without any consistent arrangement. Heterotopias result from a failure of neurons to properly migrate along their radial scaffolding and occupy their final position within the cortex.

Conclusions

A neutral exposition of neuroscience is a fantasy. Any exploration is predated not only by the phenomena that we examine but also by the frame of reference that we bring into the exploration. The frame of reference or our perspective of neuroscience shapes the data that we collect and its interpretation. Data stemming from a neuronocentric perspective and one that is based on a minicolumnar point of view may provide "incommensurate and untranslatable" results [6]. A given claim is thus true or false only within the paradigm it is articulated. The lack of neuropathological findings until recent times in autism, schizophrenia, or manic depression has been only apparent within the paradigm dictated by extrapolations of the neuronal doctrine.

The rigidity of neuronocentrism has witnessed the rise and fall of many ideas within neurosciences and will continue to do so in the future. An integral paradigm will "inherently be critical of those approaches that are, by comparison, partial, narrow, shallow, less encompassing, less integrative" [81]. For the neuronal doctrine to succeed, it should be able to justify the conclusions and inferences derived from the same. Take neuroscience from the point of view of the neuronal doctrine and compare the results with a perspective stemming from the modular organization of the cortex. Then consider in this thought experiment the ultimate aim of present day stem cell research: clinical intervention based on the replacement of lost neurons. Will the addition of neuronal cells help reacquire lost function or will it translate into iatrogenenically induced heterotopias? Significant side effects from such interventions should build insight into the modular organization of the brain. Alternatively, consider experiments dealing with stereological counts of different cortical regions. Results are given in terms of concrete numbers, but what do they mean? Can they offer meaningful information without referring to the modular organization on which they depend? Consider next the case of neural networks. These networks attempt to model cortical function as a highly divergent flow of information spanning different but highly interconnected layers composed of canonical neurons. A high degree of divergence in connectivity makes it more likely that information processing occurs through parallel pathways. Since neuronal transmission is rather slow (from 1 to 10 meters/second), parallel processing in the cortex confers the advantage of speed and allows for real time decision making. However, despite their success, it is difficult to see how neural networks are biological. What cortex of what species are they trying to imitate? The existence of minicolumns as units of anatomy and physiology is based on their sparse intracortical connectivity with adjacent units. Studies of Boolean networks suggest that a limited connection for each unit leads to optimum organizational and adaptive properties. Finally, we would like to consider whether mental conditions lack neuropathology. Should we gear our research towards behaviorism and psychoanalysis? Or should we give up on the traditional logocentric approach and deconstruct the neuronal doctrine? A century of unsuccessful attempts at uncovering the pathophysiological substrates of mental conditions has deterred any incursions of neuropathologists into the field of psychiatry. A subtle but basic commonality to these failed attempts has been their emphasis on a Ptolemaic view of the neuron, a love affair *avec soi*.

The most unsatisfactory aspect of the neuronal metatheory is its superficiality, its lack of respect for any aspect of human behavior. Anything (e.g., fear, memory, and anger) can be placed on its scale, weighed and measured. Mental illnesses, as well as behaviors, tend to be culturally relative and socially construed. The neuronal doctrine is alien to the richness of the psychosocial environment and portrays only a microscopic view of neurosciences. At the beginning of this chapter I asked whether terms such as neurology, neuroscience, and neuroanatomy were appropriate or whether they were instances of misguided intentionality. Such terms are biased in favor of the neuronal metatheory. This chapter espouses one possible alternative: one based on modular organization. There is order, beauty, and boundless untapped information within the organization of the neocortex, and it is based on its modular structure.

REFERENCES

[1] Dewey J. *How We Think*. London, UK: D.C. Heath and Co.; 1909.

[2] Glaser E. *An Experiment in the Development of Critical Thinking*. New York, NY: Teacher's College, Columbia University Press; 1941.

[3] Waldeyer-Hartz W. Ueber einige neuere Forschungen im Gebiete der Anatomie des Centralnervensystems. *Deutsche medicinische Wochenschrift*1891;. 17:1213-1218, 1244-1246, 1287-1289, 1331-1332, 1350-1356.

[4] Sperry RW, Miner N, Myers RE. Visual pattern perception following sub-pial slicing and tantalum wire implantation in the visual cortex. *J Comp Physiol Psychol.* 1955;48:50-80.

[5] Dawkins R. *The Selfish Gene*. Oxford, UK: Oxford University Press; 1976.

[6] Kuhn TS. *The Structure of Scientific Revolution.* 3rd ed. Chicago, IL: University of Chicago Press; 1996.

[7] LeDoux J. *Synaptic Self: How Our Brains Become Who We Are*. New York, NY: Viking; 2002.

[8] Shepherd GM, Koch C. Introduction to synaptic circuits. In: Shepherd GM, ed. *The Synaptic Organization of the Brain.* 4th ed. New York, NY: Oxford University Press; 1998:1-36.

[9] Bodian D. The generalized vertebrate neuron. *Science.* 1962;137:323-326.

[10] Bullock TH. Neuron doctrine and electrophysiology. *Science.* 1959;129:997-1002.

[11] Brown AG. *Nerve Cells and Nervous Systems: An Introduction to Neuroscience*. 2nd ed. London, UK: Springer; 2001.

[12] Barlow HB. Single units and sensation: a neuron doctrine for perceptual psychology? *Perception.* 1972;1:371-394. Available at: http://faculty.washington.edu/sarude/BakerLab/Mindmete/Barlow.txt.

[13] Gross C, Rocha-Miranda C, Bender D. Visual properties of neurons in inferotemporal cortex of the macaque. *J Neurophys.* 1972;35:96-111

[14] Swanson LW. *Brain Architecture*. Oxford, UK: Oxford University Press; 2003.

[15] Sellstrom A, Jacobsson S. Culturing CNS neurons: A practical approach to cultured embryonic chick neurons. In: Haynes LW, ed. *The Neuron in Tissue Culture*. Chichester, UK: John Wiley and Sons; 1999:327-338.

[16] Banker G, Goslin K. Types of nerve cell cultures, their advantage and limitations. In: *Culturing Nerve Cells*. Cambridge, MA: MIT Press; 1998 chapter 2.

[17] Banker G, Goslin K. Getting started. In: *Culturing Nerve Cells*. Cambridge, MA: MIT Press; 1998:chapter 1.

[18] Hawking S. *A Brief History of Time*. 10th ed. New York, NY: Bantam Books; 1998.

[19] Dennett DC. *Consciousness Explained*. Boston, MA: Back Bay Books; 1992.

[20] Baggini J, Fosl OS. *The Philosopher's Toolkit: A Compendium of Philosophical Concepts and Methods*. Malden, MA: Blackwell Publishing; 2003:123

[21] Dennett DC. *Brainstorms*. Montgomery, VT: Bradford Books; 1978:12.

[22] Victor M, Ropper AH. Neurobiologic disorders caused by lesions in particular parts of the cerebrum. In: *Adams and Victor's Principles of Neurology*. 7th ed. New York, NY: McGraw-Hill; 2001:464.

[23] Klawans H. *Strange Behavior: Tales of Evolutionary Neurology*. New York, NY: Norton; 2000:56-72.

[24] Rotenberg J, Pearl PL. Landau-Kleffner syndrome. *Arch Neurol.* 2003;60:1019-1021.

[25] Calvin WH. *How Brains Think: Evolving Intelligence, Then and Now*. New York, NY: Basic Books; 1996.

[26] Nieuwenhuys R. The neocortex: an overview of its evolutionary development, structural organization and synaptology. *Anat Embryol.* 1994;190:307-337.

[27] Scott Kelso JA. *Dynamic Patterns: The Self-Organization of Brain and Behavior*. Cambridge, MA: MIT Press; 1995.

[28] German DC, White CL III, Sparkman DR. Alzheimer's disease: neurofibrillary tangles in nuclei that project to the cerebral cortex. *Neuroscience.* 1987;21:305-312.

[29] Ishii T. Distribution of Alzheimer's neurofibrillary changes in the brain stem and the hypothalamus of senile dementia. *Acta Neuropathol.* 1966;6:181-187.

[30] Jellinger K. Quantitative changes in some subcortical nuclei in aging, Alzheimer's disease and Parkinson's disease. *Neurobiol Aging.* 1987;8:556-561.

[31] Saper CB, German DC, White CL III. Neuronal pathology in the nucleus basali and associated cell groups in senile dementia of the Alzheimer's type: possible role in cell loss. *Neurology.* 1985;35:1089-1095.

[32] Armstrong RA, Myers D, Smith CUM. Alzheimer's disease: size class frequency distributions of senile plaques: do they indicate when a brain tissue was affected? *Neurosci Lett.* 1991;127:223-226.

[33] de Lacoste M-C, White CL. The role of cortical connectivity in Alzheimer's disease pathogenesis: a review and model system. *Neurobiol Aging.* 1993;14:1-16.

[34] Pearson RCA, Esiri MM, Hiorns RW, Wilcock GK, Powell TPS. Anatomical correlates of the distribution of the pathological changes in the neocortex in Alzheimer's disease. *Proc Natl Acad Sci U S A.* 1985;82:4531-4534.

[35] Ritchie K, Touchon J. Heterogeneity in senile dementia of the Alzheimer type: individual differences, progressive deterioration or clinical subtypes *J Clin Epidemiol.* 1992;45:1391-1398.

[36] Buldyrev SV, Cruz L, Gomes-Isla T, et al. Description of microcolumnar ensembles in association cortex and their disruption in Alzheimer and Lewy body dementias. *Proc Natl Acad Sci U S A.* 2000;97:5039-5043.

[37] Ross DW. *Introduction to Molecular Medicine*. 3rd ed. New York, NY: Springer-Verlag; 2002:20.

[38] Brodal A. *Neurological Anatomy in Relation to Clinical Medicine*. 3rd ed. Oxford, UK: Oxford University Press; 1981.

[39] Calvin WH. Cortical columns, modules and Hebbian cell assemblies. In: Arbib MA, ed. *The Handbook of Brain Theory and Neural Networks*. Cambridge, MA: MIT Press; 1995:269-272.

[40] Purves D, Riddle DR, White LE, Gutierrez-Ospina G, LaMantia AS. Categories of cortical structure. *Prog Brain Res.* 1994;102:343-355.

[41] Passingham R. *The Human Primate*. Oxford, UK: W. H. Freeman; 1982.

[42] Stensen N. *Discours sur l'anatomie du cerveau*. Paris, France: Robert de Ninville; 1669.

[43] Sejnowski TJ, Koch C, Churchland PS. Computational neuroscience. *Science.* 1988;241:1299-1306.

[44] Hofman MA. Brain evolution in hominids: are we at the end of the road? In: Falk D, Gibson KR, eds. *Evolutionary Anatomy of the Primate Cerebral Cortex*. Cambridge, UK: Cambridge University Press; 2001:113-127.

[45] Jerison HJ. *Evolution of the Brain and Intelligence*. New York, NY: Academic Press; 1973.

[46] Holloway RL Jr. Cranial capacity and neuron number: a critique and proposal. *Am J Phys Anthropol.* 1966;25:305-314.
[47] Buxhoeveden D, Casanova MF. The minicolumn and evolution of the brain: a review. *Brain Behav Evol.* 2002;60:125-151.
[48] Buxhoeveden D, Casanova MF. The minicolumnar hypothesis in neurosciences. *Brain.* 2002;125:935-951.
[49] Rakic P, Kornack DR. Neocortical expansion and elaboration during primate evolution: a view from neuroembryology. In: Falk D, Gibson KR, eds. *Evolutionary Anatomy of the Primate Cerebral Cortex*. Cambridge, UK: Cambridge University Press; 2001:30-56.
[50] Colombo JA. A columnar-supporting mode of astroglial architecture in the cerebral cortex of adult primates? *Neurobiology.* 2001;9:1-16.
[51] Colombo JA, Fuchs E, Hartig W, Marotte LR, Puissant V. "Rodent-like" and "primate-like" types of astroglial architecture in the adult cerebral cortex of mammals: a comparative study. *Anat Embryol.* 2000;201:111-120.
[52] Colombo JA, Schleicher A, Zilles K. Patterned distribution of immunoreactive astroglial processes in the striate (V1) cortex of New World monkeys. *Glia.* 1999;25:85-92.
[53] Edvinsson L, MacKenzie ET. General and comparative anatomy of the cerebral circulation. In: Edvinsson L, Krause DN, eds. *Cerebral Blood Flow and Metabolism*. Philadelphia, PA: Lippincott Williams and Wilkins; 2002:3-29.
[54] Bar T. The vascular system of the cerebral cortex. *Adv Anat Embryol Cell Biol.* 1980;59:1-62.
[55] Mchedlishvili G, Kuridze N. The modular organization of the pial arterial system in phylogeny. *J Cereb Blood Flow Metab.* 1984;4:391-396.
[56] Lierse W. Die Kapillardichte im rhinencephalon verschiedener wirbeltiere und des menschen. *Prog Brain Res.* 3:230-236; 1963.
[57] Casanova MF, Buxhoeveden D, Switala A, Roy E. Minicolumnar pathology in autism. *Neurology.* 2002;58:428-432.
[58] Casanova MF, Buxhoeveden D, Switala A, Roy E. Asperger's syndrome and cortical neuropathology. *J Child Neurol.* 2002;17:142-145.
[59] Casanova MF, Buxhoeveden D, Cohen M, Switala A, Roy E. Minicolumnar pathology in dyslexia. *Ann Neurol.* 2002;52:108-110.
[60] Casanova MF, Buxhoeveden D, Switala A, Roy E. Neuronal density and architecture (gray level index) in the brains of autistic patients. *J Child Neurol.* 2002;17:515-521.
[61] Casanova MF, Buxhoeveden DP, Brown C. Clinical and macroscopic correlates of minicolumnar pathology in autism. *J Child Neurol.* 2002;17:692-695.
[62] Casanova MF, Buxhoeveden D, Switala A, Roy E. Rett syndrome as a minicolumnopathy. *Clin Neuropathol.* 2003;22:163-168.
[63] Casanova MF, Buxhoeveden D, Gomez J. Disruption in the inhibitory architecture of the cell minicolumn: implications for autism. *Neuroscientist.* 2003;9:496-507.
[64] Cotran RS, Kumar V, Collins T. *Robbins Pathologic Basis of Disease*. Philadelphia, PA: W.B. Saunders; 1999.

[65] Braitenberg V, Schuz A. *Anatomy of the Cortex: Statistics and Geometry*. New York, NY: Springer-Verlag; 1991.

[66] Diamond I. The subdivisions of neocortex: a proposal to revise the traditional view of sensory, motor, and association areas. In: Sprague JM, Epstein AN, eds. *Progress in Psychobiology and Physiological Psychology*. New York, NY: Academic Press; 1979:1-43.

[67] Ankney CD. Sex differences in relative brain size: the mismeasure of woman, too? *Intelligence*. 1992;16:329-336.

[68] Reiss AL, Abrams MT, Singer HS, Ross JL, Denckla MB. Brain development, gender, and IQ in children: a volumetric imaging study. *Brain*. 1996;119:1763-1774.

[69] Gur RC, Turetsky BI, Matsui M, et al. Sex differences in brain gray and white matter in healthy young adults: correlations with cognitive performance. *J Neurosci*. 1999;19:4065-4072.

[70] de Courten-Myers GM. The human cerebral cortex: gender differences in structure and function. *J Neuropathol Neurol*. 1999;58:217-226.

[71] Rabinowicz T, Dean DE, Petetot JM, de Courten-Myers GM. Gender differences in the human cerebral cortex: more neurons in males; more processes in females. *J Child Neurol*. 1999;14:98-107.

[72] Futuyma DJ. *Evolutionary Biology*. 3rd ed. Sunderland, MA: Sinauer Associates; 1998.

[73] Gustafsson L. Inadequate cortical feature maps: a neural circuit theory of autism. *Biol Psychiatry*. 1997;42:1138-1147.

[74] Buxhoeveden DP, Switala AE, Roy E, Litaker M, Casanova MF. Lateralization of minicolumn structure in human planum temporale is absent in nonhuman primate cortex. *Brain Behav Evol*. 2001;57:349-358.

[75] West TG. *In the Mind's Eye*. Amherst, NY: Prometheus Books; 1997:20-81.

[76] Fawcett J, Golden B, Rosenfeld N. *New Hope for People with Bipolar Disorder*. Rocklin, CA: Prima Publishing; 2000:54.

[77] Goldberg E. *The Executive Brain: Frontal Lobes and the Civilized Mind*. Oxford, UK: Oxford University Press; 2001.

[78] Harris JC. *Developmental Neuropsychiatry, volume 1: Fundamentals*. Oxford, UK: Oxford University Press; 1995.

[79] Fisch BJ, Spehlmann R. *Fisch and Spehlmann's EEG Primer: Basic Principles of Digital and Analog EEG*. 3rd ed. Amsterdam, Netherlands: Elsevier; 1999.

[80] Hofman MA. The fractal geometry of the convoluted brain. *J Hirnforsch*. 1991;32:103-111.

[81] Wilber K. *A Theory of Everything*. Boston, MA: Shambhala; 2001.

In: Neocortical Modularity and the Cell Minicolumn
Editor: Manuel F. Casanova, pp. 57-92
ISBN 1-59454-301
© 2005 Nova Science Publishers, Inc.

Chapter IV

REFLECTIONS ON THE STRUCTURE OF THE CORTICAL MINICOLUMN

Javier DeFelipe*
Instituto Cajal (CSIC), Madrid, Spain

INTRODUCTION

When in the second half of the 19th century the detailed structure of the cerebral cortex began to be studied, the strikingly regular columnar disposition of certain myelinated fibers and neurons became evident: the radial fasciculi ("medullary rays") and the vertical aggregates of pyramidal neurons. For example, the bundles of vertical myelinated ("medullated") fibers can be seen in the early drawings and descriptions of Dejerine and Dejerine-Klumpke [1], summarized in Figure 1. This figure nicely represents the progress made during a century of research into the structure of the cerebral cortex (1790–1890), with the studies of Vicq d'Azyr, Baillarger, Kölliker, Meynert and Cajal. Interestingly, in the first half of the XIX century, there was much debate as to whether the cortical gray matter was joined or not to the underlying white matter. Indeed, in 1840 Baillarger concluded [2]:

> "En résumé, la substance blanche, au sommet des circonvolutions, est entièrement unie à la substance grise par un grand nombre des fibres. La simple juxta-position des deux substances est donc une opinion inadmissible."[a]

* Corresponding author: Javier DeFelipe, Instituto Cajal (CSIC), Avenida Dr. Arce, 37, 28002-Madrid, Spain. Tel: (+34) 91 585 4735; Fax: (+34) 91 585 4754; E-mail: defelipe@cajal.csic.es

[a] "In summary, the white matter, in the crown of convolutions is entirely joined to the gray matter through a large number of fibers. The simple juxtaposition of the two [gray and white] matters is therefore inadmissible."

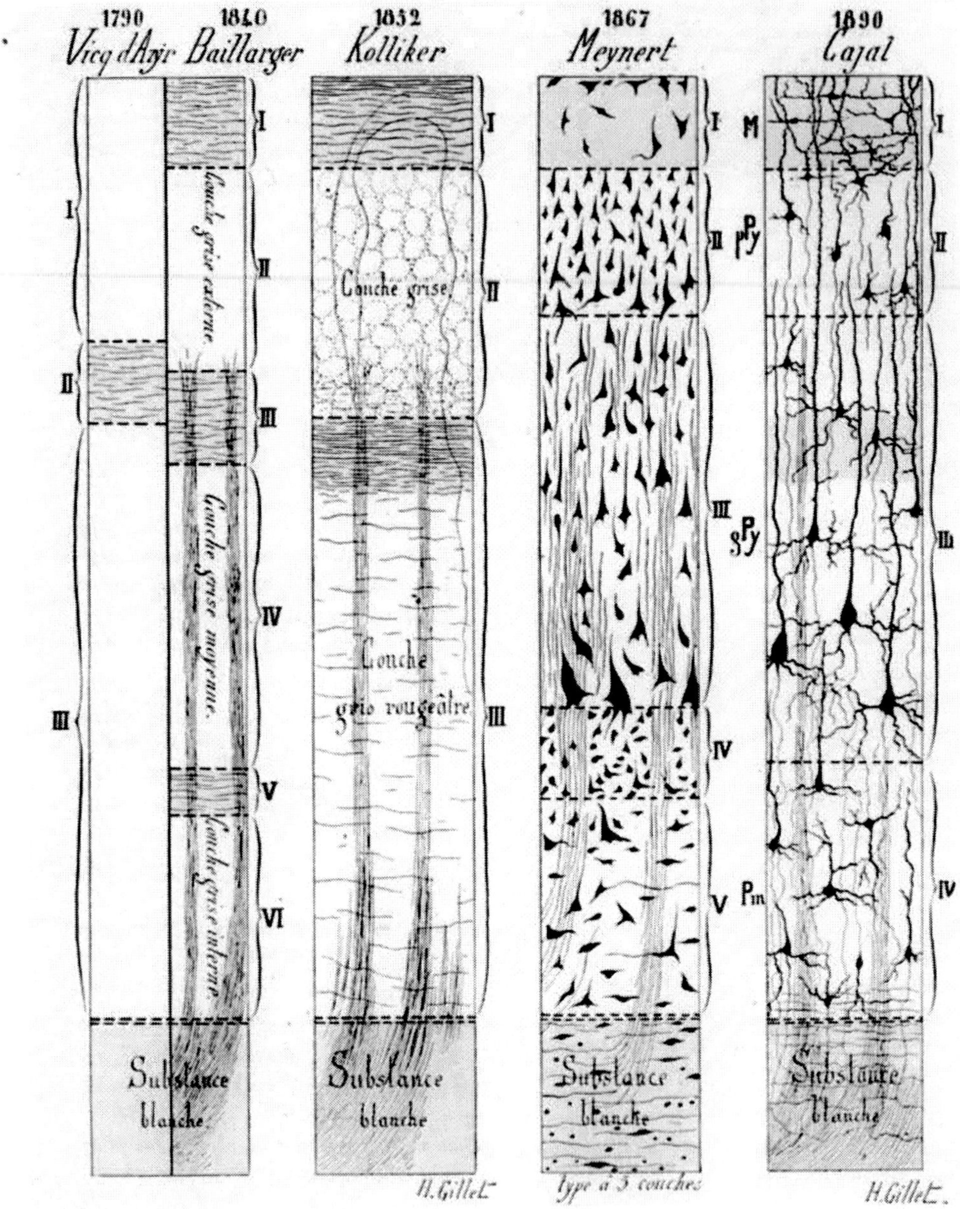

Figure 1. Drawings reflecting the progress of a century of research on the structure of the cerebral cortex (1790–1890), through the studies of Vicq d'Azyr, Baillarger, Kölliker, Meynert and Cajal. Taken from Dejerine and Dejerine-Klumpke [1].

Baillarger described these fibers as "*rangées de fibres verticales*" (rows of vertical fibers) and thus, the radial fasciculi were described as early as 1840 (Figure 1). In the drawings of Meynert [3] (Figures 1, 2A–B) it was clear that the pyramidal cells contribute to these bundles and form small vertical aggregates. However, it was not until after the introduction of the method of Weigert [5] to stain myelin (Figure 2D) that regional variations in the staining pattern of myelinated fibers could be observed as well as in the morphology of the radial bundles (e.g., the number of myelinated fibers that made up the bundles and the thickness and length of the bundles). This generated considerable interest in the myeloarchitecture of the cerebral cortex, the principal early contributions being made by Kaes [6], Bechterew [7], Edinger [8], and Flechsig [9]. One of the most detailed and systematic studies of human cortical myeloarchitecture was published by Kaes in his book *Die Grosshirnrinde des Menschen in ihren Massen und ihrem Fasergehalt* [10]. Although it was clear that pyramidal cell axons formed part of the myelinated bundles, the precise origin of these bundles remained uncertain. Indeed, it was necessary to wait five decades for the experimental demonstration by Nauta and Bucher [11] that the radial fasciculi originate in the cerebral cortex. These authors made experimental lesions in the gray matter of the rat cerebral cortex and they found that massive degeneration of radial fasciculi only occurred beneath and around the superficial cortical lesions, demonstrating that the radial fasciculi were made up mainly of efferent axons arising from nearby cells.

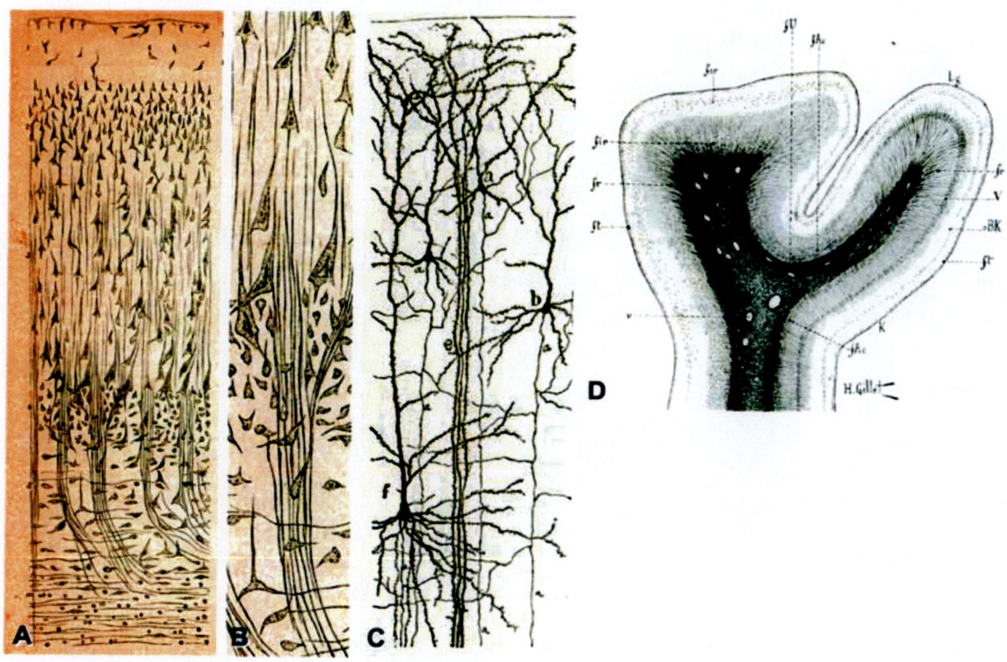

Figure 2. *A, B*: Meynert's [3] low and high magnification drawings taken from a section of the cerebral cortex, fixed with potassium dichromate and stained with carmine. These drawings show that the pyramidal cells form small vertical aggregates and contribute to the bundles of myelinated axons. *C*: Drawing made by Cajal [4] of tissue stained by the Golgi method to illustrate the bundles of apical dendrites (*e*) (© Herederos de Santiago Ramón y Cajal). These bundles of dendrites were also an indication of the vertical pyramidal cell grouping. *D*: Drawing taken from Dejerine and Dejerine-Klumpke [1] to illustrate the staining pattern of myelinated fibers in the human cerebral cortex using the method of Weigert. In this figure the topographic regularity of the radial bundles of myelinated axons is clearly visible.

After the studies of Meynert, the vertical or columnar disposition of neurons was further emphasized by a number of authors. Among these, Schlapp who produced the first complete cortical cytoarchitectonic map of the macaque monkey (Figure 3) [12,13]. Cajal, in his studies of the human cerebral cortex also described this vertical disposition of neurons. For example, in his description of the cytoarchitecture of the human motor cortex, he said [14]:

> "En sentido vertical o radial, las células están mucho menos separadas, constituyendo a menudo series radiales que son ya aparentes en la zona segunda, acentuándose mucho desde la cuarta en adelante. En ciertos puntos, se ven pirámides tan próximas que se diría se hallan en contacto longitudinal."[b]

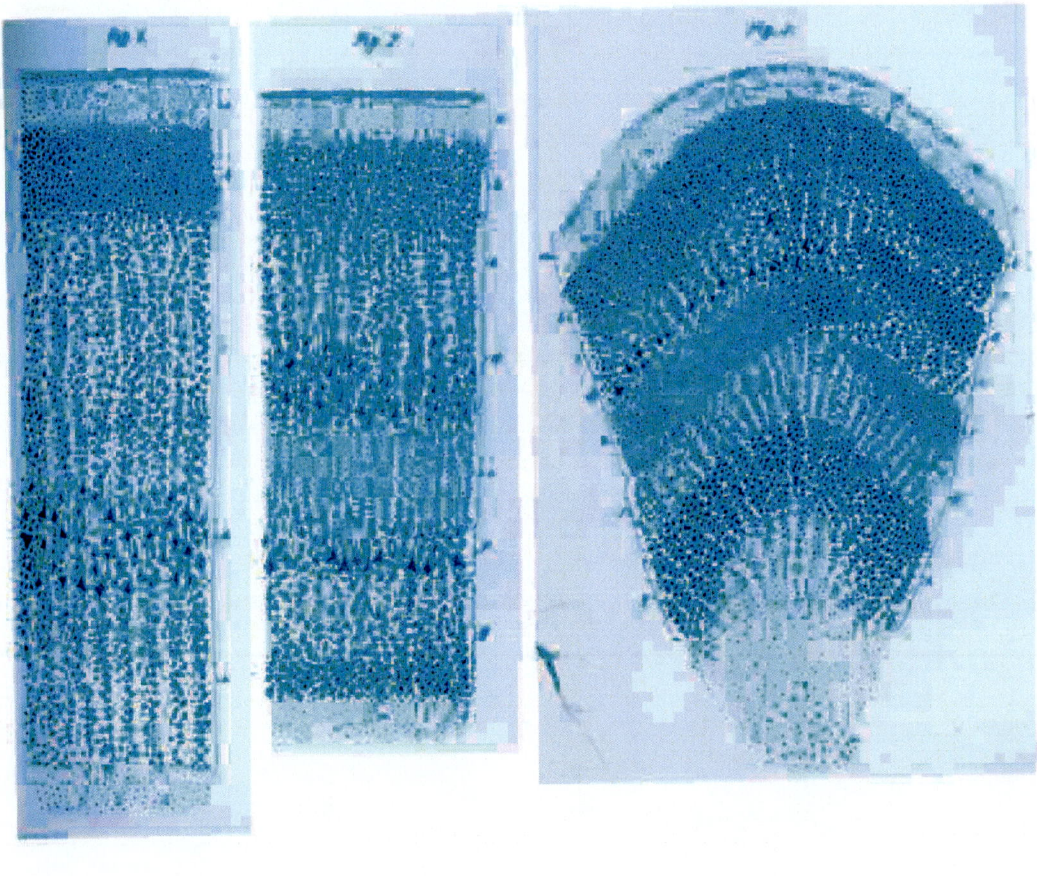

Figure 3. Drawings of the three main cortical types in Nissl-stained sections of the macaque monkey, according to Schlapp [12] (*left*, frontal; *middle*, parieto-temporal; *right*, occipital). Notice the vertical or columnar disposition of the neurons.

[b] "In the vertical or radial direction, the cells are much less separated, often forming radial series that are already evident in the second layer, being very accentuated from the fourth [layer down to deeper layers]. At certain points, pyramids are seen [which are] so close that one could say they are in contact longitudinally."

Furthermore, Cajal often described and illustrated bundles of apical dendrites when using the Golgi method (*e* in Figure 2C), which was also an indication of vertical pyramidal cell grouping [4]:

> "Los tallos radiales de las pirámides grandes, suben reunidos en fascículos apretados hasta lo alto de la zona segunda, en donde divergen para asaltar separadamente la capa plexiforme."[c]

Thanks to the use of the Golgi method, it was possible to trace the first circuits in the cerebral cortex (Figure 4, left), but without considering the above columnar features of the cortical organization nor their possible functional significance [17]. For example, Foster and Sherrington produced an excellent description of the vertical bundles of myelinated fibers and the columns of gray matter in their textbook of physiology [18], implying a columnar organization of the cortex but without including any functional considerations:

> "The lower part of [layer III to layer V], like the polymorphous layer below [layer VI], is split up into columns by the medullary rays of vertically disposed fibres; but these medullary rays diminish upwards (or increase downwards), the cosntituent fibres spreading away from the ray into the columns of gray matter, so that in the upper part of the layer the rays are far less distinct. This dispersion of a medullary ray will readily be understood if it is remembered that the fibers constituting it are on the one hand the axon of pyramidal (and other) cells, on their way to the white matter, and on the other hand axons of cells in distant parts on their way to terminate by synapses in some part or other of the cortex."

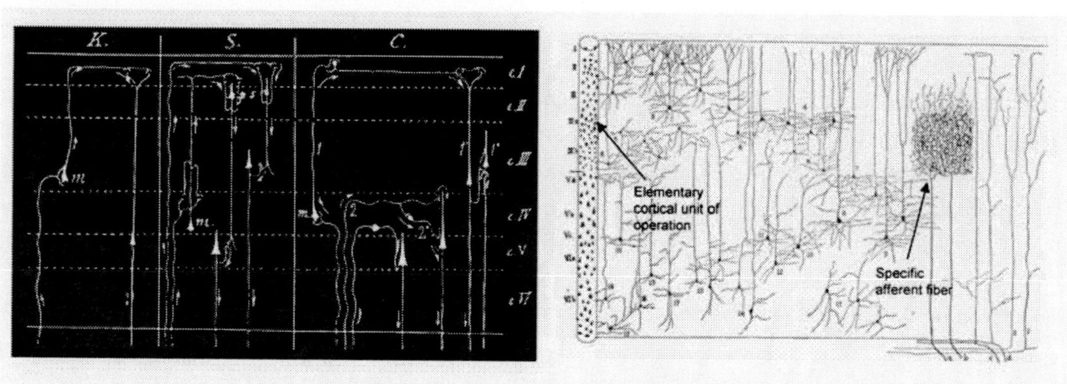

Figure 4. *Left*; Early circuit diagrams of the cerebral cortex, based on studies using the Golgi method, after Kölliker (K), Schaffer (S) and Cajal (C). *Right*, drawing made by Lorente de Nó to introduce the concept of the elementary cortical unit of operation. See text for further details. From Bonne [15] *(left)* and Lorente de Nó [16] *(right)*.

However, it was not until 1938 that Rafael Lorente de Nó introduced the fundamental concept of the *elementary cortical unit of operation*. He proposed that the cortex is made up of a huge number of elementary units, not simply juxtaposed but also overlapping. Moreover

[c] "The [apical dendritic] shafts of the large pyramids ascend together in tight bundles to the upper part of the second layer, where they diverge in order to reach separately the plexiform layer."

he suggested that these units would consist of small cylinders formed by vertical chains of neurons that crossed all cortical layers and that had specific afferent fibers as their axes [16]:

> "The small strip reproduced on the left of figure 63 [Figure 4, right] is the vertical section of a cylinder having a specific afferent fibre like an axis. All the elements of the cortex are represented in it, and therefore it may be called an elementary unit, in which theoretically, the whole process of the transmission of impulses from the afferent fibre to the efferent axon may be accomplished."

This hypothesis passed almost unnoticed until the pioneering experimental studies of Mountcastle [19,20], who presented physiological evidence for the columnar organization in the somatic sensory cortex of the cat and monkey. This organization was later confirmed, both anatomically and physiologically, in a number of cortical areas by numerous investigators, the work of Hubel and Wiesel [21] in the visual cortex of the cat and monkey was the most detailed and convincing corroboration of this organization [22-26].

Mountcastle proposed two types of vertical organization (Figure 5): the macrocolumn and the minicolumn [22,23]. The *macrocolumn* is the basic processing unit and consists of a cylinder of cortical tissue the width of which varies according to the spread of specific individual afferent fibers entering the cortex (300 to 600 μm in diameter, depending on the cortical area and/or species). This macrocolumn, commonly refered to simply as "column," would therefore be the equivalent to the elementary cortical unit of operation of Lorente de Nó. The *minicolumn* is the basic modular subunit in the cortex, representing the smallest functional unit of cortical organization, the ensemble of several minicolumns making up the macrocolumns. These minicolumns are formed by a vertically oriented group of interconnected cells, which are contained in a vertical cylinder of tissue with a diameter of approximately 25 to 50 μm (depending on the cortical area and/or species). Accordingly, Mountcastle [23] defined the macrocolumn as a complex processing and distributing unit that links a number of inputs to a number of outputs via overlapping internal processing chains (minicolumns). In addition to the obvious interest in examining the functional and anatomical features of minicolumn organization, recently interest has been renewed through the suggestion that alterations in the minicolumns are associated with certain common brain disorders, such as Alzheimer's, autism, and schizophrenia [26-29].

Finally, remarkable differences can be seen in Nissl-stained sections from different cortical regions and species, particularly with regards to neuron density and the cytoarchitectonic organization, including differences in the size and distribution of the vertical aggregates of neurons (Figure 6). Therefore, in this chapter, I shall deal with certain general structural characteristics of the minicolumn, introducing some comparative aspects between humans and other species.

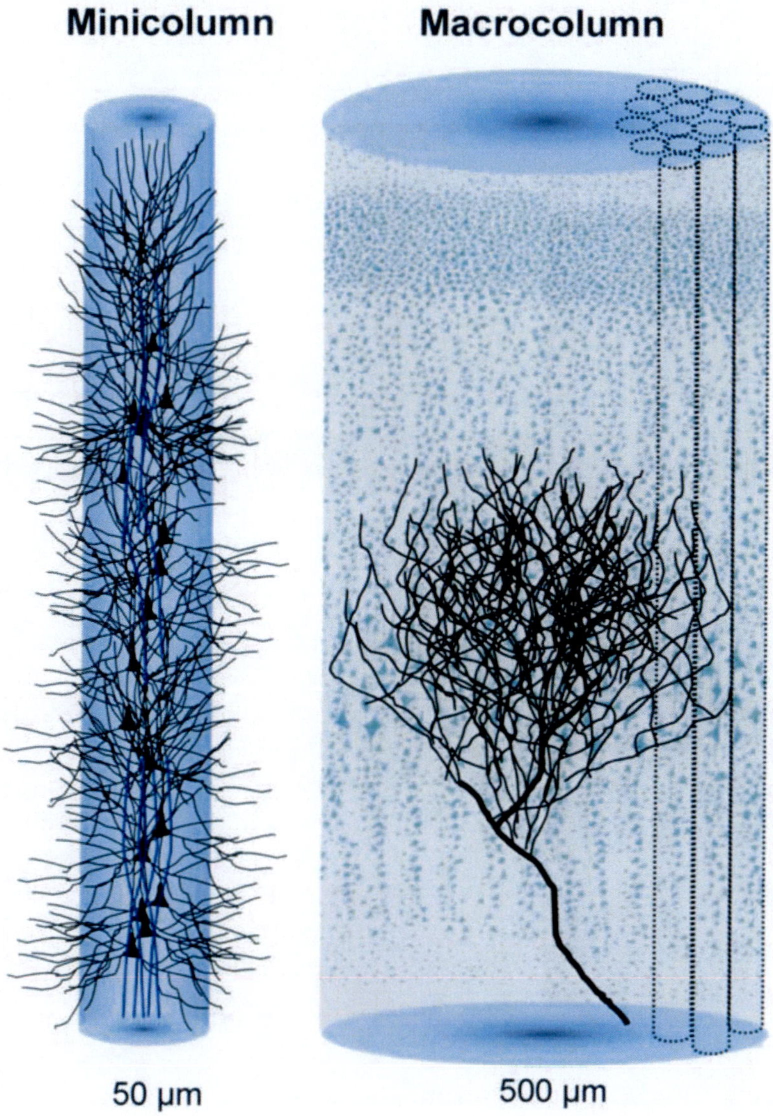

Figure 5. Schematic representation of a minicolumn and a macrocolumn. See text for further details.

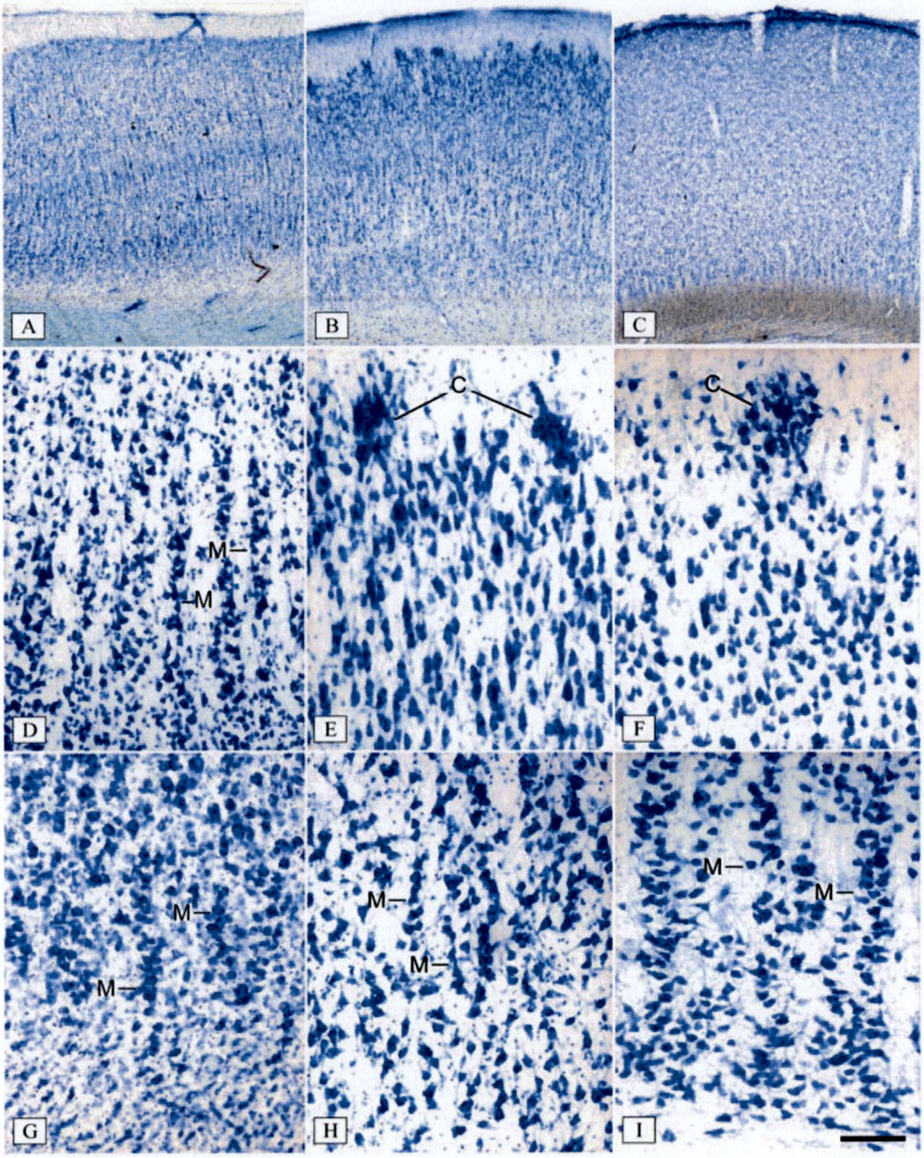

Figure 6. Variations in neuron density, cytoarchitectonic organization, and in the size and distribution of vertical aggegates of neurons. *A*, *B*, and *C*, Low-power photomicrographs of 100 μm thick vibratome sections stained with thionin from (*A*) Brodmann's area 21 of the human, (*B*) the occipital cortex of the giraffe, and (*C*) the bill representation in the primary somatosensory cortex of the platypus. *D–I*, High-power magnification images showing differences in the size and distribution of vertical aggregates of neurons or minicolumns (M) in layers II–III (*D–F*) and V–VI (*G–I*) of the human area 39 (*D*), of the giraffe occipital (*E, H*) and dorsal parietal (*F, I*) cortex, and of the platypus somatosensory cortex (*G*). C in *E* and *F* indicates the typical clusters of neurons in layer II of the giraffe [30]. Note the prominent minicolumns in layer III of area 39 of the human (*D*). In the giraffe, minicolumns are not present (or they are very hard to recognize) in layers II–III, both in the occipital (*E*) and dorsal parietal (*F*) cortex, whereas they are readily visualized in layer V of the occipital (*H*) cortex and especially, in the dorsal parietal (*I*) cortex. In the platypus, minicolumns are only present in layer VI, and they are short and relatively thick. Scale bar: 710 μm in *A*, *B*, and *C*; 100 μm in *D–I*.

NEURONAL COMPONENTS OF THE MINICOLUMN: GENERAL FEATURES

Types of Neurons

In the neocortex, there are two main classes of neurons: *spiny neurons* and *aspiny nonpyramidal neurons*. In turn, spiny neurons can be divided into two major subclasses, the pyramidal cells and the spiny nonpyramidal cells.

Pyramidal cells are the most abundant cortical neurons (70–85 % of the total population) and they are located in all layers except layer I. They constitute the vast majority of projection neurons and the main source of cortical excitatory synapses [24,31-36]. Pyramidal cells are commonly subdivided according to their projection site and the pattern of their terminal axonal arborization. In general, those pyramidal cells projecting to the subcortical nuclei are located in layers V–VI, whereas those projecting to other ipsi- or contralateral cortical areas are found mainly in layers II–III. However, depending on the cortical area and species, certain corticocortical connections originate from pyramidal cells located in layers V–VI. There is also a laminar pattern in the distribution of the terminal axonal arborization of corticocortical pathways, which can be grouped into three main types: columnar (all layers are similarly innervated); multilaminar (several layers are equally innervated, while other layers are mainly devoid of connections); and unilaminar (mainly a single layer is innervated).

Spiny nonpyramidal cells are, with some exceptions, short axon cells or spiny interneurons and they are located in the middle layers (especially in layer IV). Various types are recognized on the basis of their dendritic morphologies, axonal arborization and laminar connections. The axons of these cells terminate primarily within layer IV where their parent cell bodies are located, or alternatively in the layers above or below. The typical spiny nonpyramidal cell is the spiny stellate cell, which is a small neuron with round soma that send off spiny dendrites at all angles. Spiny stellate cells have been described chiefly in the primary visual cortex, somatosensory cortex and in the auditory cortex, where they are rather numerous [37].

Aspiny nonpyramidal neurons (smooth interneurons) are short axon cells with dendrites that are smooth or with only sparse spines. They are found in all layers and represent the vast majority of short axon cells (15–30 % of the total population of neurons). In this chapter, I shall refer to smooth or sparsely spiny nonpyramidal cells as “smooth interneurons.” A wide morphological variety of these cells exist and while the majority of smooth interneurons are recognized by their axonal arborization patterns, some of them are identified by their somato-dendritic morphology [17,38-40].The axons of smooth interneurons are found near the parent cell, but some have axonal collaterals that may run in the horizontal or vertical dimension (ascending and/or descending).

Types of Synapses and Connections

At the electron microscope level, there are two major morphological types of synapses corresponding to Gray's types I and II [41], respectively: asymmetrical and symmetrical synapses [42]. Asymmetrical synapses are characterized by a prominent postsynaptic density whereas symmetrical synapses have a very thin postsynaptic density. The proportion of asymmetrical synapses varies between approximately 80–90 %, depending on the cortical layer area and species, the remainder being symmetrical [30].The vast majority of axon terminals forming asymmetrical synapses originate from spiny neurons (pyramidal and spiny nonpyramidal cells) or extrinsic cortical afferents, whereas most axon terminals establishing symmetrical synapses originate from the smooth interneurons. Pyramidal neurons and spiny stallate cells establish synapses mainly with the dendritic spines of other spiny neurons, and with dendritic shafts of both spiny and smooth interneurons. Smooth interneurons, however, form synapses with dendritic shafts and the somata of both spiny and smooth interneurons, and with the dendritic spines and axon intial segments of pyramidal neurons.

Smooth interneurons can also be grouped by their synaptic connectivity. With the exception of chandelier cells that establish synapses exclusively with the axon initial segment of pyramidal cells, the other types of smooth interneurons form synapses at more than one post-synaptic region with both pyramidal and nonpyramidal cells (dendritic shafts, spines, somata or axon initial segments). However, distinct types of smooth interneurons show different preferences for certain postsynaptic regions (Figure 7, left). On the basis of the preferred postsynaptic region on pyramidal neurons, four different groups of smooth interneurons can be recognized: axo-dendritic cells or cells forming synapses only or almost exclusively on dendritic shafts and dendritic spines (e.g., double bouquet cells); axo-somatodendritic cells or cells forming multiple synapses with both the dendrites and somata but with a preference for somata (e.g., various types of basket cells); axo-dendrosomatic cells or cells forming multiple synapses with both the dendrites and somata, but with a preference for dendrites (e.g., various types of basket cells); and axo-axonic cells or cells forming synapses only with the axon initial segment (chandelier cells) [30,43-47]. In addition, smooth interneurons are not only connected by chemical synapses (unidirectional connections), but they may also form electrical synapses with particular types of other interneurons through dendro-dendritic gap junctions (unidirectional or bidirectional) [48-54].

Excitatory and Inhibitory Neurons and Synapses: Neurochemical Characteristics

In the cerebral cortex, glutamate and γ-aminobutyric acid (GABA) are the major excitatory and inhibitory neurotransmitters, respectively. Since spiny neurons and the major cortical afferent systems are excitatory and likely to be glutamatergic, and many smooth interneurons are GABAergic, it is generally assumed that axon terminals forming asymmetrical synapses are excitatory, and those forming symmetrical synapses are inhibitory [55-57]. In summary, there are two major morphological and functional groups of neurons one made up by the population of spiny neurons which form asymmetrical synapses and are excitatory; the other is formed by the smooth interneurons which form symmetrical inhibitory synapses.

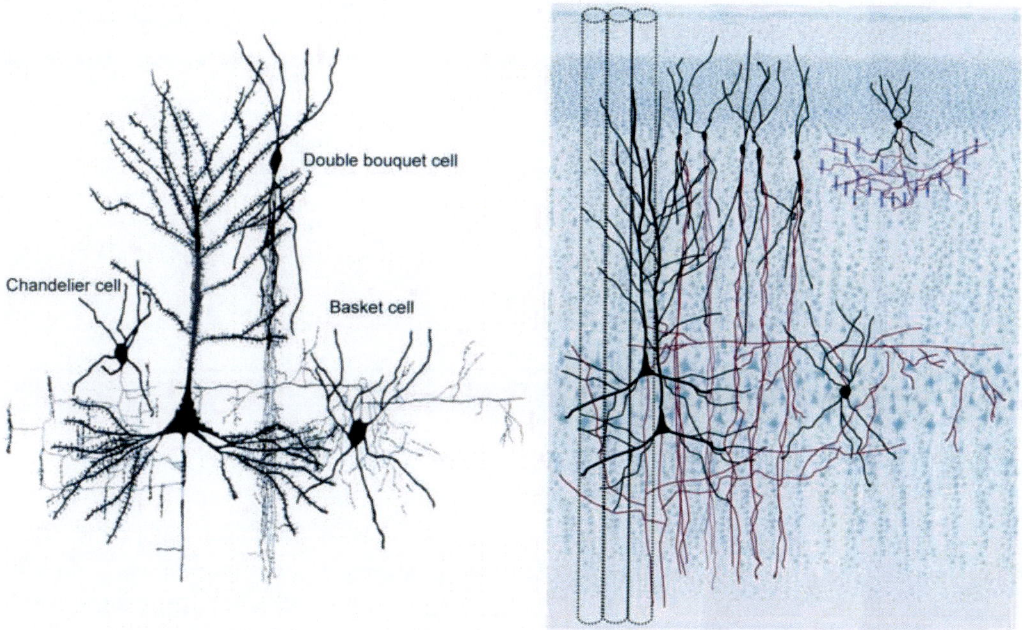

Figure 7. *Left*, Drawing to illustrate the synaptic relationships between double bouquet cells, chandelier cells and large basket cells with pyramidal cells. These cells represent the best characterized types of smooth interneurons in terms of morphology and neurochemistry. *Right*, Drawing to illustrate the relationship between minicolumns and the extent of the dendritic and axonal arborization of double bouquet cells, chandelier cells, large basket cells and pyramidal cells.

Nevertheless, a wide variety of other neurotransmitters, neuroactive peptides and calcium-binding proteins also exist in the cerebral cortex. The most common neurotransmitters (or their synthesizing enzymes) are nitric oxide synthase (NOS), tyrosine hydroxylase (TH), and choline acetyltransferase (ChAT). The most frequently found peptides are somatostatin (SOM), cholecystokinin (CCK), neuropeptide Y (NPY), vasoactive intestinal polypeptide (VIP), tachykinins (TK). The major calcium-binding proteins are represented by calbindin (CB), parvalbumin (PV) and calretinin (CR). With few exceptions, the majority of these compounds are found in smooth interneurons that are mostly GABAergic. However, the second neurotransmitter or neuroactive peptide may have an excitatory function. Indeed, it has been shown that the presence or absence of a number of these molecules in a given smooth interneuron can be correlated with its physiological properties. Therefore, a characteristic of smooth interneurons is their anatomical and molecular diversity, which may influence the effects they produce on targets depending on both their synaptic connections and their neurochemical profile [17,30,47,58-68].

Columnar Arrangement of Cortical Neuronal Elements

As mentioned in the introduction, the radial bundles of myelinated axons and the grouping of neurons in vertically oriented clusters or columns was established anatomically in the earliest studies of cortical organization. However, there are two other anatomical dispositions, which have only been highlighted or discovered more recently, but that also appear to be clearly associated with the minicolumnar organization. These are the vertical bundles of apical dendrites and the double bouquet cell axons that will be dealt with below.

Vertical Bundles of Apical Dendrites

After the description of the dendritic bundles by Cajal, little or no attention was given to this anatomical disposition until the 1970's when dendritic bundles or clusters were described in detail. This resurgence in interest is mainly the result of the studies of Peters and Walsh [69] in the rat somatosensory cortex and of Fleischhauer et al [70] in the sensory-motor cortex of the rabbit and cat. Later studies in different areas of the mice, rat, rabbit, cat and monkey cortex suggested that the bundles of apical dendrites are common features of cortical organization, although variability in the size and number of dendrites that form the bundles exists both between cortical areas and species [71-80]. In general, the vertical dendritic organization is as follows (Figures 8, 9A). The apical dendrites of pyramidal neurons located at different levels of layer V associate closely, forming prominent dendritic bundles, and ascend towards the pial surface. Apical dendrites from pyramidal cells in layers II–III are added mostly to the periphery of these bundles. At this level, the apical dendrites of layer V and layer II–III pyramidal neurons start to produce terminal tufts that end in layer I. Apical dendrites from pyramidal cells in layer VI are not added to these bundles but rather constitute separate bundles that ascend to layer IV where their terminal tufts form. Thus, the core of the long dendritic bundles running from layer V to layers II–III is made up mainly of the apical dendrites of pyramidal neurons from layer V. However, variations to this general pattern are observed (Figure 9). In certain cortical areas, where numerous pyramidal cells are found in layer IV, a third system of apical dendritic bundles extends from these pyramidal neurons to layer II. This has been described in the mouse primary motor cortex and in area 17 of the monkey visual cortex [77,80]. Furthermore, in other cortical areas and species, such as the rabbit motor cortex, the bundles in layer II/III are separated from the dendritic bundles from layer IV/V because the latter terminate in the upper part of layer IV, while layer II/III bundles begin in the middle of layer II/III (Figure 9B) [76].

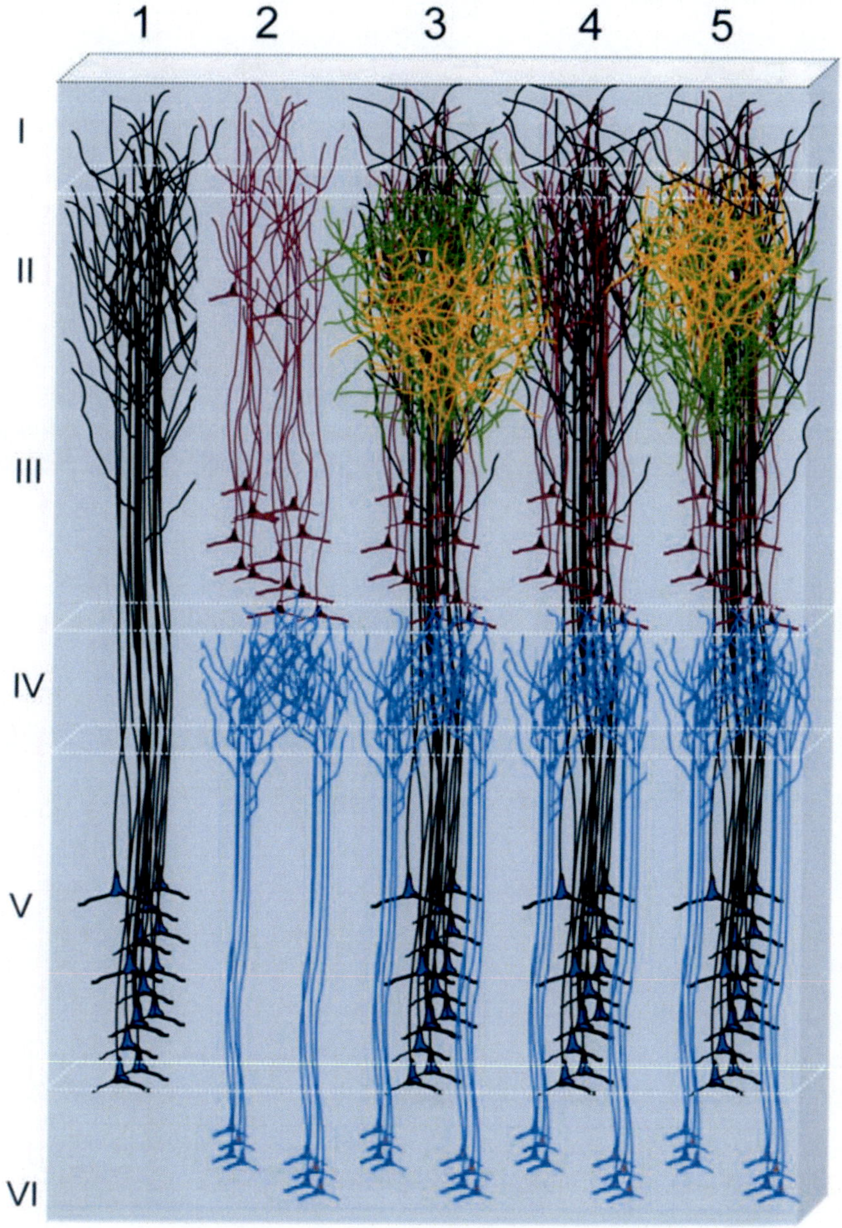

Figure 8. Schematic representation of dendritic bundles and their connections with excitatory (green) and inhibitory (yellow) focal axonal arborizations. 1: apical dendritic bundles of layer V pyramidal neurons (black). 2; apical dendrites of layers II–III (red) and layer VI (blue) pyramidal cells. In 3, 4 and 5 the apical dendrites of pyramidal neurons from layers II–III, V and VI are represented together. One of the possible functions of dendritic bundling is to connect axons with rather small, well-localized foci in the cortex (apical dendritic bundles), and with somewhat wider areas (that include the collateral branches). See text for further details.

The centre-to-centre distance between dendritic bundles of layer V pyramidal neurons varies depending on the cortical area and species. For example, this distance was estimated to be 31 μm in the mouse primary motor cortex, whereas in the hollows and walls of the primary somatosensory cortex it is 25 μm and 22 μm, respectively. Furthermore, in the rat primary somatosensory cortex, this distance is 50 μm, whereas in area 17 of the rat, cat and monkey it is 60 μm, 56 μm, and 31 μm, respectively [78,80]. In addition, there are large variations in the size and numerical composition of the bundles, which basically depends on the size and packing density of the layer V pyramidal neurons [72,73,81]. In general, there are less than 15 thick apical dendrites (originating from layer V pyramidal cells) and a variable but smaller number of thinner apical dendrites that are added to the bundle during its ascension. In order to emphasize the regional differences within the same species, Fleischhauer and Detzer [73] highlighted the amazing example of the dendritic bundling in the *gyrus genualis* of the cat (area 32 of Winkler and Potter [82]), where the bundles are made up by 50 or more thick dendrites. This was compared, with the visual cortex, in which these bundles consist of less than 10 dendrites.

Furthermore, as pointed out by Fleischhauer [81], not only does the number of apical dendrites that make up the bundles vary, but differences of a more fundamental nature exist. One of the most striking examples can be seen in the sensorimotor cortex of the cat (areas 3a and 4) [71]. In this region, the apical dendrites of layer V pyramidal neurons do not ascend straight towards the pial surface, but after a short vertical ascension, they bifurcate just above layer V where a large number of U-shaped secondary dendrite branches are observed (Figure 9C). The secondary (or tertiary) branches of neighboring columns of pyramidal cells cross one another and after initially ascending obliquely, they ascend vertically forming dendritic bundles in layer III. At this level, the apical dendrites of layer III pyramidal neurons are joined peripherally. Therefore, dendritic bundling have a complex organization that show dramatic variations in different areas and/or species.

Function of Dendritic Bundling

A possible function of dendritic bundling might be to establish particular patterns of connectivity with common afferent inputs (Figure 8). Apical dendrites receive both excitatory and inhibitory synapses and therefore, they may represent small, regularly distributed vertical postsynaptic spots for excitatory and inhibitory connections. In addition, apical dendrites give rise to a rich system of collateral branches and as a consequence, in the region of the bundle considerable overlapping of collateral branches belonging to the bundle would occur. This anatomical disposition would serve to connect the dendrites with axons at some distance from the bundle, while preserving spatial precision. Thus, dendritic bundling might serve to connect axons with rather small, well-localized spots of the cortex (apical dendritic bundles) and with somewhat wider areas (that include the collateral branches). Another possible and appealing function for dendritic bundling, may derive from the electrical coupling of apical dendrites through dendrodendritic gap junctions. This is based on the fact that dendrites are very closely packed in the bundles, normally from 1 μm apart to direct membrane apposition [83]. According to quantitative studies in tangential sections through layer IV of the area parietalis in the rabbit [84], approximately 38 % of a total of 819 dendrites were in contact with each other. The length of the membrane apposition varied from 0.3 μm to 6 μm, the average being 1.3 μm (n = 167 contacts). If such electrical coupling existed, Roney et al. [83] proposed that bundling could serve as an averaging mechanism, unifying the neurons involved in this assembly.

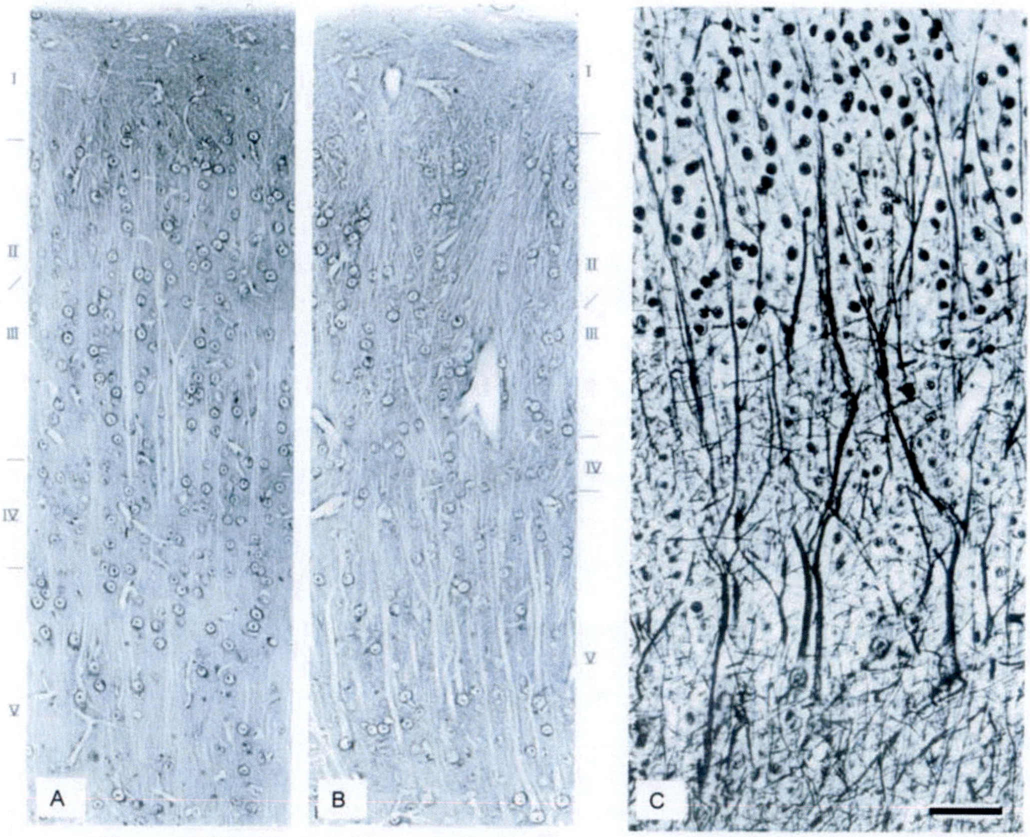

Figure 9. Photomicrographs showing different patterns of dendritic bundling in the cerebral cortex of the rabbit (*A*, *B*) and cat (*C*). *A*, *B*, dendritic bundles in the visual (*A*) and motor (*B*) cortex of the rabbit; Klüver-PAS stained 10 μm paraffin sections. *C*, Dendritic pattern in area 3a of the cat; Bodian impregnation. The apical dendrites of layer V pyramidal neurons bifurcate just above layer V where a large number of U-shaped secondary dendrite branches are observed. Scale bar: 50 μm in *A* and *B*, and 56 μm in *C*. *A* and *B* taken from Schmolke and Viebahn [76]; *C* taken from Fleischhauer [71].

Double Bouquet Cells

Cajal described several types of double bouquet cells (*células bipenachadas* in Spanish; bitufted cells in English), with different dendritic and axonal morphologies [85]. One of them was characterized by the tightly intertwined bundles of its axon that produced long descending vertical collaterals (cells E and F in figure 11 of Cajal [86]). However, instead of giving a different name to this particular cell type, like for example Szentágothai [87,88], who called them "*cells with horsestail-shaped axons*," Jones's [38] "*type 3*," and Valverde [40,89] who used "*cells with axons forming vertical bundles*," a number of authors, including ourselves, have preferred to apply the term "double bouquet cell" only to those neurons with axons forming such vertical bundles irrespective of their somato-dendritic morphology [17]. While the vast majority of axons surpass the size limit for the minicolumn, the peculiarity of double bouquet cell axons is that they fit well within these limits (Figure 7, right). Since until recently the only way to visualize these neurons was by Golgi staining or after intracellular injections of markers and therefore, their abundance and distribution remained a mystery. However, when it was subsequently shown that they could be labeled by CB immunocytochemistry [90,91], they were seen to be so numerous and regularly distributed that they formed a widespread microcolumnar structure in the monkey cortex [92,93]. In the visual and somatosensory cortex, a mean of 10 double bouquet cell axons were found in a field of 10,000 μm^2 from tangential sections through layer III (range from 7 to 15) with a center-to-center spacing of 15 μm to 30 μm. The mean width of the cross-sectioned double bouquet cell axonal arborizations was 9 μm (from 5 μm to 15 μm). The number of axonal collaterals that made up each double bouquet cell axon varied depending on the layer examined. It ranged from as few as 3 in the deepest part of the course of the axon, to as many as 10 or 15 in the upper part [92].

Double bouquet cells contain GABA and certain subpopulations also express CR, as well as the peptides somatostatin and tachykinin [92,94-100]. Moreover, the density and morphology of these double bouquet cell subpopulations varies in different areas of the macaque and human neocortex [98] (also Ballesteros-Yáñez et al., Journal of Comparative Neurology, in press). In several areas of the monkey cerebral cortex (visual, somatosensory, temporal and auditory), it has been shown that double bouquet cell axons form symmetrical synapses with small dendritic shafts (57 % to 62 %) and spines (38 % to 43 %) [91,92,94,101]. Moreover, double bouquet cell axons establish a rather similar microcolumnar structure and synaptic connectivity in the human cerebral cortex as to that found in the monkey [99,100]. A mean number of 12 double bouquet cell axons can be found in a field of 10 000 μm^2 in the temporal cortex, with a mean diameter of 12 μm (range 5 μm to 20 μm) and a mean center-to-center spacing of 30 μm. The distribution and proportion of synapses was 59 % on dendritic shafts and 41 % on spines. Thus, double bouquet cells are likely to participate in similar synaptic circuits in monkeys and humans.

Finally, while the origin of the dendritic shafts on which double bouquet cell axons form synapses is unknown, some of the postsynaptic spines belong to pyramidal cells and, possibly to spiny stellate cells. In addition, these spines form asymmetrical synapses with excitatory axons [91,100], and because double bouquet cells are very abundant and establish hundreds of inhibitory synapses within a very narrow column of cortical tissue, it is likely that many spines will form symmetrical synapses. This contrasts with the classic view that the majority of dendritic spines (80 % to 90 %) only form one asymmetrical excitatory synapse. Indeed, when spines establish synapses with two separate axon terminals, only rarely is this second synapse symmetrical [34]. However, pyramidal cells display thousands of spines and they are much more numerous than double bouquet cells. Therefore, it is conceivably that in a random examination of dendritic spines mainly those spines not innervated by these neurons would be included. Based on the orientation of the double bouquet cell axons parallel to the pyramidal apical dendrites, the postsynaptic spines should arise from basal dendrites and oblique branches of the apical dendrites. All of these observations led us to propose that double bouquet cells form synapses with a "special" type of spine capable of forming synapses with both excitatory and inhibitory axon terminals, and that they must be particularly abundant in the side branches of apical and basal dendrites of pyramidal cells [99].

Relationship between Double Bouquet Cell Axons and Radial Fasciculi

The regularity in the spacing of double bouquet cell axons is one of their most impressive characteristics (Figure 10A), since these neurons are the only type of interneuron that has such a regular distribution. Moreover, this pattern is strikingly similar to that revealed by the radial fasciculi (Figure 10B) and indeed, it has been shown that the myelinated axon bundles and double bouquet axons overlap on a one-to-one basis [93,100] (also Ballesteros-Yáñez, Journal of Comparative Neurology, in press). As such, these neurons can act on groups of pyramidal cells located in different layers within the minicolumns. All of these features have prompted double bouquet cells to be considered as key elements of the cortcal minicolumn (Figure 11) [17,25,92,93,100,102].

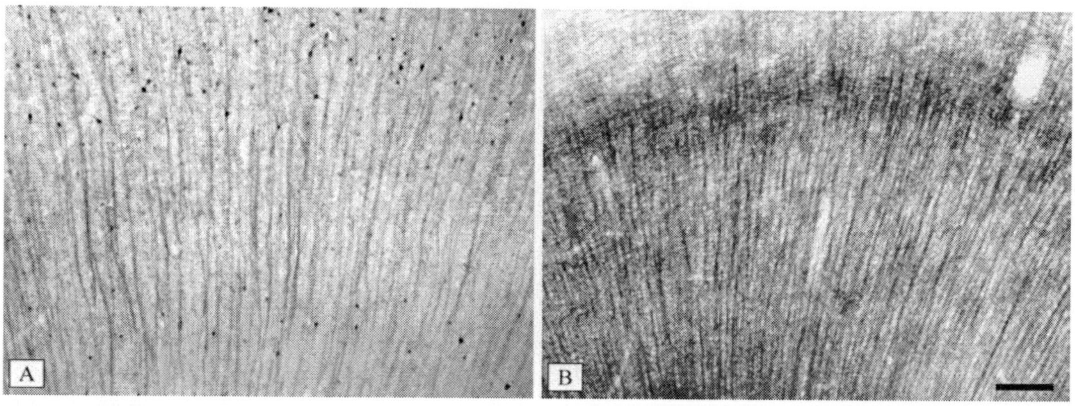

Figure 10. Photomicrographs from the human temporal cortex, showing the similarity in the distribution of double bouquet cell axons and bundles of myelinated axons. These bundles originate from pyramidal cells that form small vertical aggregates. *A*, double bouquet cell axons immunostained for calbindin. *B*, bundles of myelinated axons (myelin staining). The different density of the bundles of myelinated axons compared to the double bouquet cell axons is an artefact introduced by the procedure for staining myelin (Gallyas'method), which produces more shrinking of the tissue than immunocytochemical staining techniques. Scale bar: 175 μm.

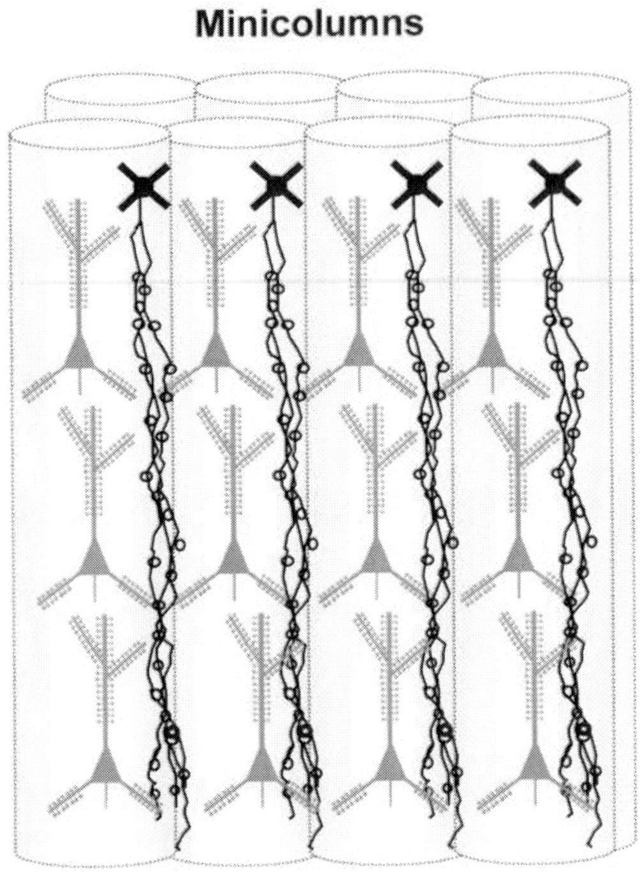

Figure 11. Diagram showing the microcolumnar structure formed by double bouquet cells and their relationship with pyramidal cells.

It is important to note that so far, the microcolumnar system formed by double bouquet cells has only clearly been demonstrated in the monkey and human neocortex. In other mammalian species, these cells are less numerous or may even be absent. For example, in a recent study of the frontal, parietal and occipital areas of different mammals, we found that these double bouquet cell axons were present in carnivores and primates but not in a number of rodents, lagomorphs or artiodactyls (Ballesteros-Yáñez et al., unpublished findings, 2004). Furthermore, relatively few double bouquet cell axons are found in carnivores, and only in the occipital cortex. We concluded that while these smooth interneurons may be an important element in the microcolumnar organization of primates, this is not necessarily the case in other mammalian species. Thus, differences in the morphology, abundance or distribution of double bouquet cells may represent one fundamental difference in the cortical microorganization between primates and other species [17] (also Ballesteros-Yáñez, Journal of Comparative Neurology, in press). A possible explanation for these differences in double bouquet cell distribution is the differential expression of transcription factors during GABAergic neurogenesis. Two distinct programs maybe responsible for the species-specific generation of smooth GABAergic interneurons in the human neocortex [103]. In one of these, the transcription factors Dlx1/2 and Mash1 are specifically expressed in the cells originating in the ventricular and subventricular zones of the dorsal telencephalon that migrate radially across the intermediate zone to the cerebral cortex. The other lineage of GABAergic neurons express Dlx1/2 but not Mash1, and they originate in the ganglionic eminence of the ventral telencephalon from where they migrate tangentially across the intermediate zone to the cerebral cortex. However, all or almost all GABAergic neurons in rodents originate in the ganglionic eminence and migrate tangentially to the cerebral cortex [104-106]. Thus, we proposed [17,30] that in the human neocortex, double bouquet cells might originate in the ventricular/subventricular zone from the GABAergic lineage expressing Dlx1/2 and Mash1. These neurons may migrate radially along common pathways as radial units or as the ontogenetic columns that form the pyramidal cell modules [107]. This could therefore represent a mechanism by which the complementary microcolumnar structures formed by double bouquet cells and pyramidal cell modules might be constructed in the neocortex of primates.

Synaptology of the Minicolumn

Are all pyramidal neurons and fmooth interneurons within the minicolumn innervated equally by excitatory and inhibitory synapses? If we consider the columnar organization of the input connections, the differences in connectivity between neighboring neurons (cells whose somata are located within 50 μm and 100 μm), and the combinations of the interlaminar connections of both pyramidal and nonpyramidal neurons, it is clear that within the minicolumn, neurons in different layers do not process the same information [24,31-33,36,108-115]. Hence, the possible quantitative differences in the excitatory and inhibitory inputs and what we know about the precise mapping of these inputs should be considered.

Since the vast majority of synapses are found in the dendritic compartment of the neurons, an initial and relatively easy approach to estimate the average number of synapses on each neuron is to divide the synaptic densities in the neuropil by the corresponding neuronal density. While it is certain that a large proportion of the dendritic arbor of a neuron is located near the soma, some dendritic segments, especially the apical dendrites of pyramidal cells, may cross several layers. Thus, the synapse/neuron ratio in a given layer is not an accurate estimate of the number of synapses received by neurons in that layer and it should be taken as an index of "general" connectivity. We have recently used this ratio to compare the synaptology between different neocortical layers in humans, rats and mice [30]. Remarkably, laminar differences in the ratios of asymmetrical and symmetrical synapses per neuron were found, both within species and between different species, when the number of neurons, asymmetrical and symmetrical synapses was analyzed in the human, rat and mouse neocortex (Figure 12). However, these laminar differences in the synapse/neuron ratio do not provide information about the precise origin of these synapses. The complexity of the synaptic circuitry is the major limitation in resolving this issue. A given neuron is innervated by thousands of synapses and the origin of many of them is unknown, particularly those located in the distal dendrites. This is because distal dendrites are not usually labeled and it is extremely difficult and time-consuming to follow a distal dendrite back to its parent cell soma in serial electron microscope sections. Furthermore, it is impossible to trace all the axon terminals forming synapses with a neuron back to their origins. In addition, the synaptic relationships among cortical neurons are highly divergent, partially due to the fact that any given smooth interneuron or pyramidal cell forms relatively few synapses with other neurons (maximally in the order of tens). The same is also true of the extrinsic cortical afferent fibers [34]. Since many types of cortical neurons and extrinsic cortical afferent fibers may innervate a given neuron, many of the details of cortical circuitry remain unknown. However, in spite of this pessimistic overview, we will see that some methods exist that allow us to study certain fundamental aspects of cortical circuits in detail.

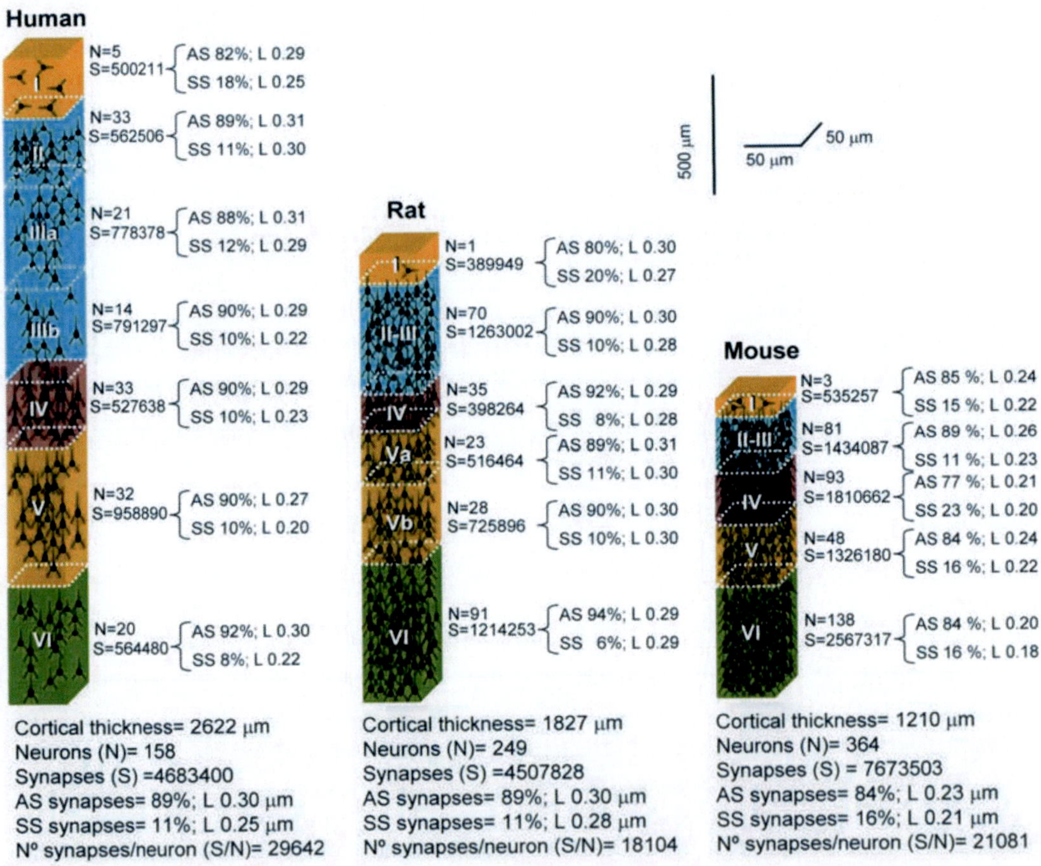

Figure 12. Comparison of the thickness of layers, number of neurons and of the synaptic profiles within cubes of cortical tissue (50 μm wide by 50 μm thick) from the pial surface to the white matter in the human (anterolateral temporal cortex; T2-T3), rat (hindlimb area of the somatosensory cortex) and mouse (barrel cortex). L, cross-sectional length of synaptic junctions; AS, asymmetrical synapses; SS, symmetrical synapses. Values taken from DeFelipe et al. [30]

Synapses on Pyramidal Cells

Excitatory Synapses

Axon terminals forming asymmetrical (excitatory) synapses with pyramidal cells are absent from the soma, axon initial segment and proximal dendritic shafts (at least in the first 20 μm). These synapses are exclusively located in the distal dendritic shafts and spines (see Alonso-Nanclares et al. [116,117] and references therein). Moreover, the great majority of these synapses are formed with spines [34,45,118]. Hence, spines represent the main postsynaptic sites to establish relationships with other pyramidal cells, spiny nonpyramidal cells and the major cortical afferent systems, all of which form asymmetrical synapses (see above). It seems that all spines receive at least one asymmetrical synapse [119-124]; and therefore, the number of excitatory synaptic inputs to the pyramidal neuron can be estimated by counting the number of dendritic spines. Using intracellular horseradish peroxidase injections, Larkman [125] analyzed the spines on pyramidal cells in layers II/III and layer V of the rat visual cortex. In layer V, two classes of pyramidal cells were distinguished, thick cells characterized by a thick apical dendrite that formed its terminal arbor in layer I, and slender cells that were characterized by a thin apical trunk that neither reached layer I nor formed a terminal arbor. The mean number of spines per cell was 7965 for layer II/III cells, 8647 for slender layer V cells and 14 932 for thick layer V cells. Similarly, Elston [126] compared the basal dendritic arbors of layer III and V pyramidal neurons injected with Lucifer yellow in area 7m and in the superior temporal polysensory area of the macaque monkey. He found that the basal dendritic field of layer III pyramidal cells in area 7m had significantly less dendritic spines (2243) than layer V pyramidal cells (4535). However, the basal dendritic fields of pyramidal neurons in layer III and V of the superior temporal polysensory area had a similar number of dendritic spines (3585 and 3324, respectively). In addition, the complexity and size of the dendritic arbor (branching pattern and length of dendrites), and the size and density of the pyramidal cell dendritic spines varies considerably between the different cortical layers, areas and species [127-131]. These features have important consequences for the functional processing of information from a pyramidal neuron. For example, differences in the number of spines indicate differences in the number of excitatory inputs they receive. Differences in the total length, number of branches and the diameter of the dendrites, or in the size of the spines, affect the electrical, biochemical and biophysical properties of the neuron [129,132-134]. Therefore, variations in these parameters reflect differences in the complexity of cortical circuits between different layers, cortical areas and species.

Inhibitory Synapses

As commented above, axon terminals that form symmetrical (inhibitory) synapses with pyramidal cells are located in all regions of the pyramidal neuron: soma, dendrites (shafts and spines) and axon initial segment. Moreover, different types of smooth interneurons differentially innervate these regions, these neurons being the major source of symmetrical synapses. Thus, one way to try to address the question of whether all pyramidal neurons within the minicolumn are similarly innervated by inhibitory synapses is by examining the synaptology of different populations of pyramidal cells located in different layers of the same minicolumn. For instance, chandelier cells are the major source of axon terminals that establish synapses with the axon intial segment of pyramidal neurons. Therefore, if there are few or no axo-axonic synapses on the initial axon segment of a given population of pyramidal cells, they are not innervated by chandelier cells. In contrast, the presence of numerous axo-axonic synapses would indicate extensive innervation by chandelier cells. Similarly, the somata of pyramidal cells is a major target for basket cells and the differences in the number of axo-somatic synapses would reflect differences in basket cell innervation.

Thus, previously characterized layer III (callosal cells), layer II–III (ipsilateral corticocortical cells) and layer VI (corticothalamic cells) pyramidal cells were analyzed by electron microscopy, comparing the number of synapses on the initial axon segments and somata in each of these populations [135,136]. We found that the total number of axo-axonic synapses varied from 16 to 23 for the axon initial segments of callosal neurons, from 22 to 28 for those of ipsilateral corticocortical neurons, and from 1 to 5 in corticothalamic cells. Axonal boutons were frequently seen joined by cytoplasmic bridges in the case of callosal and ipsilateral corticocortical neurons, whereas the axon terminals in corticothalamic axon initial segments were more frequently isolated or at a relatively large distances. These observations indicated that while callosal and ipsilateral corticocortical neurons were innervated by chandelier cells, corticothalamic neurons were not. Furthermore, we found that callosal neurons had a significantly higher density of axo-somatic synapses than corticothalamic neurons (mean number of synapses per 10 μm^2: 1.96 and 1.06, respectively). Similarly, the neurons projecting to different targets outside area VI of the macaque monkey have significantly different numbers of inhibitory synapses on their somata [137]. In addition, the laminar location of the cell is not significant in determining the differences in somatic synapses. Therefore, different populations of pyramidal neurons are differentially innervated by smooth interneurons irrespective of the layer in which they are located.

Synapses on Smooth Interneurons: Excitarory and Inhibitory Synapses

There is relatively little information regarding the inputs to smooth interneurons compared to the data available on pyramidal cells, due to the technical difficulties in studying these neurons [47]. To characterize the different types of interneurons their axons must be labeled and then their inputs studied using two or more different techniques in the same preparation. For instance, intracellular labeling of individual neurons and/or Golgi staining may be coupled to anterograde tracing to label excitatory afferent inputs (cortico-cortical or thalamo-cortical), or to other techniques such as immunocytochemistry to label inhibitory GABAergic inputs [138-143]. Another method to identify synaptic inputs to smooth interneurons involves first performing simultaneous intracellular recordings of two or more adjacent neurons to examine their synaptic connections. Subsequently, intracellular labeling is carried out to map the contacts at the light microscope level in combination with electron microscopy to confirm the synaptic nature of the contacts [53,61,113,144,145]. These methods are certainly useful to explore the synaptic connections of individual neurons, and to trace successive links in a local circuit. However, the time-consuming electron microscope techniques, the difficulty of applying correlative light and electron microscopic techniques, and the problems in distinguishing clear synapses due to the masking by labeled processes, make these methods impractical for examining large numbers of individual neurons in detail. Therefore, in most of studies relatively few cells are analyzed, a limitation when generalizing from these observations [30].

Another approach is to use dual immunocytochemical staining to study the possible synaptic connections between given populations of cells. For example, we have used immunocytochemistry for CB, PV and CR to label populations of smooth interneurons in the primary and secondary visual area, and the cytoarchitectonic TE area of the temporal cortex in the macaque monkey. We found variations in the frequency of presumptive inhibitory CB-, CR- and PV-positive multiterminals (three or more contacts) in contact with the somata and proximal dendrites of neurons labeled for CB, CR or PV, depending on the calcium-binding protein [98]. The percentage of labeled neurons receiving contacts from other calcium-binding protein neurons ranged from 22 % to 85 %. However, there was remarkable constancy in the patterns of connectivity in different areas for any given combination (the differences were less than 15 %). We concluded that differences exist in the connections between different types of smooth interneurons, and that the similarities found for different combinations in the three cortical areas examined might be attributed to general functional requisites of interneuronal circuitry. Nevertheless, it is important to bear in mind that none of these calcium-binding proteins label a single type of neuron, but rather a variety of particular types (for example, PV labels chandelier cells and basket cells, among others, but not double bouquet cells). In addition, the distal dendrites are often not labeled and thus, such studies are restricted to the somata and proximal dendrites. Thus, the data obtained from these dual immunocytochemical staining studies is only relevant to the connectivity of the perisomatic region. Another method to study connectivity involves combining intracellular recordings of single neurons with focal neuronal stimulation by uncaging glutamate with light (photostimulation-based mapping of functional inputs) [146-148]. These experiments have further emphasized the complexity of cortical circuits, revealing that inputs to individual smooth interneurons are generated from wide variety of sources and that distinct types of smooth interneurons within a cortical layer may receive different information. However, the input patterns are often similar for neurons of the same type. In summary, some general principles of connectivity have been uncovered, but detailed data regarding excitatory and inhibitory inputs to smooth interneurons are relatively scarce to date.

Are All Types of Smooth Interneurons Present in Each Layer of the Minicolumn?

We do not know how many types of smooth interneurons inhabit the neocortex, but given the great diversity of anatomical, molecular and physiological types of neurons, it is likely that dozens or even hundreds of different types exist. Of course, most interneurons in layers II–VI, such as chandelier cells, basket cells, double bouquet cells, Martinotti cells and the great variety of different types of axo-somatic neurons are not present in layer I. The question remains as to what occurs in the rest of the layers? Within a 50 μm wide by 50 μm thick minicolumn of tissue from the pial surface to the white matter, there is a total of approximately 158 neurons the human temporal cortex, and 249 and 364 neurons in the rat and mouse somatosensory cortex, respectively (Figure 12). Assuming that in primates at least 25 % are GABAergic neurons, while in rodents this percentage is only 15 % or less [30], there would be respectively 40, 37, and 55 smooth interneurons in these minicolumns. These numbers appear to be too low to include all types of such interneurons. Indeed, if we consider individual layers in the human cerebral cortex, within such a minicolumn, there would be approximately 3 and 5 smooth interneurons in layers IIIb and VI, respectively. Nevertheless, since the axonal arborization of the vast majority of smooth interneurons surpasses the limits of the minicolumn size (Figure 7, right), perhaps it would be more appropriate to consider the number of smooth interneurons within the macrocolumn, (which is approximately 500 μm wide by 500 μm thick from the pial surface to the white matter). In this macrocolumn, there would be a total number of 15 854, 24 885, and 36 395 neurons, respectivel [30]. Considering the above percentages of GABAergic neurons, in these macrocolumns there would be a total of 3963, 3733, and 5459 smooth interneurons in the human, rat and mouse neocortex, respectively. This is now a sufficiently high number that all types of smooth interneurons might be represented.

The experiments described in the previous sections do not imply differences in the neuronal types that are localized in a given layer, despite indicating differences in the connectivity of different layers or cortical areas. For example, the fact that the corticothalamic neurons in layer VI of the cat visual cortex were not innervated by chandelier cells, whereas callosal neurons in layers III are [136], does not mean that in layer VI there are no chandelier cells. Indeed, other non-corticothalamic cells located in this layer might be innervated by chandelier cells. Similarly, other non-callosal populations of pyramidal cells located in layer III may not be innervated by chandelier cells. Therefore, it raises the question of how can we study the laminar distribution of smooth interneurons?

There are three main methods to label smooth interneurons: the Golgi method, intracellular labeling, and immunocytochemistry. The later has the advantage that instead of labeling only occasional types of smooth interneurons as with the Golgi method or intracellular labeling, the staining obtained with immunocytochemistry is far more widespread and consistent. Furthermore using immunocytochemical techniques the chemical characterization of neurons through double labeling is relatively easy. Of course, the absence of immunostaining may indicate the lack of expression and not the absence of a given type of neuron. Nevertheless, the expression, or failure to express, a given neurotransmitter, peptide or calcium-binding protein by a particular type of smooth interneuron has important functional consequences [51,53,63,65,68]. Therefore, immunocytochemistry provides us with valuable information regarding the distribution and neurochemical profile of particular types of neurons. One disadvantage is that so far, no antigen has been identified to label a single morphological neuronal type, but rather various subpopulations of neurons are labelled. For example, in the human neocortex, the most characteristic type of smooth interneuron stained for PV are chandelier cells, while for CB double bouquet cells are more characteristic. Nevertheless, both PV and CB are found in a variety of other types of smooth interneurons [59]. Furthermore, there may be a some overlap since some chandelier cells in layers V and VI of the human temporal cortex are CB-positive and double bouquet cells can also be labeled for CR. However, no double bouquet cells are PV-positive nor are any chandelier cells labeled for CR [100,149].

Laminar Distribution and Frequency of Different Types of Smooth Interneurons

Bearing in mind the aforementioned limitations, through immunocytochemistry it has been possible to study the laminar distribution and abundance of various types of smooth interneurons [150-155]. These studies have shown that particular types of smooth interneurons may be distributed in two major patterns: columnar (where smooth interneurons are homogeneously distributed throughout layers II–III); and multilaminar (smooth interneurons inhabit two or more layers with a similar density, mostly avoiding or being a relatively less conspicuous in other layers). For example, in the human temporal neocortex it has been shown that neurons immunoreactive for TH, nNOS, NPY, SOM, PV, CB, and CR show marked differences in their laminar distribution and in their density [154-156]. Neurons expressing nNOS and NPY are distributed in a columnar manner, those containing SOM, PV, CB, and CR have a multilaminar pattern (they are more abundant in layers II–III), whereas neurons labeled for TH are only located in layers V–VI. In layer I, very few or no neurons are stained for nNOS, SOM, NPY or PV, although neurons expressing CB and CR can be found. Regarding the density of these neurons, CR-ir neurons show a 61 % higher density than nNOS-ir neurons, and 88 % higher than NPY-ir neurons.

Moreover, if we consider the co-expression of different markers and their laminar distribution, further subdivisions in the columnar dimension can be established. For example, it has been estimated that approximately 25 % of neurons labeled for TH also express nNOS, and that 27 % of nNOS-ir neurons also contain TH [156]. Since TH expressing neurons are only located in layers V–VI, whereas nNOS-ir neurons are found in all layers, neurons expressing nNOS in layers V–VI may differ from those in the layers above due to the pressence of TH. There are also examples of laminar differences in the distribution of particular subtypes of smooth interneurons. In the human temporal neocortex, a subpopulation of chandelier cells in layers V and VI also express CB, whereas chandelier cells expressing the polysialylated form of the cell-surface glycoprotein NCAM (PSA-NCAM) are very numerous in layers II and III, but they can also be found occasionally in deeper layers [149,157]. Furthermore, differences also exist in the density and distribution of smooth interneurons in different cortical areas [98,151,155,158,159]. For example, when the density of PV-ir, CB-ir, and CR-ir neurons in layer III of various cortical areas of the owl and monkey was compared (including the premotor cortex, the primary motor cortex, the somatosensory areas 3a, 3b, 1, and 2, the primary visual area, the second visual area, the dorsolateral visual area, the caudal and rostral divisions of inferotemporal cortex, and the dorsolateral and orbital prefrontal cortex), significant differences were detected in 128 of all 234 possible pair-wise comparisons between areas [155]. In summary, it is possible that all types of smooth interneurons are present within a macrocolumn but not in a minicolumn. Moreover, a specific or preferential laminar distribution of different subtypes of smooth interneurons exists.

Summary and Conclusions

Collectively, the studies described in this chapter indicate that the anatomically defined minicolumn is a rather complex element of the cortical information processing circuit. It consists of assemblies of microcircuits established by discrete and regularly distributed vertical aggregates of pyramidal neurons. It is clear that not all known types of interneurons are present within a minicolumn. However, a given interneuron in a minicolumn does not only establish synapses with other cells of its minicolumn, but also with cells located in adjacent minicolumns. The axonal aborization of double bouquet cells in the minicolumn is similar to the distribution of vertical aggregates of pyramidal neurons in the primate neocortex. Therefore, they appear to be key elements of the minicolumnar organization in primates. Furthermore, the pyramidal cell axon collaterals that make up the vertical aggregates by far surpass the size of the parent minicolumn. Thus, its seems clear that the general mechanisms of intracortical information processing are through the interactions of the minicolumns within a given macrocolumn and with other minicolumns belonging to distant macrocolumns. While many properties of the microcircuits within the minicolumn are stereotypical between cortical regions and species, others are unique to a given area or a set of areas within a given species, or even across orders. However, the question still remains as to what is the basic building block of minicolumnar organization or the constitutive basic microcircuit? Moreover, we have still to resolve which modifications are the results of evolutionary adaptations of excitatory and inhibitory circuits to particular functions? And how much information obtained by studying of non-human mammals can be applied to investigate the emergence of sophisticated cognitive functions in humans? Unfortunately, the gigantic task that is underway, of identifying all the elements of the macrocolumns in the functionally distinct areas of the human, is likely to be insufficient. This is in part due to the fact that some fundamental experimental data on the functional and anatomical organization cannot be obtained in humans for obvious ethical reasons. Thus, meaningful data must be obtained from experimental animals that can be used in computational models to analyze the functional complexity of circuits in the human neocortex. A starting point is to try to identify the basic microcircuits thought to be common to all species, and the variations specific to the human neocortex.

References

[1] Dejerine JJ, Dejerine-Klumpke AM. *Anatomie des centres nerveux, t. 1: Methods générales d'étude-embryologie-histogérèx et histologie-anatomie du cerveau.* Paris: Rueff ; 1895.

[2] Baillarger J. Recherches sur la structure de la couche corticale des circonvolutions du cerveau. *Mémoires de l'Académie royale de médecine.* 1840;8:149-183.

[3] Meynert T. Vom Gehirne der Säugethiere. In: Stricker S, Arnold J, ed. *Handbuch der Lehre von den Geweben des Menschen und der Thiere, v. 1.* Leipzig: Verlag von Wilhelm Engelmann; 1871:694-808.

[4] Cajal SR. Estudios sobre la corteza cerebral humana, III: estructura de la corteza acústica. *Revista Trimestral Micrográfica*. 1900;5:129-183. Translated in: DeFelipe J, Jones EG. *Cajal on the Cerebral Cortex*. New York: Oxford University Press,1988.

[5] Weigert C. Über eine neue Untersuchungsmethode des Centralnervensystems. *Centralblatt für die medicinischen Wissenschaften*. 1882;20:753-757, 772-774.

[6] Kaes T. Beiträge zur Kenntniss des Reichtums der Grosshirnrinde des Menschen an markhaltigen Nervenfasern. *Archiv für Psychiatrie und Nervenkrankheiten*. 1893;25:695-758.

[7] Bechterew W. *Die Leintungsbahnen im Gehirn und Rückenmark: Ein Handbuch für das Studium des Nervensystems* (Weinberg V, tr.) Leipzig: Besold; 1894.

[8] Edinger L. *Vorlesungen über den Bau der nervösen Zentralorgane des Menschen der Thiere*. 5th ed. Leipzig: Vogel, 1896.

[9] Flechsig P. Neue Untersuchungen über die Markbildung in den menschlichen Grosshirnlappen. *Neurologisches Centralblatt*. 1898;17:977-996.

[10] Kaes T. *Die Grosshirnrinde des Menschen: in ihren Massen und ihrem Fasergehalt: Ein gehirnanatomischer Atlas*. Jena: G. Fischer; 1907.

[11] Nauta WJH, Bucher VM. Efferent connections of the striate cortex in the albino rat. *Journal of Comparative Neurology*. 1954;100:257-286.

[12] Schlapp M. Der Zellenbau der Grosshirnrinde des Affen Macacus Cynomolgus. *Archiv für Psychiatrie und Nervenkrankheiten*. 1898;30:583-607.

[13] Kemper TL, Galaburda AM. Principles of cytoarchitectonics. In: Peters A, Jones EG, eds. *Cellular Components of the Cerebral Cortex*. New York: Pleum Press; 1984:35-57. Cerebral Cortex; v. 1.

[14] Cajal SR. Estudios sobre la corteza cerebral humana, II: estructura de la corteza motriz del hombre y mamíferos superiores. *Revista Trimestral Micrográfica*. 1899;4:117-200. In: DeFelipe J, Jones EG, trs. *Cajal on the Cerebral Cortex*. New York: Oxford University Press; 1988.

[15] Bonne C. L'écorce cérébrale, duexième partie: Cytologie, variations régionales et zoologiques de l'écorce cérébrale revue et complétée par le Dr. M. Lefébure. Paris: A. Storck; 1906. *Revue Générale d'Histologie*; t. 2 fasc. 6.

[16] Lorente de Nó R. Architectonics and structure of the cerebral cortex. In: Fulton JF, ed. *Physiology of the Nervous System*. New York: Oxford University Press; 1938:291-330.

[17] DeFelipe J. Cortical interneurons: from Cajal to 2001. *Progress in Brain Research*. 2002;136:215-238.

[18] Foster M, Sherrington CS. *A Text Book of Physiology, Part III: The Central Nervous System*. 7th ed. London: Macmillan; 1897.

[19] Mountcastle VB. Modality and topographic properties of single neurons of cat's somatic sensory cortex. *Journal of Neurophysiology*. 1957;20:408-434.

[20] Powell TPS, Mountcastle VB. Some aspects of the functional organization of the cortex of the postcentral gyrus of the monkey: a correlation of findings obtained in a single unit analysis with cytoarchitecture. *Bulletin of the Johns Hopkins Hospital*. 1959;105:133-162.

[21] Hubel DH, Wiesel TN. Functional architecture of macaque monkey cortex. *Proceedings of the Royal Society of London, Series* B. 1977;198:1-59.

[22] Mountcastle VB. An organizing principle for cerebral function: the unit module and the distributed system. In: Mountcastle VB, Edelman GM. *The Mindful Brain*. Cambridge, MA: MIT press; 1978:7-50.

[23] Mountcastle VB. The columnar organization of the neocortex. *Brain*. 1997;120;701-722.

[24] Jones EG. The columnar basis of cortical circuitry. In: Willis WD, ed. *The Clinical Neurosciences*. New York: Churchill Livingstone; 1983:357-383.

[25] Jones EG. Microcolumns in the cerebral cortex. *Proceedings of the National Academy of Sciences of the United States of America*. 2000;97:5019-5021.

[26] Buxhoeveden DP, Casanova MF. The minicolumn hypothesis in neuroscience. *Brain*. 2002;125:935-951.

[27] Buldyrev SV, Cruz L, Gomez-Isla T, et al. Description of microcolumnar ensembles in association cortex and their disruption in Alzheimer and Lewy body dementias. *Proceedings of the National Academy of Sciences of the United States of America*. 2000;97:5039-5043.

[28] Casanova MF, Buxhoeveden DP, Switala AE, Roy E. Minicolumnar pathology in autism. *Neurology*. 2002;58:428-432.

[29] Casanova MF. Modular concepts of brain organization and the neuropathology of psychiatric conditions. *Psychiatry Research*. 2003;118:101-102.

[30] DeFelipe J, Alonso-Nanclares L, Arellano JI. Microstructure of the neocortex: comparative aspects. *Journal of Neurocytology*. 2002;31:299-316.

[31] Jones EG. Anatomy of cerebral cortex: columnar input-output organization. In: Schmitt FO, Worden FG, Adelman G, Dennis M, eds. *The Cerebral Cortex*. Cambridge, MA: MIT Press; 1981:199-235.

[32] Jones EG. Laminar distribution of cortical efferent cells. In: Peters A, Jones EG, eds. *Cellular Components of the Cerebral Cortex*. New York: Pleum Press; 1984:521-553. Cerebral Cortex; v. 1.

[33] Felleman DJ, Van Essen DC. Distributed hierarchical processing in the primate cerebral cortex. *Cerebral Cortex*. 1991;1:1-47.

[34] DeFelipe J, Fariñas I. The pyramidal neuron of the cerebral cortex: morphological and chemical characteristics of the synaptic inputs. *Progress in Neurobiology*. 1992;39:563-607.

[35] Lund JS, Yoshioka T, Levitt JB. Substrates for interlaminar connections in area V1 of the macaque monkey cerebral cortex. In: Peters A, Rockland KS, eds. *Primary Visual Cortex in Primates*. New York: Plenum Press; 1994:37-60. Cerebral Cortex; v.10.

[36] Lund JS. Anatomical organization of macaque monkey striate visual cortex. *Annual Review of Neuroscience*. 1988;11:253-258.

[37] Lund JS. Spiny stellate neurons. In: Peters A, Jones EG, eds. *Cellular Components of the Cerebral Cortex*. New York: Pleum Press; 1984:255-308. Cerebral Cortex; v. 1.

[38] Jones EG. Varieties and distribution of non-pyramidal cells in the somatic sensory cortex of the squirrel monkey. *Journal of Comparative Neurology*. 1975;160:205-268.

[39] Fairén A, DeFelipe J, Regidor J. Non pyramidal neurons: General account. In: Peters A, Jones EG, eds. *Cellular Components of the Cerebral Cortex*. New York: Pleum Press; 1984:201-253. Cerebral Cortex; v. 1.

[40] Valverde F. The organizing principles of the primary visual cortex in the monkey. In: Peters A, Jones EG, eds. *Visual Cortex*. New York: Plenum Press; 1985:207-257. Cerebral Cortex; v. 3.

[41] Gray EG. Axo-somatic and axo-dendritic synapses of the cerebral cortex: an electron microscopic study. *Journal of Anatomy*. 1959;93:420-433.

[42] Colonnier M. Synaptic patterns on different cell types in the different laminae of the cat visual cortex: an electron microscope study. *Brain Research*. 1968;9:268-287.

[43] Somogyi P, Freund TF, Cowey A. The axo-axonic interneuron in the cerebral cortex of the rat, cat and monkey. *Neuroscience*. 1982;7:2577-2607.

[44] Peters A, Jones EG, eds.*Cellular Components of the Cerebral Cortex*. New York: Plenum Press, 1984. Cerebral Cortex; v. 1.

[45] White EL. *Cortical Circuits: Synaptic Organization of the Cerebral Cortex: Structure, Function and Theory*. Boston, MA: Birkhäuser; 1989.

[46] Peters A, Palay SL. The morphology of synapses. *Journal of Neurocytology*. 1996;25:687-700.

[47] DeFelipe J, Alonso-Nanclares L, Blatow M, Caputi A, Monyer H. Anatomical and molecular heterogeneity of cortical GABAergic interneurons. In: Grillner S, Graybiel A, eds. *Micorcircuits: The Interface Between Neurons and Global Brain Function*: 93rd Dahlem Workshop. Cambridge, MA: The MIT Press; 2005:In press.

[48] Gibson JR, Beierlein M, Connors BW. Two networks of electrically coupled inhibitory neurons in neocortex. *Nature*. 1999;402:75-79.

[49] Tamás G, Buhl EH, Lorincz A, Somogyi P. Proximally targeted GABAergic synapses and gap junctions synchronize cortical interneurons. *Nature Neuroscience*. 2000;3:366-371.

[50] Galarreta M, Hestrin S. Electrical synapses between GABA-releasing interneurons. *Nature Reviews Neuroscience*. 2001;2:425-433.

[51] Galarreta M, Hestrin S. Electrical and chemical synapses among parvalbumin fast-spiking GABAergic interneurons in adult mouse neocortex. *Proceedings of the National Academy of Sciences of the United States of America*. 2002;99:12438-12443.

[52] Amitai Y, Gibson JR, Beierlein M, et al. The spatial dimensions of electrically coupled networks of interneurons in the neocortex. *The Journal of Neuroscience*. 2002;22:4142-4152.

[53] Blatow M, Rozov A, Katona I, et al. A novel network of multipolar bursting interneurons generates theta frequency oscillations in neocortex. *Neuron*. 2003;38:805-817.

[54] Fukuda T, Kosaka T. Ultrastructural study of gap junctions between dendrites of parvalbumin-containing GABAergic neurons in various neocortical areas of the adult rat. *Neuroscience*. 2003;120:5-20.

[55] Houser CR, Vaughn JE, Hendry SHC, Jones EG, Peters A. GABA neurons in the cerebral cortex. In: Jones EG, Peters A, eds. Functional Properties of Cortical Cells. New York: Plenum Press; 1984:63-89. *Cerebral Cortex*; v. 2.

[56] Peters A. Synaptic specificity in the cerebral cortex. In: Edelman GM, Gall WE, Cowan WM, eds. *Synaptic Function*. New York: John Wiley; 1987:373-397.

[57] Ribak CE, Roberts RC. GABAergic synapses in the brain identified with antisera to GABA and its synthesizing enzyme, glutamate decarboxylase. *Journal of Electron Microscopy Technique*. 1990;15:34-38.

[58] DeFelipe J. Neocortical neuronal diversity: chemical heterogeneity revealed by co-localization studies of classic neurotransmitters, neuropeptides, calcium binding proteins and cell surface molecules. *Cerebral Cortex*. 1993;3:273-289.

[59] DeFelipe J. Types of neurons, synaptic connections and chemical characteristics of cells immunoreactive for calbindin-D28K, parvalbumin and calretinin in the neocortex. *Journal of Chemical Neuroanatomy*. 1997;14:1-19.

[60] Jones EG. GABAergic neurones and their role in cortical plasticity in primates. *Cerebral Cortex*. 1993;3:361-372.

[61] Thomson AM, Deuchars J. Synaptic interactions in neocortical local circuits: dual intracellular recordings *in vitro*. *Cerebral Cortex*. 1997;7:510-522.

[62] Somogyi P, Tamás G, Lujan R, Buhl EH. Salient features of synaptic organisation in the cerebral cortex. *Brain Research: Brain Research Reviews*. 1998;26:113-135.

[63] Kawaguchi Y, Kubota Y. GABAergic cell subtypes and their synaptic connections in rat frontal cortex. *Cerebral Cortex* 1997;7:476-486.

[64] Morrison JH, Hof PR, Huntley GW. Neurochemical organization of the primate visual cortex. In: Bloom FE, Björklund A, Hökfelt T, eds. *The Primate Nervous System, Part II.* Amsterdam: Elsevier; 1998:299-433. Handbook of Chemical Neuroanatomy; v. 14.

[65] Gupta A, Wang Y, Markram H. Organizing principles for a diversity of GABAergic interneurones and synapses in the neocortex. *Science*. 2000;287:273-278.

[66] Silberberg G, Gupta A, Markram H. Stereotypy in neocortical microcircuits. *Trends in Neurosciences.* 2002;25:227-230.

[67] Kawaguchi Y, Kondo S. Parvalbumin, somatostatin and cholecystokinin as chemical markers for specific GABAergic interneuron types in the rat frontal cortex. *Journal of Neurocytology.* 2002;31:277-287.

[68] Monyer H, Markran H. Molecular and genetic tools to study GABAergic interneuron diversity and function. *Trends in Neurosciences.* 2004;27:90-97.

[69] Peters A, Walsh TM. A study of the organization of apical dendrites in the somatic sensory cortex of the rat. *Journal of Comparative Neurology.* 1972;144:253-268.

[70] Fleischhauer K, Petsche H, Wittkowski W. Vertical bundles of dendrites in the neocortex. *Zeitschrift für Anatomie und Entwicklungsgeschichte.* 1972;136:213-223.

[71] Fleischhauer K. On different patterns of dendritic bundling in the cerebral cortex of the cat. *Zeitschrift für Anatomie und Entwicklungsgeschichte*. 1974;143:115-126.

[72] Feldman ML, Peters A. A study of barrels and pyramidal dendritic bundles in the cerebral cortex. *Brain Research*. 1974;77:55-76.

[73] Fleischhauer K, Detzer K. Dendritic bundling in the cerebral cortex. *Advances in Neurology*. 1975;12:71-77.

[74] Escobar MI, Pimienta H, Caviness VS Jr, Jacobson M, Crandall JE, Kosnik KS. Architecture of apical dendrites in the murine neocortex: dual apical dendritic systems. *Neuroscience*. 1986;17:975-989.

[75] Peters A, Kara DA.The neuronal composition of area 17 of rat visual cortex, IV: the organization of pyramidal cells. *Journal of Comparative Neurology*. 1987;260:573-590.

[76] Schmolke C, Viebahn C. Dendritic bundles in lamina II/III of the rabbit neorcortex. *Anatomy and Embryology*. 1986;173:343-348.

[77] Peters A, Sethares C. Organization of pyramidal neurons in area 17 of the monkey visual cortex. *Journal of Comparative Neurology*. 1991;306:1-23.

[78] Peters A, Yilmaz E. Neuronal organization in area 17 of cat visual cortex. *Cerebral Cortex*. 1993;3:49-68.

[79] White EL, Peters A. Cortical modules in the posteromedial barrel subfield (Sm1) of the mouse. *Journal of Comparative Neurology*. 1993;334:86-96.

[80] Lev DL, White EL. Organization of pyramidal cell apical dendrites and composition of dendritic clusters in the mouse: emphasis on primary motor cortex. *European Journal of Neuroscience*. 1997;9:280-290.

[81] Fleischhauer K. Cortical architectonics: the last 50 years and some problems today. In: Brazier MAB, Petsche H, eds. *Architectonics of the Cerebral Cortex*. New York: Raven Press; 1978:99-117.

[82] Winkler C, Potter A. *An Anatomical Guide to Experimental Researches on the Cat's Brain*. Amsterdam: Versluys; 1914.

[83] Roney KJ, Scheibel AB, Shaw GL. Dendritic bundles: survey of anatomical experiments and physiological theories. *Brain Research: Brain Research Reviews*. 1979;1:225-271.

[84] Latz H. *Quantitative Messungen an Dendritenbündeln in der Hirnrinde des Kaninchens*. [Inaugural dissertation] Bonn: Med Fakultät, 1975.

[85] DeFelipe J, Jones EG. *Cajal on the Cerebral Cortex*. New York, NY: Oxford University Press; 1988.

[86] Cajal SR. Estudios sobre la corteza cerebral humana, I: corteza visual. *Revista Trimestral Micrográfica*. 1899;4:1-63. In: DeFelipe J, Jones EG, trs. *Cajal on the Cerebral Cortex*. New York: Oxford University Press; 1988.

[87] Szentágothai J. Synaptology of the visual cortex. In: Jung R, ed. *Handbook of Sensory Physiology, Vol. VII/3: Central Visual Information*, Part B. Berlin: Springer-Verlag; 1973:269-324.

[88] Szentágothai J. The "module-concept" in cerebral cortex architecture. *Brain Research*. 1975;95:475-496.

[89] Valverde F. The organization of area 18 in the monkey: a Golgi study. *Anatomy and Embryology*. 1978;154:305-334.

[90] Hendry SHC, Jones EG, Emson PC, Lawson DE, Heizmann CW, Streit P. Two classes of cortical GABA neurons defined by differential calcium binding protein immunoreactivities. *Experimental Brain Research*. 1989;76:467-472.

[91] DeFelipe J, Hendry SHC, Jones EG. Synapses of double bouquet cells in monkey cerebral cortex visualized by calbindin immunoreactivity. *Brain Research*. 1989;503:49-54.

[92] DeFelipe J, Hendry SHC, Hashikawa T, Molinari M, Jones EG. A microcolumnar structure of monkey cerebral cortex revealed by immunocytochemical studies of double bouquet cell axons. *Neuroscience*. 1990;37:655-673.

[93] Peters A, Sethares C. The organization of double bouquet cells in monkey striate cortex. *Journal of Neurocytology*. 1997;26:779-797.

[94] de Lima AD, Morrison JH. Ultrastructural analysis of somatostatin-immunoreactive neurons and synapses in the temporal and occipital cortex of the macaque monkey. *Journal of Comparative Neurology*. 1989;283:212-227.

[95] DeFelipe J, Jones EG. High resolution light and electron microscopic immunocytochemistry of co-localized GABA and calbindin D-28k in somata and double bouquet cell axons of monkey somatosensory cortex. *European Journal of Neuroscience.* 1992;4:42-60.

[96] Ferrer I, Tuñon T, Soriano E, et al. Calbindin immunoreactivity in normal human temporal cortex. *Brain Research*. 1992;572:33-41.

[97] Hayes TL, Lewis DA. Nonphosphorylated neurofilament protein and calbindin immunoreactivity in layer III pyramidal neurons of human neocortex. *Cerebral Cortex.* 1992;2:56-67.

[98] DeFelipe J, González-Albo MC, del Río MR, Elston GN. Distribution and patterns of connectivity of interneurons containing calbindin, calretinin, and parvalbumin in visual areas of the occipital and temporal lobes of the macaque monkey. *Journal of Comparative Neurology.* 1999;412:515-526.

[99] del Río MR, DeFelipe J. A light and electron microscopic study of calbindin d-28k immunoreactive double bouquet cells in the human temporal cortex. *Brain Research.* 1995;690:133-140.

[100] del Río MR, DeFelipe J. Double bouquet cell axons in the human temporal neocortex: relationship to bundles of myelinated axons and colocalization of calretinin and calbindin D-28k immunoreactivities. *Journal of Chemical Neuroanatomy.* 1997;13:243-251.

[101] Somogyi P, Cowey A. Combined Golgi and electron microscopic study on the synapses formed by double bouquet cells in the visual cortex of the cat and monkey. *Journal of Comparative Neurology.* 1981;195:547-566.

[102] DeFelipe J. Microcircuits in the brain. In: Mira J, Moreno-Díaz R, Cabestany J, eds. *Biological and Artificial Computation: From Neuroscience to Technology*. Berlin: Springer; 1997:1-14. Lecture Notes in Computer Science; v. 1240.

[103] Letinic K, Zoncu R, Rakic, P. Origin of GABAergic neurons in the human neocortex. *Nature*. 2002;417:645-649.

[104] Tan SS, Kalloniatis M, Sturm K, Tam PPL, Reese BE, Faulkner-Jones B. Separate progenitors for radial and tangential cell dispersion during development of the cerebral neocortex. *Neuron*. 1998;21:295-304.

[105] Anderson S, Mione M, Yun K, Rubenstein JLR. Differential origins of neocortical projection and local circuit neurons: role of Dlx genes in neocortical interneuronogenesis. *Cerebral Cortex*. 1999;9:646-654.

[106] Marin O, Rubenstein JL. Cell migration in the forebrain. *Annual Review of Neuroscience*. 2003;26:441-446.

[107] Rakic P. Evolving concepts of cortical radial and areal specification. *Progress in Brain Research.* 2002;136:265-280.

[108] Lund JS. Excitatory and inhibitory circuiting and laminar mapping strategies in the primary visual cortex of the monkey. In: Edelman GM, Gall WE, Cowan WM, eds. *Signal and Sense: Local and Global Order in Perceptual Maps.* New York: Wiley-Liss; 1990:51-82.

[109] Lund JS, Yoshioka T, Levitt JB. Comparison of intrinsic connectivity in different areas of macaque monkey cerebral cortex. *Cerebral Cortex.* 1993;3:148-162.

[110] Gilbert CD. Circuitry, architecture, and functional dynamics of visual cortex. *Cerebral Cortex.* 1993;3:373-386.

[111] Rockland KS. Elements of cortical architecture: hierarchy revisited. In: Rockland KS, Kaas JH, Peters A, eds. *Extrastriate Cortex in Primates.* New York: Plenum Press; 1997:243-293. Cerebral Cortex; v. 12.

[112] Thomson AM, Morris OT. Selectivity in the inter-laminar connections made by neocortical neurones. *Journal of Neurocytology.* 2002;31:239-246.

[113] Thomson AM, West DC, Wang Y, Bannister AP. Synaptic connections and small circuits involving excitatory and inhibitory neurons in layers 2-5 of adult rat and cat neocortex: Triple intracellular recordings and biocytin labeling in vitro. *Cerebral Cortex.* 2002;12:936-953.

[114] Schubert D, Kötter R, Zilles K, Luhmann HJ, Staiger JF. Cell type-specific circuits of cortical layer IV spiny neurons. *The Journal of Neuroscience.* 2003;23:2961-2970.

[115] Karube F, Kubota Y, Kawaguchi Y. Axon branching and synaptic bouton phenotypes in gabaergic nonpyramidal cell subtypes. *Journal of Neuroscience.* 2004;24:2853-2865.

[116] Alonso-Nanclares L, White EL, Elston GN, DeFelipe J. Synaptology of the proximal segment of pyramidal cell basal dendrites. *European Journal of Neuroscience.* 2004;19:771-776.

[117] Alonso-Nanclares L, Minelli A, Melone M, Edwards RH, DeFelipe J. Perisomatic glutamatergic axon terminals: A novel feature of cortical synaptology revealed by vesicular glutamate transporter 1 immunostaining. *Neuroscience.* 2004;123:547-556.

[118] Peters A, Palay SL, Webster H deF. *The Fine Structure of the Nervous System: Neurons and their Supporting Cells.* New York: Oxford University Press; 1991.

[119] Jones EG, Powell TPS. Morphological variations in the dendritic spines of the neocortex. *Journal of Cell Science.* 1969;5:509-529.

[120] Peters A, Kaiserman-Abramof IR.The small pyramidal neuron of the rat cerebral cortex: the synapses upon dendritic spines. *Zeitschrift für Zellforschung und mikroskopische Anatomie.* 1969;100:487-506.

[121] Peters A, Kaiserman-Abramof IR. The small pyramidal neuron of the rat cerebral cortex: the perikaryon, dendrites and spines. *American Journal of Anatomy.* 1970;127:321-355.

[122] White EL, Hersch SM. Thalamocortical synapses of pyramidal cells which project from SmI to MsI cortex in the mouse. *Journal of Comparative Neurology.* 1981;198:167-181.

[123] White EL, Hersch SM. A quantitative study of thalamocortical and other synapses involving the apical dendrites of corticothalamic projection cells in mouse SmI cortex. *Journal of Neurocytology*. 1982;11:137-157.

[124] Feldman ML. Morphology of the neocortical pyramidal neuron. In: Peters A, Jones EG, eds. *Cellular Components of the Cerebral Cortex*. New York: Pleum Press; 1984:123-200. Cerebral Cortex; v. 1.

[125] Larkman AU. Dendritic morphology of pyramidal neurones of the visual cortex of the rat, III: spine distributions. *Journal of Comparative Neurology*. 1991;306:332-343.

[126] Elston GN. Interlaminar differences in the pyramidal cell phenotype in cortical areas 7m and STP (the superior temporal polysensory area) of the macaque monkey. *Experimental Brain Research*. 2001;138:141-152.

[127] Elston GN, Tweedale R, Rosa MGP. Cortical integration in the visual system of the macaque monkey: large scale morphological differences of pyramidal neurones in the occipital, parietal and temporal lobes. *Proceedings: Biological Sciences*. 1999;266:1367-1374.

[128] Elston GN. Cortical heterogeneity: implications for visual processing and polysensory integration. *Journal of Neurocytology*. 2002;31:317-335.

[129] Elston GN. Cortex, cognition and the cell: new insights into the pyramidal cell and prefrontal function. *Cerebral Cortex*. 2003;13:1124-1138.

[130] Elston GN, DeFelipe J. Spine distribution in cortical pyramidal cells: a common organizational principle across species. *Progress in Brain Research*. 2002;136:109-133.

[131] Benavides-Piccione R, Ballesteros-Yáñez I, DeFelipe J, Yuste R. Cortical area and species differences in dendritic spine morphology. *Journal of Neurocytology*. 2002;31:337-346.

[132] Konur S, Rabinowitz D, Fenstermaker VL, Yuste R. Systematic regulation of spine sizes and densities in pyramidal neurons. *Journal of Neurobiology*. 2003;56:95-112.

[133] Kasai H, Matsuzaki M, Noguchi J, Yasumatsu N, Nakahara H. Structure-stability-function relationships of dendritic spines. *Trends in Neurosciences*. 2003;26:360-368.

[134] Tsay D, Yuste R. On the electrical function of dendritic spines. *Trends in Neurosciences*. 2004;27:77-83.

[135] Fariñas I, DeFelipe J. Patterns of synaptic input on corticocortical and corticothalamic cells in the cat visual cortex, I: the cell body. *Journal of Comparative Neurology*. 1991;304:53-69.

[136] Fariñas I, DeFelipe J. Patterns of synaptic input on corticocortical and corticothalamic cells in the cat visual cortex, II: the axon initial segment. *Journal of Comparative Neurology*. 1991;304:70-77.

[137] Lund JS, Griffiths S, Rumberger A, Levitt JB. Inhibitory synapse cover on the somata of excitatory neurons in macaque monkey visual cortex. *Cerebral Cortex*. 2001;11:783-795.

[138] White EL. Identified neurons in mouse SmI cortex which are postsynaptic to thalamocortical axon terminals: a combined Golgi-electron microscopic and degeneration study. *Journal of Comparative Neurology*. 1978;181:627-662.

[139] Somogyi P. The study of Golgi stained cells and of experimental degeneration under the electron microscope: a direct method for the identification in the visual cortex of three succesive links in a neuron chain. *Neuroscience*. 1978;3:167-180.

[140] Somogyi P, Hodgson AJ, Smith AD. An approach to tracing neuron networks in the cerebral cortex and basal ganglia: combination of Golgi staining, retrograde transport of horseradish peroxidase and anterograde degeneration of synaptic boutons in the same material. *Neuroscience*. 1979;4:1805-1852.

[141] Somogyi P. Synaptic connections of neurones identified by Golgi impregnation: characterization by immunocytochemical, enzyme histochemical, and degeneration methods. *Journal of Electron Microscopy Technique*. 1990;15:332-351.

[142] White EE, Benshalom G, Hersch, SM. Thalamocortical and other synapses involving nonspiny multipolar cells of mouse SmI cortex. *Journal of Comparative Neurology*. 1984;229:311-320.

[143] Freund TF, Somogyi P. The section-Golgi impregnation procedure, 1: description of the method and its combination with histochemistry after intracellular iontophoresis or retrograde transport of horseradish peroxidase. *Neuroscience*. 1983;9:463-474.

[144] Tamás G, Somogyi P, Buhl EH. Differentially interconnected networks of GABAergic interneurons in the visual cortex of the cat. *Journal of Neuroscience*. 1998;18:4255-4270.

[145] Wang Y, Gupta A, Toledo-Rodriguez, Wu CZ, Markram H. Anatomical, physiological, molecular and circuit properties of nest basket cells in the developing somatosensory cortex. *Cerebral Cortex*. 2002;12:395-410.

[146] Dantzker LJ, Callaway EM. Laminar sources of synaptic input to cortical inhibitory interneurons and pyramidal neurons. *Nature Neuroscience*. 2000;3:701-707.

[147] Sawatari A, Callaway EM. Diversity and cell type specificity of local excitatory connections to neurons in layer 3B of monkey primary visual cortex. *Neuron*. 2000;25:459-471.

[148] Callaway EW. Cell type specificity of local cortical connections. *Journal of Neurocytology*. 2002;31:231-237.

[149] del Río MR, DeFelipe J. Colocalization of parvalbumin and calbindin d-28k in neurons including chandelier cells of the human temporal neocortex. *Journal of Chemical Neuroanatomy*. 1997;12:165-173.

[150] Condé F, Lund J, Jacobowitz DM, Baimbridge KG, Lewis DA. Local circuit neurons immunoreactive for calretinin, calbindin D-28k or parvalbumin in monkey prefrontal cortex: distribution and morphology. *Journal of Comparative Neurology*. 1994;341:95-116.

[151] Kondo H, Hashikawa T, Tanaka K, Jones EG. Neurochemical gradient along the monkey occipito-temporal cortical pathway. *NeuroReport*. 1994;5:613-616.

[152] Gonchar Y, Burkhalter A. Three distinct families of GABAergic neurons in rat visual cortex. *Cerebral Cortex*. 1997;7:347-358.

[153] Gabbott PLA, Bacon SJ. Local circuit neurons in the medial prefrontal cortex (areas 24a,b,c, 25 and 32) in the monkey, II: quantitative areal and laminar distributions. *Journal of Comparative Neurology*. 1996;364:609-636.

[154] González-Albo MC, Elston GN, DeFelipe J. The human temporal cortex: characterization of neurons expressing nitric oxide synthase, neuropeptides, calcium-binding proteins, and their glutamate receptor subunit profiles. *Cerebral Cortex.* 2001;11:1170-1181.

[155] Elston GN, González-Albo MC. Parvalbumin-, calbindin-, and calretinin-immunoreactive neurons in the prefrontal cortex of the owl monkey (*Aotus trivirgatus*): a standardized quantitative comparison with sensory and motor areas. *Brain, Behavior and Evolution.* 2003;62:19-30.

[156] Benavides-Piccione R, DeFelipe J. Different populations of tyrosine hydroxylase-immunoreactive neurons defined by differential expression of nitric oxide synthase in the human temporal cortex. *Cerebral Cortex.* 2003;13:297-307.

[157] Arellano JI, DeFelipe J, Muñoz A. PSA-NCAM immunoreactivity in chandelier cell axon terminals of the human temporal cortex. *Cerebral Cortex*. 2002;12:617-624.

[158] Kritzer M, Cowey A, Somogyi P. Patterns of inter- and intralaminar GABAergic connections distinguish striate (V1) and extrastriate (V2, V4) visual cortices and their functionally specialized subdivisions in the rhesus monkeys. *Journal of Neuroscience.* 1992;12:4545-4564.

[159] Dombrowski SM, Hilgetag CC, Barbas H. Quantitative architecture distinguishes prefrontal cortical systems in the rhesus monkey. *Cerebral Cortex.* 2001;11:975-988.

Acknowledgements

I am grateful to Alberto Muñoz for his helpful comments on the manuscript and to Inmaculada Ballesteros-Yáñez for assitance with the prepration of the figures. This work was supported by grants DGCYT PM99-0105, BFI2003-02745 and the 'Comunidad de Madrid' (08.5/0027/2001.1).

In: Neocortical Modularity and the Cell Minicolumn
Editor: Manuel F. Casanova, pp. 93-116
ISBN 1-59454-301
© 2005 Nova Science Publishers, Inc.

Chapter V

THE CELL COLUMN IN COMPARATIVE ANATOMY

Daniel Buxhoeveden
Medical College of Georgia, Augusta, GA
Manuel F. Casanova*
University of Louisville, KY

INTRODUCTION

DeFelipe [1] points out that as long ago as 1938, Lorente de Nó [2] described an "*elementary cortical unit of operation,*" viewing the cortex as consisting of small vertical cylinders consisting of chains of cells that crossed several layers. He also stated, "*All the elements of the cortex are represented in it, and therefore it may be an elementary unit in which, theoretically, the whole process of the transmission of impulses from the efferent fibre to efferent axons may be accomplished.*" Mountcastle later rediscovered the columnar hypothesis on the basis of his physiological studies [3.4], identifying the minicolumn as the most basic unit in cortical organization. While the presence of such a basic anatomical element would seemingly provide an ideal source for comparative anatomical work, this has not occurred.

Comparative anatomy seeks to determine morphological differences and similarities between organisms in an evolutionary context. Many features of the brain have been utilized including nuclei, cell populations, and gross anatomical structures. Yet with few exceptions the cell column has not been among them. Studying minicolumns yields a key benefit: they represent genetically determined units creating a fundamental organization of cells and fibers in the neocortex. These columns are refined by environmental cues, making them an ideal locus for study of the interaction between the genetic blueprint and selection pressures. A

* Corresponding author: Manuel F. Casanova, MD, Gottfried and Gisela Kolb Endowed Chair in Psychiatry, University of Louisville, Department of Psychiatry, 500 South Preston St., A Bldg., Rm. 217, Louisville, KY 40292. Tel: (502)852-4077; Fax: (502)852-4078; E-mail: M0CASA02@louisville.edu

vertical component to cortical organization is certainly a part of the makeup of the neocortex in one manner or another. Thus, minicolumnar research entails a holistic approach to the anatomical placement of cells, synapses, and fibers within cortical tissue. The translaminar interconnectivity within minicolumns subsumes the local circuits of each layer including the functional specificity of cell types. This vertical element may provide the most comprehensive view of cortical circuitry [5].

Nonetheless, minicolumn study is often difficult and sometimes contentious. The term "cell column" (Table 1) refers specifically to the array of cortical cells as seen in Nissl stain tissue. Strictly speaking, the term infers little more than the vertical pattern of cells viewed microscopically as described by Vernon B. Mountcastle [4]. The minicolumn is a subunit of a larger functional unit, the macrocolumn [6-8]. The larger cortical column is more widely studied because, in some occasions, it is easier to detect and measure, and performs a more obvious functional role. The layer 4 barrel, for instance, is readily visible even without staining and has a one to one correspondence with a facial whisker and barreloids in the thalamus.

Table 1. Glossary

Cell column	The vertical arrangement of cells as seen in cell stained material. Usually refers to pyramidal cells in layers III, V, VI, but at lower magnification can include layer 4 as well.
Cortical column	Typically refers to the larger macrocolumn.
Functional column	Usually refers to the macrocolumn. However this can be confusing since functionality has been shown to occur at the microcolumn level.
Vertical cell array	Another phrase for cell column. Refers specifically to a line or vertical array of neurons as seen in a cell body stain. It is more neutral in tone in that it does not imply anything more than the observation of a pattern.
Minicolumn / Microcolumn	The smallest functional column or unit in the cortex. The terms are interchangeable. The use of this term generally imputes the presence of functional properties.
Macrocolumn	The larger unit of function such as a barrel column composed of many minicolumns.
Segregate	Used to refer to larger macrocolumn units usually as seen in metabolic studies.
Barrel column	A specialized form of macrocolumn found in rodents, marsupials, and lagomorphs. Consists of the layer 4 barrel in addition to the infra-and-supragranular layers.
Radial column	Synonymous with cell columns or ontogenetic cell columns in developing fetal cortex.
Ontogenetic column	Cell columns present in the earliest fetal cortex [15].

By contrast, the functional activity of a minicolumn is subtle and more difficult to detect. Considering present knowledge, minicolumns are grouped within macrocolumns, though their functions are only partly understood. At the same time, one should not view them as isolated self-contained units that repeat identically throughout cortex. Rather, as a basic unit of the cortex they may function as a modifiable template. Given their heterogeneity, the repetitive nature of minicolumns does not require the presence of clone-like elements throughout the cortex [9]. It is the template which is repetitive, not the specific configuration of every minicolumn. This paradigm has a parallel in a comparison of barrel columns with ocular dominance columns; they are not precisely the same but they share underlying features. Moreover, both overlay a horizontal organization onto a vertical one.

Making minicolumns useful in comparative neurology raises several issues. The minicolumn must be a "real" anatomical entity present in a sufficient number of cortical areas to reward study. One must prove that, to some extent, they function as a fundamental physiological unit. Yet they not need function independently. Even if one limits their role to part of the macrocolumn (rather than displaying functional independence), alterations in their morphology reflect significant changes in the microcircuit of the macrocolumn. Finally, after meeting the above criteria, research needs techniques to reliably detect and measure them.

In order to measure minicolumns they must exist as physiological or anatomical entities. The issues surrounding vertical columns include their ubiquity, their existence anatomically or as physiological units formed on the basis of lateral inhibition, their anatomy and physiology, and the degree to which they are stereotypic [10-12]. Additionally, the question arises whether they are secondary or primary patterns of cortical organization. The following section responds to these issues with physiological and anatomical evidence for the existence of the minicolumn.

THE VERTICAL CELL COLUMN IN THE FETAL CORTEX

Studies of cortical development provide a major argument for existence of the minicolumn. During the earliest phases of fetal development, a near homogeneous vertical column of cells emerges. It represents the first anatomical organization of cortex (Figure 1). These early cell arrays are known as ontogenetic or radial cell columns [13-15]. The radial unit hypothesis states that the developing neocortex consists primarily of these cell arrays. These radial columns also involve a strong genetic component [16]. A comparative study by Gressens and Evrard [17] reported that the neuronal-glial unit (consisting of the radial glia cells and migrating neurons) is conserved in a variety of animals including the mouse, rat, hamster, cat, and human fetus. The presence of ontogenetic columns in many mammals infers it is a generalized feature of the mammalian cortex, though many of its aspects remain unclear.

While no one has finally confirmed that the ontogenetic cell columns give rise to the adult cell column, research strongly suggests that they do [8,18]. When Krmpotic-Nemanic et al. [18] performed a qualitative study of ontogenetic cell columns through time, they concluded they were the same as those found in the adult brain. We provide a similar analysis in a series of micrographs taken in fetal and post-natal material (Figure 2). The earliest brain examined is 18 gestational weeks (GW). At this age the tight linear organization of cells is quite evident and appears essentially homogenous throughout the section. It is only with maturation that the cortex begins to manifest cytoarchitectonic differentiation. This infers that cytoarchitectonic differences that arise from this near uniform linear distribution of cells. The onset of lamination disrupts the vertical appearance at around 26 GW, especially in layer III.

However, the vertical cell columns re-appear with later development as seen in the late gestational weeks and postnatal material (Figure 2). The tightly packed cell columns in pre-lamination cortex are not only the earliest pattern in the cortex. They are the arrangement around which later fiber connections will manifest. Therefore, one might reasonably suppose that the vertical organization is the primary template around which other types of cortical organization form and not the other way around.

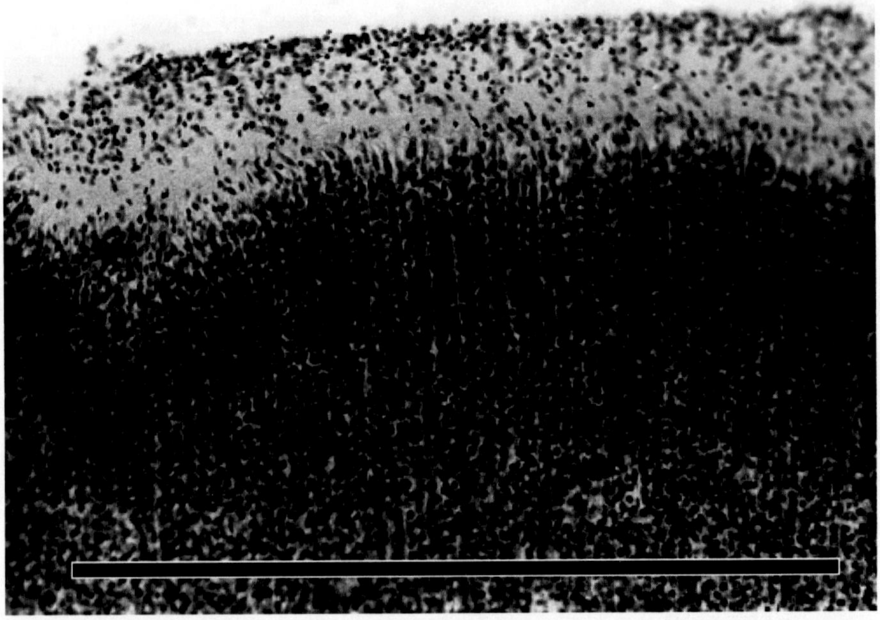

Figure 1. 18 week fetal cortex: Note the highly vertical arrays of neurons with very little space between them. The scale bar measures.

In addition to the emergence of ontogenetic cell columns during development, other indicators of vertical organization appear. For one, the distribution of callosal axon terminals occurs in discrete patches by the end of the first postnatal month in cat visual cortex. From the beginning synaptic boutons are distributed in radial columns whose diameter increases with age [19]. On a larger scale, McKinstry et al. [20] demonstrated the vertical orientation of the fetal cortex. They applied water diffusion anisotropy in a diffusion tensor imaging (DTI) study in living human infants aged 26 GW to 40 GW. They found that the apparent diffusion of water in cortex is oriented radially at 26 GW based on the predominant vertical placement of neuronal constituents. At 36 GW it dropped off. Water diffusion properties are strongly influenced by tissue microstructure including cells and fibers. Thus by 36 weeks the clear radial orientation detected by DTI is blurred by the proliferation of axons and dendrites. This loss is due to the addition of fiber systems, which redirects water displacement more uniformly in all directions.

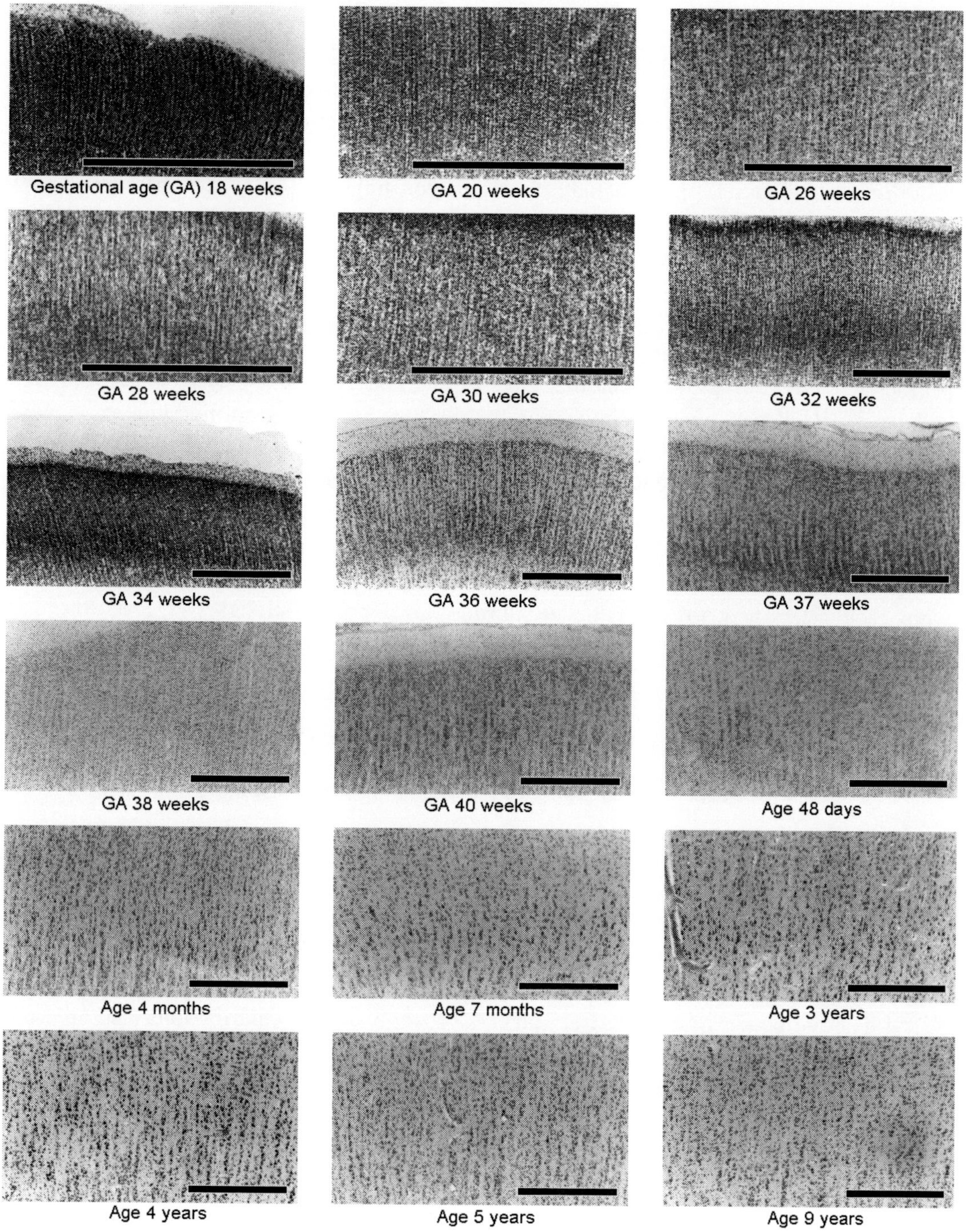

Figure 2. Cell column development from 18 weeks *in utero* to 9 years of age. All scalebars are 500 μm long.

Studies of cortical development in rats also confirm the shape and function of minicolumns. Lohmann and Koppen [21] describe the development of pyramidal dendritic and axonal bundles in the developing rat V1. Vertical bundles were clearly present at birth and had an initial center-to-center spacing of 18 μm. The authors noted that in the ensuing weeks the axonal and dendritic bundles grew "in parallel with regard to their center-to-center distances, diameters, and number of elements up to their adult values around postnatal day 90." Interestingly, at that point they report values of 50.1 μm for axons and 52.6 μm for dendrite bundles. This corresponds perfectly with reports by others in rat V1 using different measuring techniques [22]. The study clearly demonstrated not only the early presence of these vertical bundles. It also shows their origination from the same neurons present at birth and developed in accordance with the maturational process. The initial vertical bundles developed from intracortical axons observed at time of birth. Also notable was the clustering of dendrites and axons into bundles after lamination. When the authors tracked the center-to-center spacing of the two bundles through development, they found that they developed in parallel. Curtetti et al. [23] explain that three to four dendritic bundle systems show up very early in rat V1 development. With ageing the distance between dendritic bundles increases while the morphology and distribution remain stable. This was also reported for the developing ontogenetic cell column, axons bundles, and dendritic bundles [18,21,24].

Developmental studies have traced the presence and size of columnar cell arrays through adulthood [18-21,24]. These studies show that the center-to-center spacing distances increase in relationship to neocortical area and volume [21,22]. The correspondence of these elements with each other and to cortical size during development strongly suggests they are anatomically and functionally related.

Evidence for Narrow Vertical Organization in the Components of the Neocortex

The vertical orientation of cortical elements proliferating in the adult cortex provides the anatomical basis of columnar organization. Apical dendrites from pyramidal cells form tightly-knit bundles that vertically traverse the cortical lamina. These bundles repeat at minicolumn-size intervals. Existing studies show areal and species-specific differences in regards to these bundles, making them a good topic for comparative anatomy. The largest apical dendrite bundles originate from layers V though smaller contributions also appear in layers VI and IV. For comparative purposes, apical dendrite bundles have been described in monkey areas 17 and 18, the prefrontal cortex, and the cingulate gyrus [25-27]. Peters et al. [26] report that area 18 and 17 varied in their apical dendrite systems. Area 18 had two tiers, dendritic tufts formed by pyramidal cells in layers IV, V, and VI, which did not reach layer I. Another arose from layers II and III where the apical dendrite tufts reached layer I. In area 17, the apical dendrites of layer V formed discrete clusters that were joined by those cells in layers II/III and all of the apical dendrites form apical tufts in layer I. Reiterative apical dendrite bundles have been reported in cat area 41 [28], mouse S1 barrel cortex 29,30], rabbit V1 and M1 [31-34], rat areas 3, 17, and 32 [21,28,35-37], and all cortical areas in the lesser hedgehog [38] Viebahn [34] examined vertical apical dendrite bundles in rabbit neocortex in 12 neocortical areas. Ichinohe and Rockland [39] additionally reported finding that dendrites from GABAergic neurons were co-localized with those of apical dendrites in the rat retrosplenial cortex. In all areas apical dendrites were bundled in layers IV, II, and III. They also found evidence of differences in the structure of the bundles, especially between motor and occipital cortex. It is important to note that no one observed apical dendrite bundles in three-layered entorhinal cortex or the hippocampus, nor were they present in the cerebral cortex of a turtle (*Trachemys scripta elegans*).

Several researchers portray vertically-oriented fiber architecture during development. Curtettti et al. [23] describe up to four types of dendritic bundles in developing rat visual cortex. One originates in layer V and extends to the supragranula layers but does not co-mingle with the apical dendrites in II/III. Another type resembling those reported above joins the apical dendrites in the supragranula layers. A third type is formed by neurons located within the supragranular layers. They also report layer VI to IV dendrite bundle as described by Peters and Kara [40]. They conclude that the dendritic bundles in cortex are "highly conserved through species," [26,33,38] cortical areas [30,35,41], and age [42]. Curtetti et al. [23] further comment that "Even if their function in cortical physiology remains unclear, their highly organized distribution and their early electrical coupling are suggestive of a functional role within cortical columns." They also suggest that dendritic bundles may represent morphological units underlying the organization of cortical columns as described by Mountcastle [8]. Wahle and Meyer [43] also describe vertically oriented fiber architecture during development.

In addition to dendrites, axons also form narrow bundles in repeating vertical patterns. Kenan-Vaknin et al. [44] described vertically descending axon bundles in human visual *association* cortex in layers II/III that are 20 μm in diameter and spaced 15 μm apart. The horizontal spread of the axons occurred in layers II, III, and V. The double bouquet cell projects their axons as narrow vertical bundles as well [45], with spacing distances within the minicolumn range. In addition to the well known axon bundles, double bouquet cells also project very long descending dendrites, some 1800 μm 2000 μm long, which ramify in "claw-shaped" patterns in layer V [46]. The same authors report on the basis of calbindin immunoreactivity the presence of vertically oriented fibers in layers III and V/VI that were between 8 μm and 10 μm thick separated by immunonegative spaces about 20 μm to 40 μm wide in human temporal cortex [46]. These apparently correspond to the double bouquet axon bundles reported by DeFelipe et al. [45] and are similar in center-to-center spacing. DeFelipe et al. [45] found reiterative center-to-center spacing of double bouquet axon bundles ranging from 15 μm 30 μm in regions of the brain including auditory, motor, and visual cortex in four species of *Macaca* (*M. fascicularis, M. mulatta, M. fuscata, M. nemestrina*). The differences in size could be related to species differences or cortical regions within species. Del Río and DeFelipe [47] reported double bouquet axon bundles with a mean spacing of about 30 μm in human temporal cortex as well. In an earlier study, DeFelipe and Jones [48] found two types of putative inhibitory interneurons with vertical projections in sensory motor cortex, and three types in area 17 in monkey cortex. Somogyi et al. [49] describe a vertical configuration for GABA neurons in V1 of *Macaca mulatta* cortex. They found that a GABA vertical neuron system that passes throughout layers V to II can influence those in layer VI. The axon bundles were highly restricted laterally to within 20 μm and 50 μm. Peters and Sethares [50] described the myelinated axon bundles that originated in the supragranular layers and became thicker as they descended into the infragranula lamina until they entered the white matter. They demonstrated a mean center-to-center spacing of 23 μm in area 17 in monkey cortex. Dem′ianenko [51] reports that pyramidal cells in prefrontal cortex of *Macaca mulatta* have vertical connections for recurrent and collateral axons. These links unite the pyramidal cells both in horizontal and minicolumn-size vertical directions.

Researchers have used different methods to measure the vertical arrangement of (essentially) pyramidal cells in human brain in the cingulate cortex [52], the superior temporal sulcus [53], the temporal lobe [47], and area 22 [54-57], and area 17 (Casanova et al., unpublished data, 2003). Von Bonin and Mehler [58] examined cell arrays in one human brain in areas 4, 17, 7, and 40. They have also been measured in nonhuman primates [24,59,60] and mouse brain (Casanova et al., unpublished data, 2004). Lohmann and Koppen [21] describe seeing pyramidal cells aggregating their axons and dendrites into bundles that "stood completely in register to each other." They state that neurons which group their axons also group their apical dendrites so that a "vertical pyramidal cell cluster probably resembles and input as well as an out module." The authors describe these units as the structural correlates of the physiological columns of Mountcastle. The authors point out that the spacing of 30 μm for dendritic bundles in monkey V1 corresponds almost exactly to the orientation column size postulated by Hubel and Wiesel [61,62].

Other features of the cortex display vertical orientation including cell soma of basket cells [63], GABAergic interneurons [48], and dendrites of non-pyramidal cells [64]. However, these do not necessarily represent a single column nor are they necessarily known to be reiterative. Budd and Kisvarday [65] and Kozloski et al. [66] show that local connections and synapses are highly specific and stereotypic and determined in each animal, tending to fall within the microcircuit dimensions. Kozloski et al. [66] found precisely determined cortical microcircuits in mouse layer V cortex, showing that local connectivity is not probabilistic or random. The position of the targeted neurons appeared "remarkably precise, indicating robust developmental control of circuit information."

The hard wiring that can account for vertical physiological responses across layers is well documented [8]. It consists of incoming afferents to layer 4, which are passed on to cells directly above them in the supragranular layers. They are then sent down to the infragranular layers, with recurrent connections between them. Necessarily, a time delay results. Thus, all the layers are vertically organized. The inhibitory interneurons embedded within the cortex can enhance activation in one column while damping it in another, creating contrast. Even these cells are not located randomly. They appear in close proximity to pyramidal cells and are oriented vertically along with their dendrites [48,49,63,64,66]. Furthermore, they demonstrate patterns of periodicity in the cortex rather than the randomness one would expect if they were positioned according to a pattern related to columns [67].

Tanaka [68] describes experiments by Thomson and Deuchars [69] which suggest pyramidal cells have two kinds of connections based on their axon collaterals. Both provide similar response properties in a minicolumn size range. One kind consists of pyramidal cells located within a region that is from about 50 μm to 100 μm wide. They are tightly connected by synapses on either the basal dendrites or proximal part of the apical dendrites. This connection apparently causes them to discharge together. The other are the apical dendrite bundles described by Peters and Yilmaz [70] which, in Tanaka's view, corresponds to the minicolumn Mountcastle describes. Interestingly, pyramidal cells located farther apart are probably connected by synapses at the distal part of the apical dendrites. In the closely related connections, the EPSPs are large and sharp-rising, while the more distant connections are said to be small, slow-rising and long lasting. Tanaka concludes that in inferotemporal cortex (area TE), an area that represents the final stage of the ventral visual cortical pathway that begins in V1, "cells within minicolumns compose a unit by receiving common inputs and exciting each other, and nearby minicolumns send long-lasting but weak excitatory inputs to each other. The focus of activation may move from one minicolumn to another, through interaction with distant activation foci in TE or interaction with other brain sites."

A recent paper reported evidence for small-scale anatomical modularity in various regions of rat, cat, and monkey cortex [71]. They found a pattern at the borders of layers I and II by double-labeling immunocytochemistry. The authors describe a honeycomb pattern of walls and hollows composed of distinct afferent and dendritic systems. This pattern, which does not extend into layer III, is suggestive of a lamina-specific substructure within larger cortical columns. They found this pattern in numerous areas of the rat brain including V1 and S1 barrel cortex. The same pattern was confined to layer II with a mean center-to-center spacing of around 80 μm versus the barrel columns size which is typically over 300 μm. In rat V1 the mean spacing was also 80 μm, and ranged from 50 μm to 120 μm, the same as in barrel cortex. This is within range of the minicolumn size reported on the basis of layer V apical dendrite bundles and pyramidal cell arrays, though somewhat larger. The means reported for layer V apical dendrite bundles in diverse studies are typically around 50 μm to 60 μm and include areas 3,17, 32, and S1 [21,28,35-37,40].

Ichinohe et al. [71] replicated the MAP2-ir apical dendrite bundles reported elsewhere and suggested the presence of several subpopulations. The layer V apical dendrite bundles apparently go up to the hollows. They noted that two of these bundles beginning in layer V frequently merged within one honeycomb hollow. This suggests that the two cell columns merge anatomically. It partly explains the accounts of functional microcolumnar activity occurring at sizes two or three times that of a single cell column, but considerably smaller than a macrocolumn. A second subpopulation of apical dendrites consists of thinner ones that end in the honeycomb walls in layer II. Those which originate in the superficial layers are not stained by MAP2. Evidence appears of parallel systems and a high degree of connectional selectivity. The cortico-cortical (CC) terminations may target dendrites of layer II pyramidal cells, whereas the thalamocortical (TC) terminations contact distal apical dendrites of deeper neurons in III and V. In layer II, the TC terminals target the distal dendrites tufts of the deeper pyramidal cells, i.e., the apical dendrite bundles arising from layers V and III. The CC targets apical dendrites of the superficial pyramidal cells and with PV-ir neuropil. They report that in layer Ia both dendritic populations are accessible to the TC terminals. Because apical dendrites bundles in rats also extend from layer V into layer II, TC information processing probably proceeds vertically along the cells in that group. The interaction between lamina specific function and vertical ones is critical to understanding columns. Lamina specific functionality is well known and in the context of columns reveals a complex microcircuit organization. The honeycomb pattern was also detected with cytochrome oxidase (CO). The CO patches had the same mean spacing distances (~80 μm, range of 50 μm to 124 um) as the PV-ir honeycombs. However, other stains such as AChe, NADPH-d, or MBP did not reveal the pattern. These patterns are not confined to the rat brain. They were also present in cat V1 and auditory cortex in monkey brain, leading the authors to identify them as a basic feature of neocortical organization.

In addition to cells and fiber bundle modularity, some research suggests that the architecture of astroglial processes supports the columnar structure in cortex [72,73]. The author describes a close spatial relationship between pyramidal cell columns as determined by MAP2-ir, and astroglial processes (GFAP-Ir lattice). The non-random distribution of the interlaminated astroglial process contributed to the modularity of the cortex. They found that GFAP-ir astroglial patterns in new world monkeys had a size frequency distribution similar to the spacing distances of apical dendrite bundles reported by Peters et al. [50,74] The author argues that glia is intimately interactive with neurons in terms of growth, fate, and function. It also supports columnar structure, both at the micro and macro level. Columns should be therefore be mirrored by similarly organized glia components. The author proposes a "columnar-based neuron-glial interaction" that could be achieved by apposing astroglial cable-like processes with apical dendrites of neurons. This would provide a spatial orientation column-like resolution of neuron ionic/molecular requirements and reduce volume operations in favor of more discrete columnar ones.

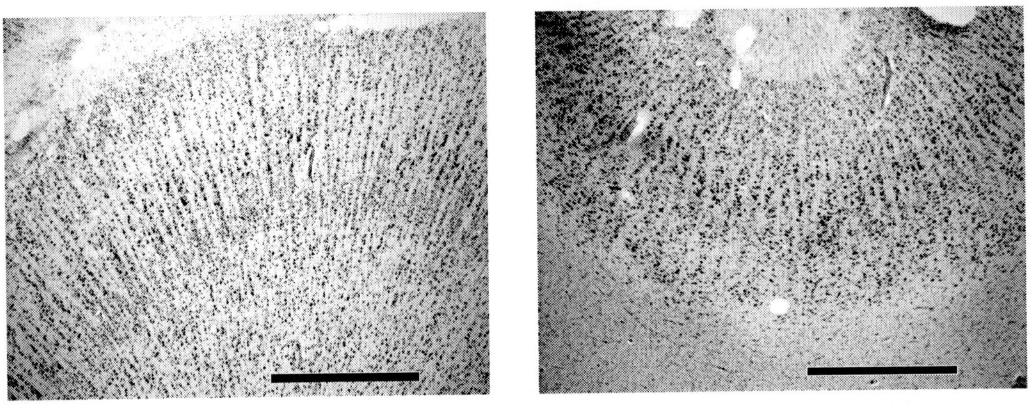

Figure 3. Gyri (left) and sulci (right): While greatly deformed and highly variable in depth, it is clear that the vertical pattern of the cells remains intact in both extremes. The scale bars measure 1000 μm.

Interconnections within the gyri and sulci also support the vertical anatomical organization of minicolumns. Within a gyrus, cell arrays and corresponding myelin bundles clearly follow the bend in the cortex, so that lines of cells or myelin bundles follow the curving of the gyrus at increasingly sharp angles. The cell arrangements must be interconnected physically, tying them together vertically. Thus, they remain unified when the cortex bends or folds. Cell arrays and myelin bundles maintain their linearity within the cortex in a gyrus or a sulcus (Figure 3). In a gyrus the columns fan out, remaining closer together at the base than at the top. In gyri the cortex becomes thicker and the cells thin out while maintaining their orientation to each other. In a sulcus, the opposite occurs. As the cortex becomes compressed, so do the cell columns. In both cases the cell and myelin columns remain identifiable. Cells must have a strong anatomical interconnection under diverse mechanical stresses in order to maintain their vertical pattern. The glue that helps shape the vertical orientation of both the cells and major fiber systems combines the dendritic systems. These systems weave together pyramidal cells across the horizontal layers along with the vertical axons that form in bundles.

Physiological Evidence at the Minicolumnar Level

Some have argued that evidence for a minicolumnar organization in the cortex is vague or does not exist. An objective consideration would seem to provide a sound basis for their functionality. While few dispute the evidence for the larger macrocolumn, the physiology of these units appears uncertain in some areas of the cortex [12]. Furthermore, ocular dominance columns are absent in some species altogether [75,76].

An assortment of studies using different techniques provide evidence for the physiological basis of microcolumns. The small-scale at which minicolumns operate, coupled with small dissimilarities between them, present surmountable challenges. Predictably, the amount of activity localized in one minicolumn at any given moment is considerably less than that of a macrocolumn. However, the macrocolumn is not a monolithic unit of function in which all of the neurons and local circuits respond uniformly to a given stimuli. It is recognized that cells within larger modules respond to similar but not identical features [68]. Since macrocolumns consist of many thousands of cells, some form of sub-macrocolumn level of activity occurs since all cells do not respond simultaneously under all conditions. For example, Panzeri et al. [77] explain that barrel column neurons sharing very similar response neurons still show only a small amount of redundancy. Low firing rates cause each spike to carry nearly independent information. Thus, observers should not view seemingly disparate response properties between closely situated neurons as the lack of a shared anatomical foundation. The lack of conformity to response properties can be the byproduct of temporal phasing which overlie a "hardwired" anatomical connectivity between neurons in a column or neighboring column.

Nerve regeneration experiments have shown that single minicolumns are responsible for specific areas of cutaneous input in cortex of owl, squirrel, and macaque monkey [78,79]. Researchers find it difficult to isolate specific minicolumns physiologically because overlap occurs in the receptive fields between neighbors. In, nerve regeneration experiments peripheral nerve fibers are cut and allowed to regenerate to different locations on the skin. As a result, the locations of the receptive fields on the skin became widely displaced. When minicolumns receive information from widely separated regions of the skin, adjoining columns no longer share similar properties. Subsequent electrophysiology recordings (area 3b and 1) clearly distinguish minicolumns in a size range between 40–60 μm. Studies using different methods over the years have repeatedly confirmed this size range.

A number of researchers have shown that cells organized in a vertical, columnar-sized space (40–50 μm) display individually specific responses to peripheral stimulation. Some used microelectrode single cell recordings to conduct a series of experiments in somatosensory cortex of monkey brain (*Macaca mulatta and Macaca fascicularis*) and cat [80-84]. These experiments demonstrated that the response property of neurons shifted within a narrow vertical array that is minicolumn in size. Tommerdahl et al. [85] (1993) argue that this evidence, along with the findings of McCasland and Woolsey [86], support the concept of the two classes of columns, mini- and macro-. Both of them participate in the neocortical response to peripheral stimulation. McCasland and Woolsey [86], found smaller minicolumnar-size variations in metabolic columns of barrel cortex, a specialized form of macrocolumn found in the somatosensory cortex of rodents. These "receptive field" minicolumns reported by electrophysiology are presumably the same as the "radially oriented cords of neurons evident in Nissl-stained sections." They are also within the size range reported for vertical "cell cords" in Nissl-stained tissue [24,52,54-56,59,60].

Orientation columns of minicolumn size are a well established part of primary visual cortex [61,62] and have been demonstrated in V5 (area MT) as well [87,88]. A recent paper based on microelectrode studies demonstrates their presence in V3 of the macaque brain [89]. The authors show that vertical columns extending across the entire cortex are responsible for orientation selectivity, and disparity-selection as well. They conclude that V3 participates in the analysis of three-dimensional form. Orientation preference changed by 36 degrees in a single step between two consecutive recording sites that were 100 μm apart. Adams and Zeki [89] also devised a test distinguishing between a clustering of cells with similar response properties versus the organization of cells into vertical columns extending from white matter boundary to the cortical surface. The test measured an index of the number of cell type changes per mm measured parallel to the cortical surface. The authors concluded that cells tuned for disparity were indeed organized into columns and not simply clustered.

Direct evidence also correlates anatomical cell columns seen in Nissl stain tissue with physiological units. Tommerdahl et al. [85] directly compared physiological responses with Nissl-stain vertical columns. In this study, within-2-DG-module periodicity corresponded to the size of minicolumns as reported in somatosensory cortex. Most importantly, they matched their results with pyramidal cell columns in Nissl-stained slices. As a result, they confirmed the presence of identical spatial frequencies, demonstrating for the first time that the metabolic discontinuities and cell column arrays were one and the same. In another experiment, Kohn et al. [36] applied electrical stimulation to the VI/white matter border in a rat brain using spectral analysis to measure the metabolic response. The IOS response revealed radially oriented spatial variations in the intensity of optical signals with a periodicity of 30–60 μm/cycle, which is within the range of a typical minicolumn. Optical density patterns obtained on Nissl stained tissue from the same slice used in the IOS experiment, revealed "the same orientation and precisely the same spatial frequency as those seen in the IOS" [36]. The optical density methods used in a Nissl-stain section are very similar to those applied by other authors to detect cell dense vertical orientations [52,54,59,60]. Thus, these experiments directly correlate physiological minicolumnar activity with the cell arrays found in Nissl-stained tissue.

Rao et al. [90] provide evidence of minicolumnar organization in the prefrontal cortex of the monkey (*Macaca mulatta*) in working memory. Their paper focuses on iso-and-cross-directional mechanisms relationships between minicolumns. This study describes functional minicolumns in prefrontal associational cortex in monkeys and their role within the context of the macrocolumn.[4] The authors propose that each minicolumn functions in response to 5

[4] See also references [6,7,8].

degree increments of isodirectional tuning, while cross-directional tuning occurs between the larger macrocolumn. Each minicolumn connects to a minicolumn in the adjacent macrocolumn by sending inhibitory signals. Pyramidal cells within minicolumn size distances were responsible for isodirectional tuning. Minicolumns were said to maintain a functional organization for iso-directional relationships among neurons inside a single functional macrocolumn. They further regard the probable anatomical substrate for the circuit to be the apical dendrite bundles as described by Peters and Kara [40]. Neurons recorded at the same site shared similar angles of tuning regardless of the direction of the cue stimulus. They point out that earlier studies seemed to contradict this due to methodological issues, the problem revolving around the proper resolution required to distinguish activity at the level of the minicolumn. The small size of these structures creates problems in regards to the sampling radius of electrodes. The authors conclude they recorded from within one or between two adjacent microcolumns, providing evidence that individual microcolumns performed isodirectional tuning. This model is supported by Thomson and colleagues [91,92]. The latter found considerable inhibitory connections between FS cells and pyramidal cells within distances of 50–250 μm.

Rao et al. [90] describe the anatomical basis for the macrocolumns as based on the spatial size of afferents to the principal sulcus from the contralateral hemisphere, and the basket cells which project to nearby iso-oriented sites at 100 μm to 400 μm and more distant ones (i.e., between macrocolumns) of 400 μm 800 μm [93]. Budd and Kisvarday [65] also show that most lateral inhibitory connections from basket cells (in cat V1) are formed within neurons in nearest-neighbor columns. The basket cells provide isotropic connectivity within a 50 μm radius of the cell. Outside of this zone the pattern of anisotropic connectivity more strongly targets some sectors than others. Rao et al. [90] conclude that "the evidence supports a microcolumnar organization of the functionally grouped neurons in prefrontal cortex, which serve to enhance the resolution of stimulus encoding and/or retrieval in the working memory processes."

Evidence for Minicolumns in Diverse Regions of Cortex

Critics sometimes cite evidence showing the adult minicolumn is restricted to a very few regions of the cortex, essentially the primary sensory ones. However, studies of minicolumns are often buried in articles with other headings or as part of studies focused primarily on macrocolumns. The majority of articles reported below do not have the word "minicolumn" or "microcolumn" in their headings. Collecting relevant data often requires organizing disparate information from various sources. The reports of vertical organization in many regions of the cortex are more extensive than some believe, as described in table 2.

Table 2. Studies on Anatomical Aspects of Vertical Organization of the Cortex

Cortical area	Investigators
M1	von Bonin and Mehler [58], Schmolke and Viebahn [32], Thomson and Deuchars [69], DeFelipe et al. [45]
V1	von Bonin and Mehler [58], Hubel and Wiesel [94], Peters and Kara [40], Feldman and Peters [95], DeFelipe et al. [45], Peters and Sethares [25,50,96] Peters and Yilmaz [70]
V5	Zeki [88], Albright [87], DeAngelis and Newsome [97]
S1	Kaas et al. [78], Favorov and Whitsel [80,81], DeFelipe et al. [45], Tommerdahl et al. [85], Holthoff and Witte [98], Kohn et al. [36]
B.A. 22	Seldon [56,57], Ong and Garey [99], Buxhoeveden et al. 59,60]
B.A. 41	Seldon [56,57],
B.A. 42	Seldon [56,57], Ong and Garey [99]
Prefrontal	Dem´ianenko [51], Sakai [27], Rao et al. [90]
B.A. 7, 19, 23b, 24b, and 31	Sakai [27], Schlaug et al. [52]
B.A. 20 and 21	Ong and Garey [99]
V2	DeFelipe et al. [45], Peters et al. [26]
TE	Tanaka [68]
Temporal lobe	del Río and DeFelipe [47,100]
Superior temporal sulcus	Buldyrev et al. [53]
V3	Adams and Zeki [89]

Cell Columns are not Visible in Some Regions of the Cortex

Cell column study is complicated by the greater clarity of their appearance in some areas than in others (Figure 4). While this difficulty may relate to cortical regions, no one has ever studied the problem systematically. The lack of an apparent (visual) vertical organization in some areas of neocortex makes the ubiquity of cell columns problematic [10]. Granular cortex and striate cortex in particular lack visible cell arrays. Paradoxically, this region contains one of the best established physiological columns in the neocortex. It also has established anatomical correlates in the form of orientation (minicolumns) and ocular dominance columns (macrocolumns) [45,50,62,70]. For a number of reasons, the lack of visually obvious cell columns does not imply their absence. Most important, the use of postmortem tissue involves many problems such as thickness of the slice and plane of cut. Tissue thickness matters when examining cell columns. If the mean cell column diameter in a given brain is roughly 40 μm, then tissue cut very thin would fail to contain a complete column. It would be dominated instead by fragments of columns and z-axis artifact. Cutting sections too thin would affect the accuracy of their center-to-center spacing in a coronal or sagittal plane.

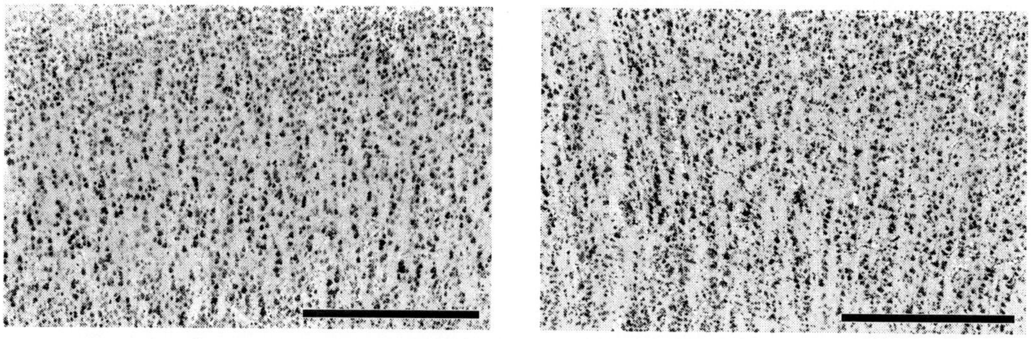

Figure 4. Note that there are fragments of columns in these micrographs where A vertical line of cells appears for a brief distance. But overall, they lack A clear and unambiguous display of isolated individual columns.

Likewise, tissue cut too thick may display an overlapping appearance and loss of distinctiveness to individual columns. The angle of cut is another concern. If cell columns are radially oriented, oblique planes of cut may distort the actual appearance. Large sections pose special problems. Because of the complex pattern of folding in the brains of higher mammals, it is almost impossible to get a large section that is free of distortion. During the cutting process cells can also be torned out of the tissue, causing gaps in cell columns.

Four criteria describe the anatomical equivalent to the minicolumn: pyramidal cell arrays, myelinated axon bundles, apical dendrite bundles, and double bouquet cell axon bundles. Peters and Sethares [50] associated the pyramidal cells found in layers III and V with the apical dendrites bundles, calling these "pyramidal cell modules." They further state, "An individual module is considered to be composed of those pyramidal cells that are contained within a cylinder of cortical tissue that extends through the depth of the cortex, with the axis of the module being represented by the clustered apical dendrites of the layer V and II/III pyramidal cells. Thus, the average diameters of the modules are equivalent to the mean center-to-center spacing of the clusters of apical dendrites. It is envisioned that these pyramidal cell modules represent the basic functional units of the neurons in cortex, so that in essence they are equivalent to the minicolumns of Mountcastle."

Electron micrographs show that apical dendrites are paired with myelin bundles, each cluster lying adjacent to the other. Furthermore, these paired bundles are also coupled with the pyramidal cell arrays which link them all together [50]. Lohmann and Koppen [21] also found evidence that the center-to-center spacing of axonal and dendritic bundles in rat visual cortex correspond to each other. Del Río and DeFelipe [47] demonstrated a direct correspondence between double bouquet axon bundles and myelinated bundles in human temporal lobe. They found a remarkable coincidence between myelinated axons bundles and double bouquet axons, as well as a strong synaptic relationship between double bouquet cells and pyramidal cells. They add that the types, distribution, and proportion of synapses formed by double bouquet cells in human temporal cortex are identical to those found in monkey V1. The authors concluded that the minicolumnar structure formed by the double bouquet cell is a common organizational device of neocortex in humans and monkeys. Lohmann and Koppen [21] also found a close correspondence between dendritic and axonal bundles, concluding that they probably arise from the same cells. Thus, all four anatomical elements are linked, each representing a minicolumn. Moreover, for the purposes of determining center-to-center spacing of minicolumns, any of these elements should be interchangeable; the presence of one should infer the existence of the others.

Since bundled axons arise from pyramidal cells, one should not conclude that cell columns are absent. With this in mind, Figure 5 shows a micrograph of a Nissl slice in which cell columns are somewhat obvious but not particularly clear, especially figure 5a. However, in the myelinated serial section just following this slice (35 μm removed), myelinated bundles can be clearly discerned. The correlation of pyramidal cells to fiber bundles in these instances makes it more difficult to deny the presence of vertical organization simply on the basis of the poor visual appearance of cell columns. Several researchers reported seeing apical dendrite bundles in mouse in two MAP2 studies [29,30]. Yet cell columns in mouse cortex are generally far less obvious than in primate cortex (Figure 6). Presumably, fiber bundles would tend to remain together under conditions that would cause cell disarray.

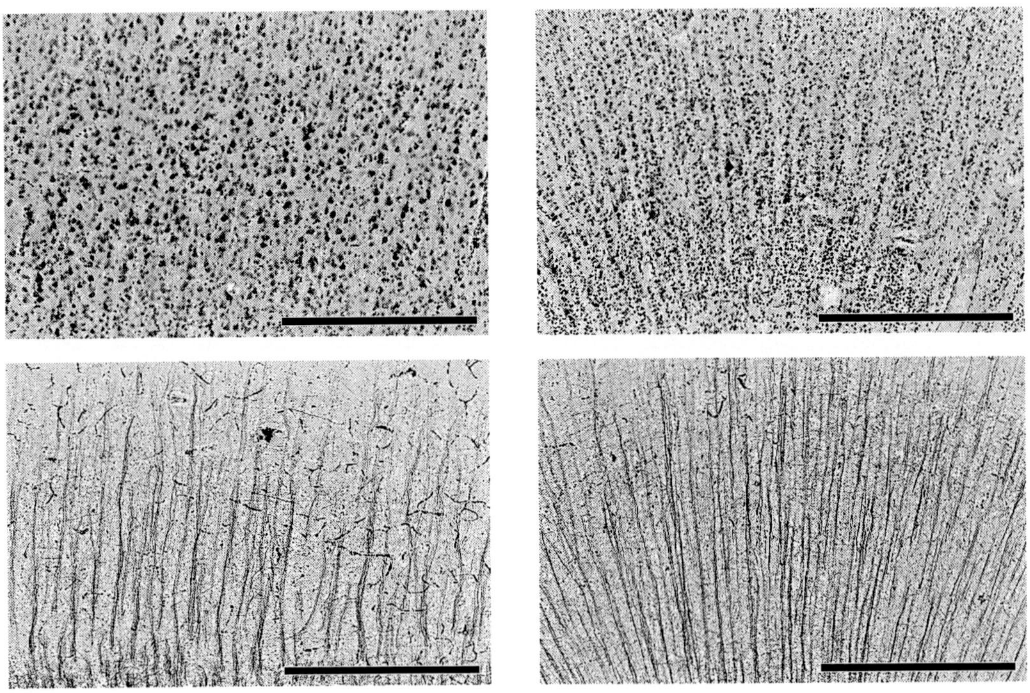

Figure 5. *Top.* The uppermost Nissl stain image has only a faint appearance of vertical organization. However, the corresponding serial myelin image is only 35 μm removed, and displays clearly delineated myelinated axon bundles. Since the bundles arise from cell soma, and send information from a vertically oriented group of cells with similar response properties, this suggest the presence of a cell column. Also see Figure 7. *Bottom.* In the Nissl image the vertical organization, while present, is not exceptional. However, it is much more obvious in the serial myelin image.

On the other hand, a particular slice may actually lack visible cell columns, an absence not caused by artifact. The typical width of a minicolumn extends beyond the mean cross-sectional width of the cells within it. Thus, space exists for the cell soma to disperse within the spatial domain of the column with a loss of a perfectly linear alignment (Figure 7). To function properly, the cells in a minicolumn need not be perfectly aligned. Rather, the cells must be located within a shared spatial field that responds to a given stimulus. One might test this by correlating the thickness (spread) of myelin or apical dendrite bundles with the verticality of the cell columns in serial sections. In the absence of artifact, one could predict that where the cell arrays are very linear (one atop another), fiber bundles would be tightly woven. At the same time, highly dispersed cell columns would also display more widely spaced and less tightly woven fiber bundles. The change in cell configuration from very linear to scattered would reflect a presumed change in organization, not unlike cytoarchitectonic differences. This change would also significantly affect, the peripheral neuropil space, among other things.

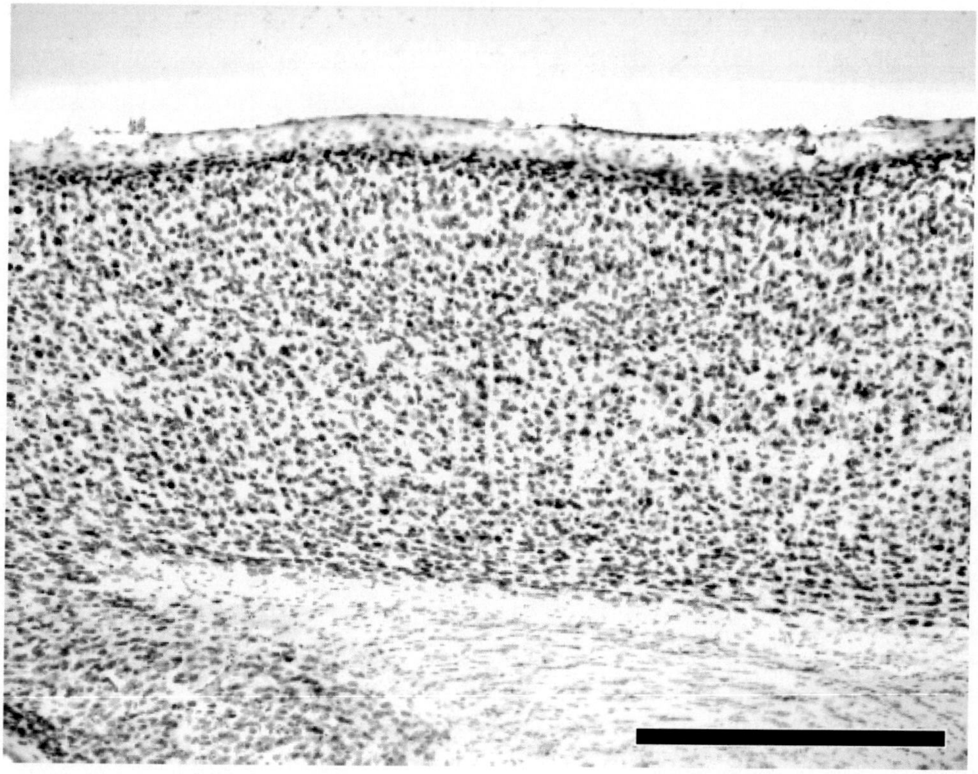

Figure 6. A columnar organization is not readily discernable in mouse cortex.

Finally, the use of computer programs has demonstrated the presence of vertical arrays in fields where the eye may not detect them. Buldyrev et al. [53] used statistical physics with computer imaging to detect microcolumns in normal, Alzheimer's disease, and Lewy Body dementia brains. They also tested the program against a randomly generated field. While the results of their findings do not generally match more typical minicolumn sizes, their approach shows the ability to detect vertical units within cortex which visual inspection misses.

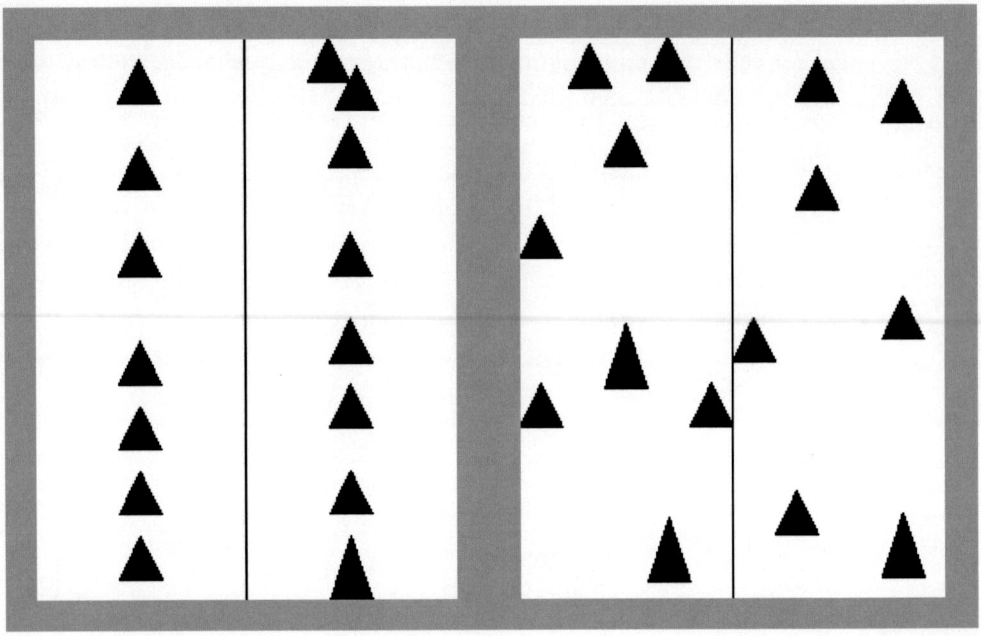

Figure 7. The cell columns on the left side appear vertical while those on the right do not. However, the surrounding space as demarcated by the box represents shared afferent fields. Therefore, even though the cells are distributed differently each would still respond to a shared stimulus and send out efferent projections from the cells within the boxes.

Conclusion

Silberberg et al. [101] reviewed microcircuits in the cortex including the minicolumn. They concluded that comparison of these units requires careful attention to the species, region, area, and age. They also pointed to the large amount of variation related to microcircuitry between brains of different species. Clearly, the variation in neuronal types and connectivity at the microcircuit level may rule out a rigid definition of the mini- or macrocolumn. That is, the minicolumn appears to be a common template rather than a stereotypical component in all brains and regions [101,102]. However, it is not possible to dismiss local or even species-specific examples of more strictly repeating configurations of minicolumns. In discussing this variation Mountcastle [102] noted that "The important point is that columnar organization depends upon a certain set of properties common to all neurons in the elementary unit, but that other properties may vary between different neurons in the same minicolumn." Mountcastle [102] emphatically denies that minicolumns are stereotypic. He provides a conceptual basis to variability upon the basic template by stating that "differences in afferent input are convolved with different intrinsic operations in different cortical areas to produce what we call different functions." Silberberg et al. [101] also conclude that despite the great range in microcircuitry, stereotypical features exist nonetheless at multiple levels indicating a deterministic basis for them [64,66,103], and that all neocortical microcircuits may be subtle variations of a common template. Perhaps, the minicolumnar "template" may more accurately be described as the shared set of properties for a set of neurons across lamina. It may be a general principle that cortical neurons with similar stimulus selection properties are found in close proximity to each other [16]. If so, the minicolumn is the vertical component of that association.

REFERENCES

[1] DeFelipe J. Cortical interneurons: from Cajal to 2001. *Progress in Brain Research.* 2002;136:215-238.

[2] Lorente de Nó R. Cerebral cortex, architecture, intracortical connections, motor programs. In: Fulton JF, ed. *Physiology of the Nervous System.* London, UK: Oxford University Press; 1938:274-301.

[3] Mountcastle VB. Modality and topographic properties of single neurons of cat's somatic sensory cortex. *Journal of Neurophysiology.* 1957;20:408-434.

[4] Mountcastle VB. An organizing principle for cerebral function: The unit module and the distributed system. In: Edelman GM, Mountcastle VB. *The Mindful Brain: Cortical Organization and the Group-Selective Theory of Higher Brain Function.* Cambridge, MA: MIT Press; 1978:7-51.

[5] Somogyi P, Tamas G, Lujan R, Buhl EH. Salient features of synaptic organization in the cerebral cortex. *Brain Research: Brain Research Reviews.* 1998;26:113-135.

[6] Favorov OV, Kelly G. Minicolumnar organization within somatosensory cortical segregates, I: development of afferent connections. *Cerebral Cortex.* 1994;4:408-427.

[7] Favorov OV, Kelly G. Minicolumnar organization within somatosensory cortical segregates, II: emergent functional properties. *Cerebral Cortex.* 1994;4:428-442.

[8] Mountcastle VB. The columnar organization of the neocortex. *Brain.* 1997;120:701-722.

[9] Buxhoeveden DP, Casanova MF. Quantitative comparison of radial cell columns in children with Down syndrome and controls. *Journal of Intellectual Disability Research.* 2002;46:76-81.

[10] Jones EG. Microcolumns in the cerebral cortex. *Proceedings of the National Academy of Sciences of the United States of America.* 2000;97:5019-5021.

[11] Purves D, Riddle DR, LaMantia A-S. Iterated patterns of brain circuitry (or how the cortex gets its spots). *Trends in Neurosciences.* 1992;15:362-368.

[12] Swindale NV. Is the cerebral cortex modular? *Trends in Neurosciences.* 1990;13:487-492.

[13] Rakic P. Neuronal migration and conduct guidance in primate telencephalon. *Postgraduate Medical Journal.* 1978;54:25-40.

[14] Rakic P. The specification of cerebral cortical areas: the radial unit hypothesis. *Science.* 1988;241:928-931.

[15] Rakic P. Defects of neuronal migration and the pathogenesis of cortical malformations. *Progress in Brain Research.* 1988;73:15-37.

[16] Reich DS, Mechler F, Victor JD. Independent and redundant information in nearby cortical neurons. *Science.* 2001;294:2566-2568.

[17] Gressens P, Evrard P. The glial fascicle: an ontogenic and phylogenic unit guiding, supplying and distributing mammalian cortical neurons. *Brain Research: Developmental Brain Research.* 1993;76:272-277.

[18] Krmpotić-Nemanić J, Kostović I, Nemanić D. Prenatal and perinatal development of radial cell columns in the human auditory cortex. *Acta Oto-laryngologica.* 1984;97:489-495.

[19] Aggoun-Aouaoui D, Kiper DC, Innocenti GM. Growth of callosal terminal arbors in primary visual areas of the cat. *European Journal of Neuroscience.* 1996;8:1132-1148.

[20] McKinstry RC, Mathur A, Miller JH, Ozcan A, Snyder AZ, Schefft GL, Almli CR, Shiran SI, Conturo TE, Neil JJ. Radial organization of developing preterm human cerebral cortex revealed by non-invasive water diffusion anisotropy MRI. *Cerebral Cortex.* 2002;12:1237-1243.

[21] Lohmann H, Köppen H-J. Postnatal development of pyramidal dendritic and axonal bundles in the visual cortex of the rat. *Journal für Hirnforschung.* 1995;36:101-111.

[22] Buxhoeveden DP, Casanova MF. The minicolumnar hypothesis in neurosciences. *Brain.* 2002;125:935-951.

[23] Curtetti R, Garbossa D, Vercelli A. Development of dendritic bundles of pyramidal neurons in the rat visual cortex. *Mechanisms of Ageing and Development.* 2002;123:473-479.

[24] Buxhoeveden DP, Lefkowitz W, Loats P, Armstrong E. The linear organization of cell columns in human and nonhuman anthropoid Tpt cortex. *Anatomy and Embryology.* 1996;194:23-36.

[25] Peters A, Sethares C. The organization of double bouquet cells in monkey striate cortex. *Journal of Neurocytology.* 1997;26:779-797.

[26] Peters A, Cifuentes JM, Sethares C. The organization of pyramidal cells in area 18 of the rhesus monkey. *Cerebral Cortex.* 1997;7:405-421.

[27] Sakai M. Dendritic bundles formed by layer VI pyramidal cells in the monkey frontal association cortex. *Experimental Brain Research.* 1985;58:609-612.

[28] Feldman ML, Peters A. A study of barrels and pyramidal dendritic clusters in the cerebral cortex. *Brain Research.* 1974;77:55-76.

[29] Escobar MI, Pimenta H, Caviness VS Jr, Jacobson M, Crandall JE, Kosik KS. Architecture of apical dendrites in the murine neocortex: dual apical dendritic systems. *Neuroscience.* 1986;17:975-89.

[30] White EL, Peters A. Cortical modules in the posteromedial barrel subfield (Sm1) of the mouse. *Journal of Comparative Neurology.* 1993;334:86-96.

[31] Fleischauer K, Hellmuth P, Werner W. Vertical bundles of dendrites in the neocortex. *Zeitschrift für Anatomie und Entwicklungsgeschichte.* 1972;136:213-223.

[32] Schmolke C, Viebahn C. Dendrite bundles in lamina II/III of the rabbit neocortex. *Anatomy and Embryology.* 1986;173:343-348.

[33] Schmolke C. The ontogeny of dendritic bundles in rabbit visual cortex. *Anatomy and Embryology.* 1989;180:371-381.

[34] Viebahn C. Correlation between differences in the structure of dendrite bundles and cytoarchitectonic patterns in the cerebral cortex of the rabbit. *Journal für Hirnforschung.* 1990;31:645-652.

[35] Gabbott PL, Bacon SJ. Local circuit neurons in the medial prefrontal cortex (areas 24a, b, c, 25 and 32) in the monkey, II: quantitative areal and laminar distributions. *Journal of Comparative Neurology.* 1996;364:609-636.
[36] Kohn A, Pinheiro A, Tommerdahl MA, Whitsel BL. Optical imaging in vitro provides evidence for the minicolumnar nature of cortical response. *Neuroreport.* 1997;8:3513-3518.
[37] Peters A, Walsh TM. A study of the organization of apical dendrites in the somatic sensory cortex of the rat. *Journal of Comparative Neurology.* 1972;144:253-268.
[38] Schmolke C, Künzle H. On the presence of dendrite bundles in the cerebral cortex of the Madagascan lesser hedgehog tenrec and the red-eared pond turtle. *Anatomy and Embryology.* 1997;196:195-213.
[39] Ichinohe N, Rockland KS. Parvalbumin positive dendrites co-localize with apical dendritic bundles in rat retrosplenial cortex. *Neuroreport.* 2002;13:757-761.
[40] Peters A, Kara D. The neuronal composition of area 17 in rat visual cortex, IV: the organization of pyramidal cells. *Journal of Comparative Neurology.* 1987;260:573-590.
[41] Lev DL, White EL. Organization of pyramidal cell apical dendrites and composition of dendritic clusters in the mouse: emphasis on primary motor cortex. *European Journal of Neuroscience.* 1997;9:280-290.
[42] Hirst E, Asante J, Price J. Clustering of dendrites in the cerebral cortex begins in the embryonic cortical plate. *Journal of Neurocytology.* 1991;20:431-438.
[43] Wahle P, Meyer G. Early postnatal development of vasoactive intestinal polypeptide- and peptide histidine isoleucine-immunoreactive structures in the cat visual cortex. *Journal of Comparative Neurology.* 1989;282:215-248.
[44] Kenan-Vaknin G, Ouaknine GE, Razon N, Malach R. Organization of layers II–III connections in human visual cortex revealed by *in vitro* injections of biocytin. *Brain Research.* 1992;594:339-342.
[45] DeFelipe J, Hendry S, Hashikawa T, Molinari M, Jones EG. A microcolumnar structure of monkey cerebral cortex revealed by immunocytochemical studies of double bouquet cell axons. *Neuroscience.* 1990;37:655-673.
[46] Ferrer I, Tunon T, Soriano E, et al. Calbindin immunoreactivity in normal human temporal neocortex. *Brain Research.* 1992;572:33-41.
[47] del Río, MR, DeFelipe J. Double bouquet cell axons in the human temporal neocortex: relationships to bundles of myelinated axons and colocalization of calretinin and calbindin D_{28k} immunoreactivities. *Journal of Chemical Neuroanatomy.* 1997;13:243-251.
[48] DeFelipe J, Jones EG. Vertical organization of γ-aminobutyric acid-accumulating intrinsic neuronal systems in monkey cerebral cortex. *Journal of Neuroscience.* 1985;5:3246-3260.
[49] Somogyi, P, Cowey, A, Halász, N, Freund, TF. Vertical organization of neurons accumulating 3H-GABA in visual cortex of rhesus monkey. *Nature.* 1981;294:761-763.
[50] Peters A, Sethares C. Myelinated axons and the pyramidal cell modules in monkey primary visual cortex. *Journal of Comparative Neurology.* 1996;365:232-255.

[51] Dem′ianenko GP. Neĭrony i neĭronnye ob″edineniia v lobnoĭ kore obez′iany [Neurons and neuronal associations in the frontal cortex in the monkey]. *Neĭrofiziologiia.* 1983;15:115-20.

[52] Schlaug G, Schleicher A, Zilles K. Quantitative analysis of the columnar arrangement of neurons in the human cingulate cortex. *Journal of Comparative Neurology.* 1995;351:441-452.

[53] Buldyrev SV, Cruz L, Gomez-Isla T, et al. Description of microcolumnar ensembles in association cortex and their disruption in Alzheimer and Lewy body dementias. *Proceedings of the National Academy of Sciences of the United States of America.* 2000;97:5039-5043.

[54] Buxhoeveden DP, Roy E, Switala AE, Casanova MF. Reduced interneuronal space in schizophrenia. *Biological Psychiatry.* 2000;47:681-683.

[55] Buxhoeveden DP, Switala AE, Roy E, Casanova MF. Quantitative analysis of cell columns in the cerebral cortex. *Journal of Neuroscience Methods.* 2000;97:7-17.

[56] Seldon HL. Structure of human auditory cortex, I: cytoarchitectonics and dendritic distributions. *Brain Research.* 1981;229:277-294.

[57] Seldon HL. Structure of human auditory cortex, II: axon distributions and morphological correlates of speech perception. *Brain Research.* 1981;229:295-310.

[58] von Bonin G, Mehler WR. On columnar arrangement of nerve cells in cerebral cortex. *Brain Research.* 1971;27:1-10.

[59] Buxhoeveden DP, Switala AE, Roy E, Litaker M, Casanova, MF. Lateralization in human planum temporale is absent in nonhuman primates. *Brain, Behavior and Evolution.* 2001;57:349-358.

[60] Buxhoeveden DP, Switala AE, Roy E, Litaker M, Casanova, MF. Morphological differences between minicolumns in human and nonhuman primate cortex. *American Journal of Physical Anthropology.* 2001;115:361-371.

[61] Hubel DH, Wiesel TN. Sequence regularity and geometry of orientation columns in the monkey striate cortex. *Journal of Comparative Neurology.* 1974;158:267-294.

[62] Hubel DH, Wiesel TN. Functional architecture of the macaque monkey visual cortex. *Proceedings of the Royal Society of London, Series B: Containing Papers of a Biological Character.* 1977;198:1-59.

[63] Marin-Padilla M. Prenatal and early postnatal ontogenesis of the human motor cortex: a Golgi study, II: the basket–pyramidal system. *Brain Research.* 1970;23:185-191.

[64] Jin X, Mathers PH, Szabo G, Katarova Z, Agmon A. Vertical bias in dendritic trees of non-pyramidal neocortical neurons expressing GAD67-GFP in vitro. *Cerebral Cortex.* 2001;11:666-678.

[65] Budd LML, Kisvarday ZF. Local lateral connectivity of inhibitory clutch cells in layer 4 of cat visual cortex (area 17). *Experimental Brain Research.* 2001;140:245-250.

[66] Kozloski J, Hamzei-Sichani F, Yuste R. Stereotyped position of local synaptic targets in neocortex. Science. 2001;293:868-972.

[67] Schwartz ML, Zheng DS, Goldman-Rakic PS. Periodicity of GABA-containing cells in primate prefrontal cortex. *Journal of Neuroscience.* 1988;8:1962-1970.

[68] Tanaka K. Columnar organization in the inferotemporal cortex. In: Rockland KS, Kaas JH, Peters A, eds. *Extrastriate Cortex in Primates*. Dordrecht, Netherlands: Kluwer Academic; 1998:469-495.

[69] Thomson AM, Deuchars J. Temporal and spatial properties of local circuits in neocortex. *Trends in Neurosciences.* 1994;17:119-126.

[70] Peters A, Yilmaz E. Neuronal organization in area 17 of cat visual cortex. *Cerebral Cortex.* 1993;3:49-68.

[71] Ichinohe N, Fujiyama F, Kaneko T, Rockland KS. Honeycomb-like mosaic at the border of layers 1 and 2 in the cerebral cortex. *Journal of Neuroscience.* 2003;23:1372-1382.

[72] Colombo JA. A columnar-supporting mode of astroglial architecture in the cerebral cortex of adult primates? *Neurobiology (Budapest, Hungary)* 2001;9:1-16.

[73] Colombo JA, Schleicher A, Zilles K. Patterned distribution of immunoreactive astroglial processes in the striate (V1) cortex of New World monkeys. *Glia.* 1999;25:85-92.

[74] Peters A, Leahu D, Moss MB, McNally KJ. The effects of aging on area 46 of the frontal cortex of the rhesus monkey. *Cerebral Cortex.* 1994;4:621-635.

[75] Adams DL, Horton JC. The representation of retinal blood vessels in primate striate cortex. *Journal of Neuroscience.* 2003;23:5984-5997.

[76] Hendrickson AE, Wilson JR, Ogren MP. The neuroanatomical organization of pathways between the dorsal lateral geniculate nucleus and visual cortex in Old World and New World primates. *Journal of Comparative Neurology.* 1978;182:123-136.

[77] Panzeri S, Petroni F, Petersen RS, Diamond ME. Decoding neuronal population activity in rat somatosensory cortex: role of columnar organization. *Cerebral Cortex.* 2003;13:45-52.

[78] Kaas JH, Nelson RJ, Sur M, Merzenich MM. Organization of somatosensory cortex in primates. In: Schmitt FO, Worden FG, Adelman G, Dennis SG, eds. *The Organization of the Cerebral Cortex*. Cambridge, MA: MIT Press; 1981:237-261.

[79] Paul RL, Goodman H, Merzenich MM. Alterations in mechanoreceptor input to Brodmann's Areas 1 and 3 of the postcentral hand area of *Macaca mulatta* after nerve section and regeneration. *Brain Research.* 1972;39:1-19.

[80] Favorov OV, Whitsel BL. Spatial organization of the peripheral input to area 1 cell columns, I: the detection of "segregates". *Brain Research.* 1988;13:25-42.

[81] Favorov OV, Whitsel BL. Spatial organization of the peripheral input to area 1 cell columns, II: the forelimb representation achieved by a mosaic of segregates. *Brain Research.* 1988;13:43-56.

[82] Favorov OV, Diamond ME. Demonstration of discrete place-defined columns—segregates—in the cat SI. *Journal of Comparative Neurology.* 1990;298:97-112.

[83] Lee CJ, Whitsel BL. Mechanisms underlying somatosensory cortical dynamics, I: *in vivo* studies. *Cerebral Cortex.* 1992;2:81-106.

[84] Lee CJ, Whitsel BL, Tommerdahl M. Mechanisms underlying somatosensory cortical dynamics, II: *in vitro* studies. *Cerebral Cortex.* 1992;2:107-133.

[85] Tommerdahl M, Favorov O, Whitsel BL, Nakhle B, Gonchar YA. Minicolumnar activation patterns in cat and monkey S1 cortex. *Cerebral Cortex.* 1993;3:399-411.

[86] McCasland JS, Woolsey TA. High-resolution 2-deoxyglucose mapping of functional cortical columns in mouse barrel cortex. *Journal of Comparative Neurology.* 1988;278:555-569.

[87] Albright TD. Direction and orientation selectivity of neurons in visual area MT of the macaque. *Journal of Neurophysiology.* 1984;52:1106-1130.

[88] Zeki SM. Functional organization of a visual area in the posterior bank of the superior temporal sulcus of the rhesus monkey. *Journal of Physiology.* 1974;236:549-573.

[89] Adams DL, Zeki S. Functional organization of macaque V3 for stereoscopic depth. *Journal of Neurophysiology.* 2001;86:2195-2203.

[90] Rao SG, Williams GV, Goldman-Rakic PS. Isodirectional tuning of adjacent interneurons and pyramidal cells during working memory: evidence for microcolumnar organization in PFC. *Journal of Neurophysiology.* 1999;81:1903-1916.

[91] Thomson AM, Deuchars J. Synaptic interactions in neocortical local circuits: dual intracellular recordings *in vitro*. *Cerebral Cortex.* 1997;7:510-522.

[92] Thomson AM, Deuchars J, West DC. Neocortical local synaptic circuitry revealed with dual intracellular recordings and biocytin-filling. *Journal of Physiology, Paris.* 1996;90:211-215.

[93] Kisvárday ZF, Kim D-S, Eysel UT, Bonhoeffer G. Relationship between lateral inhibitory connections and the topography of the orientation map in cat visual cortex. *European Journal of Neuroscience.* 1994;6:1619-1632.

[94] Hubel DH, Wiesel TN. Laminar and columnar distribution of genicular-corticol fibres in the macaque monkey. *Journal of Comparative Neurology.* 1972;158:421-450.

[95] Feldman ML, Peters A. The forms of non-pyramidal neurons in the visual cortex of the rat. *Journal of Comparative Neurology.* 1978;179:761-793.

[96] Peters A, Sethares C. Organization of pyramidal neurons in area 17 of monkey visual cortex. *Journal of Comparative Neurology.* 1991;306:1-23.

[97] DeAngelis GC, Newsome WT. Organization of disparity-selective neurons in macaque area MT. Journal of Neuroscience. 1999;19:1398-1415.

[98] Holthoff K, Witte OW. Intrinsic optical signals in rat neocortical slices measured with near-infrared dark-field microscopy reveal changes in extracellular space. *Journal of Neuroscience.* 1996;16:2740-2749.

[99] Ong WY, Garey LJ. Neuronal architecture of the human temporal cortex. *Anatomy and Embryology.* 1990;181:351-369.

[100] del Río MR, DeFelipe J. Colocalization of parvalbumin and calbindin D_{28k} in neurons including chandelier cells of the human temporal neocortex. *Journal of Chemical Neuroanatomy.* 1997;12:165-173.

[101] Silberberg G, Gupta A, Markram H. Stereotypy in neocortical microcircuits. *Trends in Neurosciences.* 2002;25:227-230.

[102] Mountcastle, VB. Introduction to the special issue: computation in cortical columns. *Cerebral Cortex.* 2003;13:2-4.

[103] Kisvárday ZF, Ferecskó AS, Kovács K, Buzás P, Budd JML, Eysel UT. One axon—multiple functions: specificity of lateral inhibitory connections by large basket cells. *Journal of Neurocytology.* 2002;31:255-264.

In: Neocortical Modularity and the Cell Minicolumn
Editor: Manuel F. Casanova, pp. 117-136 ISBN 1-59454-301
© 2005 Nova Science Publishers, Inc.

Chapter VI

ENCEPHALIZATION, MINICOLUMNS, AND HOMINID EVOLUTION

Daniel Buxhoeveden
Medical College of Georgia, Augusta, GA
Manuel F. Casanova*
University of Louisville, KY

INTRODUCTION

In general, the more closely related two species are, the more difficult it is to differentiate between them. This predictable but nonetheless frustrating fact lies at the difficulty in assigning taxonomic classifications to closely related fossils. This problem also arises regarding the evolution of the hominid brain, where size (either overall or by region) has been the most distinguishing factor. But the question remains whether the amount of brain tissue alone is enough to account for the human behavioral condition. Even those who propagate brain size as the fundamental explanation realize that reorganization is a critical part of the equation [1].

The use of brain volumes in paleoneurology would be meaningless without an adequate database for reference, and the same is true for columnar organization. To properly assess the significance and range of minicolumnar size and configuration, it is necessary to have their measurements in brains of all sizes and animals of widely diverse genera. Yet, this is far from the case. Our knowledge base about comparative minicolumnar anatomy is in its infancy. An examination of Table 1 reveals that only a few species have actually been examined, all of which have brains smaller than the majority of anthropoid primates. Certainly, none are larger or even close to those of the anthropoid apes. Of this data, the number of different

* Corresponding author: Manuel F. Casanova, MD, Gottfried and Gisela Kolb Endowed Chair in Psychiatry, University of Louisville, Department of Psychiatry, 500 South Preston St., A Bldg., Rm. 217, Louisville, KY 40292. Tel: (502)852-4077; Fax: (502)852-4078; E-mail: M0CASA02@louisville.edu

brain regions for which information is available is also extremely limited. There is more information for columns in humans and primates than for any other type of mammal, but it is less useful due to the scarcity of other mammals of diverse brain size for comparison. These gaps make it impossible to fully comprehend the meaning of minicolumn size and configuration in the human condition. Nor do we understand the potential for different approaches to columnar organization that may occur in response to diverse environments, behavioral constraints, and brain volume.

Table 1. Comparative Minicolumn Size

Width (μm)	Measurement*	Cortical areas†	Reference
Mouse			
20–40	AD	BC	Escobar et al. [2]
22–25	AD	BC	White & Peters [3]
26.3	PCA	V1	Casanova et al., unpublished findings, 2003
35.1	PCA	S1	Casanova et al., unpublished findings, 2003
Rat			
44.2	AD	32	Gabbott & Bacon [4]
50	AD	3	Peters & Walsh [5]
50	AD	3	Feldman & Peters [6]
30–40	AD	V1	Feldman & Peters [6]
55–60	AD	V1	Peters & Kara [7]
30–60	PCA	SM	Kohn et al. [8]
52.6	AD	V1	Lohmann & Köppen [9]
50.1	AB	V1	Lohmann & Köppen [9]
53.1	AD	V1	Winkelmann et al. [10]
Hedgehog (**Echinops telfairi*****)***			
32	AD	all cortex	Schmolke and Kunzle [11]
Cat			
56	AD	17	Peters & Yilmaz [12]
50–70	AD	41	Feldman & Peters [6]
28.6–55.6	PCA	3	Tommerdahl et al. [13]
40–50	SC	3	Favorov and Diamond [14]
***Rabbit*‡**			
40–50	AD	17	Fleischhauer et al. [19]
Monkey (**Macaca fascicularis, M. mulatta, M. fuscata, M. nemestrina*****)***			
15–30	DB	4, 3, 1, 17, 18	DeFelipe et al. [20]
Monkey (**Macaca mulatta*****)***			
23	MB	17	Peters and Sethares [21]
30	AD	17	Peters & Sethares [22]
36	PCA	22	Buxhoeveden et al. [23]
21	MB	18	Peters et al. [24]
23	AD	17	Peters et al. [24]
80	AD§	PFC	Sakai [25]
Monkey (**Macaca mulatta, Macaca nemestrina*****)***			
23	DB	17	Peters & Sethares [26]

Table 1. Comparative Minicolumn Size (Continued)

Width (μm)	Measurement*	Cortical areas†	Reference
Monkey (*Macaca fascicularis*)			
28.6–55.6**	PCA	3	Tommerdahl et al. [13]
Monkey (*Aotus trivirgatus, Saimiri sciureus*)			
40–60	SC	3, 1	Kaas [27]
Chimpanzee (*Pan troglodytes*)			
36.5	PCA	22	Buxhoeveden et al. [23]
Chimpanzee (*Pan paniscus*)			
35	PCA	22	Buxhoeveden, et al. [28]
Orangutan (*Pongo pygmaeus*)			
31.4	PCA	22	Buxhoeveden, et al. [28]
Gorilla (*Gorilla gorilla*)			
33	PCA	22	Buxhoeveden et al. [28]
Homo sapiens			
41.7	PCA	23b, 24b, 31, 7, 19	Schlaug et al. [29]
46.7	PCA	22	Seldon [30]
44.8	PCA	42	Seldon [30]
46.1	PCA	41	Seldon [30]
51	PCA	22	Buxhoeveden et al. [23]
31.6	PCA	V1	Casanova et al., unpublished findings, 2003
38.5–52.4	PCA	4, 9, 17, 21, 22, 40, 41, 46	Casanova et al., unpublished findings, 2003
29.8	DB	TL	del Río & DeFelipe [31]
80, 50††	PCA	STS	Buldyrev et al. [32]
35	AB	VA	Kenan-Vaknin et al. [33]
16	Nissl	V1	Morgane et al. [34]
Cetaceans (*Stenella coeruleoalba, Tursiops Truncatus*)			
19.9	Nissl	V1	Morgane et al. [34]

* AB: axon bundle; AD: apical dendrite bundle; DB: double bouquet axon bundle; MB: myelin bundle; PCA: pyramidal cell array; SC: single cell recording.

† BC: barrel cortex; SM: sensory motor; STS: superior temporal sulcus; TL: temporal lobe; VA: visual association cortex; numbers are Brodmann areas.

‡ Several studies have identified apical dendrite bundles in rabbit cortex areas V1 and M1, but did not report a center-to-center spacing distance [15–17]. Detzer [18] reports on apical dendrite bundles in mouse barrel field and area parietalis without providing a measurement.

§ Layer VI pyramidal cell bundles.

** Reported as 18–35 cycles/mm. Estimated conversion. Range only, no means given.

†† 80 μm was noted as the periodicity, while 50 μm was given as the width of each column. The method utilized does not attempt to correspond directly to pyramidal cell arrays.

Paleoneurologists are always seeking better ways to measure and elucidate the changes that occur during primate brain evolution. The behavioral traits that distinguish humans from nonhuman primates represent a challenge to neuroscience that speaks to the need of studying anatomical structures with identifiable physiological correlates. In this regard, the study of the minicolumn may be particularly helpful. It is both an anatomical configuration and an intermediary between individual cells, regional parcellations, and the cortical module (macrocolumn). This chapter briefly considers the role of the minicolumn on two interrelated aspects of brain evolution: encephalization and reorganization. It is our contention that the study of the minicolumn provides a novel view of brain evolution and a method of parcellating the cortex of different species. As with all methods and approaches, there are limitations as no single approach can encompass the entire workings of the brain.

MINICOLUMN AND CORTICAL VOLUME RELATIONSHIPS

From what is currently known about both minicolumn and brain size among diverse species, it is clear that these measurements are not correlated [35]. Minicolumns in small animals such as rabbits and rats may be larger than those in humans (Table 1). The same is apparently true for at least two types of macrocolumns: the layer IV barrel column and cytochrome oxidase blobs in V1.

Aside from the lack of correlation between minicolumnar size and brain volume, other unknowns remain. First, measurements indicative of vertical organization are available in only a handful of mammals [36]. Second, while data exist on the small end of the scale in the form of the mouse and rat, nothing is known about very large mammalian brains. After humans, the next largest brains in which cell columns have been measured are the great apes which have brain volumes about one third that of humans. The data presented in Table 1 suggest a tantalizing, but as yet undocumented, tendency to see minicolumns in nonhuman primates as absolutely (and relatively) smaller than those of other mammals, with the exception of the mouse, particularly area 17. To determine if minicolumns are in fact smaller in primates, data from additional extant primates and a sizeable population of non-primate mammals are required. No measure of minicolumns in brains larger than those of the human has ever been made.

A majority of the work on minicolumns and modules generally focuses on the stability of their size across species (Leise, 1990; Mountcastle, 1997) [37,38]. Minicolumnar size has remained relatively stable across species when compared with other brain changes, e.g., volume. When considering the size range of columns in light of the huge disparity in evolutionary time, species divergences, and brain size, the relative stability of minicolumnar morphology suggests the presence of rules that govern the size of minicolumns and macrocolumns [35]. Manger et al. [35] have argued that these rules arose due to selection for an optimal connection length.

Hypothetically, minimum and maximum size limits for microcolumns may exist because their basic elements place constraints on how small they may be. These basic elements include neurons, apical dendrites, myelinated efferents, and double-bouquet bundles; thalamic, callosal, and cortico-cortical input; dendritic arborizations and spines, synaptic contacts, as well as glia. Brain volume may not correlate with column size because neuronal elements such as cells and axons require a minimum size to function. As a result, their dimensions stay essentially similar while cortical surface area expands.

On the other hand, the maximum limit on minicolumn size may be set by metabolic efficiency and conduction speed. Cherniak [39] postulates that the spatial layout of the brain minimizes total connection costs. Long connections require a large volume of metabolically active tissue and increased conduction times, resulting in signal-propagation delays [40]. Rapid sensory reaction time is critical to survival. As the brain enlarges, the distance between cells and columns increases so that attempts to maintain interconnections result in reduced conduction time and efficiency. The use of closely interconnected modules helps to maximize efficiency by processing similar information in a particular region (at least initially) rather than having it dispersed throughout. This process maintains shorter connections and decreases metabolic requirements. In fact, the use of modules increases the efficiency of the system by replacing individual cell-to-cell connectivity with column-to-column interconnectivity. While this seems to be the case for different stages of processing, it also means that information is not passed to other more distant regions. Simply put, the relatively stable size of modules is due to the selection of optimal connection length. The range for module size and long-range connections between fields for large or small brains is evolutionarily stable [35]. But as the authors point out, only sparse data exist for large-brained mammals like humans, elephants, and whales, though evidence of module size (i.e., both macro- and minicolumns) is also restricted in humans.

The presence of similarly sized minicolumns (or macrocolumns) in brains of grossly different size creates its own disparity. If the volume of a particular region is much larger in a given brain than the relative increase in column size, then the columns in that brain become relatively smaller. A 50 μm column in a 20 cm^3 brain is relatively large compared to the same size column in a 1400 cm^3 brain. Decreasing the size of individual columns when cortical surface area is very small increases their numbers and maximizes interconnectivity. This appears to be the case in the mouse brain, though not in the rat: While still very small, the rat brain is several times larger than that of the mouse (Table 2).

Table 2. Brain Weight and Minicolumn Size

Species	Mean brain weight (g)	Mean minicolumn width (μm)
Pan paniscus	350	33
Pan troglodytes	350	36
Pongo pygmaeus	370	35
Macaca mulatta	170	36
Gorilla gorilla	500	33
Homo sapiens	1350	40–50
Mouse	0.4	22–30
Rat	2	50–60
Cat	30	50–60
Rabbit	10	40–50

The human brain is about 13 times larger than that of the monkey and over 3 times larger than the chimpanzee while its cell columns are only about a third larger. Relative to brain volume, columns in human cortex are actually smaller than those of the chimpanzee and rhesus monkey. On the other hand, the chimpanzee brain is about 4 times larger than the rhesus monkey, yet both have similar size columns. Thus, the chimpanzee columns appear relatively smaller than those of the rhesus monkey. Increased brain size allows more flexibility regarding the size of columns in particular cortical regions.

The functional operation of the mammalian brain is thought be distributed across many areas of the brain rather than being strictly modular [38]. This means that individual columns serve multiple purposes depending on how they are recruited. The visual system has orientation columns ranging from 25 μm to 50 μm wide [41], color columns that are 100 μm to 250 μm wide [42], and ocular dominance or preference columns that are 250 μm to 500 μm wide [43,44]. These columns overlap and occupy the same space. Thus, individual minicolumn modules participate in more than one type of function [7]. In this way they maximize cortical space and increase the efficiency of cortical tissue. While all of these cells and columns specialize in visual tasks, they participate in multiple aspects of information processing.

The composition of an individual minicolumn depends on many local factors. However, the functional capacity of minicolumns in a given region is partly influenced by the brain's degree of potential complexity, i.e., its interconnected pathways and regions. Cortical structures in the form of minicolumns and cortical volume exert a reciprocal effect on each other. The relationship between the size of minicolumns and brain volume may be summarized as follows. (1) Larger cell minicolumns have a potentially greater number and variety of internal elements. However, everything else being equal, larger cell minicolumns also reduce their total number and therefore the amount of interconnectivity between them. It remains undecided as to which approach is best suited to express a particular function. In general, a larger brain allows for either larger cell columns with equal amounts of interconnectivity or an increase in the number of processing units and interconnections. (2) A large brain may contain more minicolumns as well as more "complex" ones. However, to the extent that brains minimize connection distances, column size must also be restricted [39,40]. (3) A large brain may contain more and larger cortical regions. As the cortical region size increases, so does the number of columns. These changes increase the amount of information that regions can share. (4) Larger brains with more regional specializations create the opportunity for more indirect influences or secondary connections, i.e., greater integration of information from diverse sources. For example, Tpt, a cortical region within the planum temporale, may not connect directly to area 9. However, it does connect to area 46, which in turn connects to area 9 [45]. Even if a column in one area lacks a direct connection to another, it may influence it indirectly, magnifying the effects of direct connections. Therefore, the greater the number of regional specializations with direct or indirect influences, the greater their indirect influences may be also.

The relationships between cell columns and cortical volume may be studied from a number of perspectives. One approach considers minicolumnar size and cortical volume across the mammalian order. Because of the difficulty if not the total lack of homologous regions in such a study, it would only answer generalized questions about the extreme limits of column size. This would, however, yield vital information about minicolumnar variability during cortical evolution. Some basic questions such as whether minicolumns are present in all species and if they arose in the earliest cortex forms need to be addressed. Questions about changes in specific taxonomic categories would require a more targeted approach. Studies of the evolutionary relationships of more closely related organisms call for the examination of animals with established relationships and the presence of some degree of homology among cortical regions. Yet another method compares different regions of the same cortex in the same species.

Minicolumnar Configuration

There is no doubt that differences exist in the morphology of cell minicolumns. Generally, variations within a vertical column are similar to those that make any cortical tissue different from another, e.g., cell types, lamina specializations, different sources of afferent input and efferent output, etc. However, there is evidence that one potential source of variation, synaptic density, may express little variability in visual cortex in a wide variety of mammals even while synaptic number fluctuates [46]. Moreover, synaptic boutons are distributed with constant intensity along the length of the axon; in particular, bouton density does not increase as the axon approaches its terminus [47]. Not only does dendritic branching of rat single neurons display similar densities and proportion of synaptic contacts, but this stability remains even with sensory deprivation [48].

If the synaptic density remains stable, then increased total synaptic area in a minicolumn could be achieved by enhancing the amount of space provided for neuropil. It appears that changing the width of the column almost always results in an increase in the neuropil space, though this does not follow for cell density *within* the column. While it appears that narrower cell columns would also have less neuropil space, this need not be proportional. Thus, the brain can provide variations in microcircuitry by altering the proportion of space occupied by neuropil versus that occupied by cell soma and large fiber bundles.

An example of a subtle but potentially very significant variation within the internal configuration of minicolumns is found in the apical dendrite bundles of areas 17 and 18 in the rhesus monkey. While these bundles are present in both areas, their pathways are not identical [24]. Pyramidal cells in Brodmann area 18 aggregate in layer V to form clusters that reach layer IV, where they are joined by smaller apical dendrites from small layer IV pyramidal cells. Most of these form terminal tufts in layer III, and only a few reach layer I. Layer I is dominated by apical dendrite tufts from pyramidal cells in layer II/III. By contrast, the area 17 apical dendrites from layer V cells form discrete clusters that are joined by those in layers II/III and then terminate their tufts in layer I.

Minicolumns and Brain Reorganization

Brain size has been used to distinguish humans from ancestral hominids, primates, and other mammals. It is most useful for the study of fossil brains since it can easily be measured. However, it is also recognized that the relationship between brain and body size is not straightforward. Some small bodied animals have relatively large brains and vice versa. Increases in body size do not imply corresponding enlargements in brain size. Moreover, this comparison fails to explain what makes humans different. Were size the only factor, then human patients who have had an entire hemisphere removed (e.g., for epilepsy) would no longer exhibit human behavioral qualities since the resultant cortical volume would be similar to those of early ancestral hominids or of larger extant gorillas. Clearly, this does not occur because the brains of modern humans, ancestral hominids, and apes are not organized in the same way.

The relationship of column size to brain volume is especially relevant since the rise of cortical surface areas during evolution may be directly related to changes in the origin of the ontogenetic cell column [49]. Cortical genesis occurs by symmetrical and asymmetrical division. In the first phase, symmetrical division determines the total number of cell columns in the cortex. Asymmetrical division occurs in the next phase and affects the number of cells within a column and the cortical thickness [50]. Therefore, cell columns may lie at the root of cortical enlargement both regarding their number and, to a lesser extent, their size. The addition of new cell columns by cortico-genesis leads to cortical surface area enlargement while at the same time providing fertile ground for reorganization. The competition for new connectivity from thalamocortical, callosal, and corticocortical input to new cell minicolumns creates the potential for re-wiring. Thus, the concepts of reorganization and encephalization are closely related.

It is sometimes assumed that minicolumns share the same morphology among species [51]. However, no one has consistently examined this despite indications of differences across species and between different cortical regions of the brain [21,29,30,52,53]. To the extent that a generalized model exists for minicolumn organization in the mammalian brain, there is also evidence of variation across species and between different regions within the same brain [5,19,21,29,54,55].

LATERALIZATION

As Manger et al. [35] state, "There is a limited collection of tools or underlying mechanisms that are accessed by human brains so in the course of evolutionary history repetition of similar structural elements occurs." One tool brains can use to optimize their operation is to create areas of specialized function in each hemisphere. This speeds computational time by permitting local circuits to perform functions without waiting for information to cross the corpus callosum. Evolution is even thought to select against long range corticocortical connections [39,40]. Based on this logic, lateralization selects for short range intrahemispheric connections required for high resolution and time-critical tasks such as language. Manger et al. [35] suggest that modules are generated by correlated activity for both anatomical and physiological heterogeneity. Lateralization would seem to be an efficient way of changing brain function without creating entirely new areas.

While asymmetries in surface anatomical structures were well known, Seldon [30,53] was perhaps the first researcher to document laterality in the configuration of minicolumns. His work focused on cell arrays, dendrites, and axons in human auditory association cortex, specifically areas TA, TB, and TC. TB refers to area 42 of Brodmann, and TC is the primary auditory cortex also known as A1. TA is synonymous with area 22 of Brodmann, which includes an anterior and posterior portion, and is analogous to temporoparietal cortex (Tpt). In posterior TA the minicolumnar size and the neuropil interval (another way of measuring the peripheral neuropil space) were larger in the left hemisphere. Although the columns were smaller in TB and TC, they nonetheless displayed a similar left-right bias. What varied between area TA and the others was the relationship between this asymmetry and dendritic spread. In TA the dendritic expansion was only slightly less in the right hemisphere. Because the cell minicolumns are packed more tightly on the right than the left, they individually receive input from more minicolumns in the right hemisphere than in the left. On the other hand, this differs from areas TB and TC where the dendritic spread is smaller on the right side in conjunction with a smaller minicolumnar size. A sort of "compensation" occurs resulting in left-right symmetry of the dendritic contacts. In TA one afferent axon with a radius of 150 μm contacts about 450 minicolumns for the right hemisphere compared to 375 minicolumns for the left, a pattern also found in the other areas. This study may prove to be especially important because it reveals that cell minicolumns in three different but closely related cortical areas can vary morphologically and display asymmetries that are distinctive for each area.

Later studies support the presence of minicolumnar laterality in the posterior portion of area 22 of Brodmann. Galuske et al. [56] examined clusters of long-range intrinsic connections in human posterior 22. They found that clusters in the left hemisphere contained more subsystems of interconnected minicolumns than those in the right. This was based on an increase in cluster spacing on the left side compared to the right. Other studies used quantified computer imaging to examine tens of thousands of minicolumns in dozens of human brains [23,28,57]. In humans, the minicolumns and peripheral neuropil space were larger on the left side than the right. Based on this series of studies, the differences between the size of minicolumns (left *versus* right hemisphere) of posterior 22, relative to the minicolumnar size in the left hemisphere, range between 14 % and 17 % [23,30,36]. Interestingly, this approaches the 20 % asymmetry for clusters reported by Galuske et al. [56] Recent work by Anderson et al. [58] on larger myelinated axon bundles in the left hemisphere of superior posterior temporal gyrus area show that the left hemisphere in area 22 contains larger pyramidal cells with longer and wider axons (see also Hutsler and Gazzaniga [59]). These studies strongly support organizational changes in the left human superior temporal gyrus, where they are readily assimilated into differences in minicolumnar morphology.

Alternatively, when cell minicolumns were examined in homologous regions in the common chimpanzee and rhesus monkey, no evidence of significant laterality appeared [23.60]. Nonetheless, studies of this same region have revealed more basic similarities regarding lateralization between humans and apes than between humans and monkeys [61,62]. Magnetic resonance imaging (MRI) studies have found similar asymmetry of the PT in humans and in African great apes but none in Old or New World monkeys [63,64]. This demonstrates that the left-right status of minicolumns need not correspond to gross anatomical structure. Macro-anatomical structures consist of many functional subunits, each possessing different pathways and intracortical connections. Macroscopic examination of the brain at the gross anatomical level, therefore, often fails to adequately detect internal organizational differences in cortical tissue.

Several conclusions can be drawn from this data. These results distinguish cortical minicolumns in the human planum temporale from those of nonhuman primates, reflecting organizational differences. Lateralization of minicolumns may reflect intrinsic differences in the wiring of the human and nonhuman primate brains. Changing the size of minicolumns in corresponding areas of the opposite hemisphere significantly alters the connectivity pattern of dendrites as well as the distribution of the afferent input [30,53]. For example, if the width of the dendritic spread to both sides remains identical, then dendrites in the hemisphere containing smaller minicolumns will receive information from more columns. This can result in less specificity but greater spread of information between columns. Likewise, equal afferent input to both hemispheres will contact more columns in the side occupied by more columns per unit area. This process will decrease the specificity of information per column but spread information to more columns [30,53].

Evolution subtly modifies minicolumnar morphology between hemispheres to alter the anatomy and physiology of similar cortical areas without creating totally new ones. Altering minicolumnar circuitry for homologous regions of each hemisphere also exploits the complexity of a system by making minute adjustments that create profound effects. Discovering the distinctiveness of human brains is complicated by the lack of dramatic anatomical and physiological differences compared with other mammalian brains. Evolution proceeds along conservative pathways, thus requiring sophisticated methods to detect the subtle but very significant differences that lie within specific modules of the brain.

SPECIES DIFFERENCES—MORPHOLOGY

The visual cortex provides one of the best examples of species-specificity related to minicolumnar size and organization (Table 3). Rabbits and cats apparently contain very large minicolumns (based on apical dendrites) measuring between 50–60 μm in their primary visual cortex. By comparison, center-to-center spacing of apical dendrite bundles in rhesus monkey (*Macaca mulatta*) V1 results in much smaller minicolumns of around 30 μm. Strikingly, the rhesus monkey has a much larger brain but smaller V1 minicolumns [12,22]. When extrapolated to three dimensions, the columns in the cat visual cortex are actually three times larger than those of the monkey [12]. These studies alone confirm that no direct relationship exists between cortical volume and minicolumnar size. Instead, the size of minicolumns appears to relate more to function. In these studies, the authors concluded that the cell minicolumns in the monkey are more "complex" than in cats or rabbits. In area V1 primates have acquired species-specific modules to process color, form, and motion, making them different from those of rodents or cats [65]. Detailed comparisons reveal that the visual systems of monkeys display better color and visual acuity than those of cats [66]. Further evidence of the functional and anatomical differences between these species is that projections from minicolumns in V1 to extrastriate cortex in primate brains differ from those of the rodent. This research shows how functional requirements dictate minicolumnar size and why brain volume is a poor predictor of minicolumnar size. The fundamental argument used to describe these differences should also apply to the rest of the cortex. Brodmann area 17 has also been measured in human brains, and the mean minicolumnar size is very similar to that reported for monkeys. It also demonstrates a significant reduction compared to other areas of human cortex examined by the same method.

Table 3. Minicolumn Size in a Homologous Region of Cortex in Brains of Diverse Size

Species	CW (μm)	Parameter[‡‡]	Method	Source
Mouse	26.3	Cell somas	Nissl	Casanova et al. (unpublished findings, 2003)
Rat	55–60	AD	Toluidine blue	Peters & Kara [7]
Rabbit	40–50	AD	Luxol fast blue	Fleischhauer [19]
Cat	56	AD	MAP2	Peters & Yilmaz [12]
Macaca mulatta	30	AD	MAP2	Peters & Sethares [22]
Monkeys[§§]	15–30	DB	Immuno	DeFelipe et al. [20]
Macaca mulatta	23	MB	Myelin	Peters & Sethares [21]
Homo sapiens	29.8	DB	Immuno	del Río & DeFelipe [31]
Homo sapiens	31.6	Cell somas	Nissl	Casanova et al. (unpublished findings, 2003)

[‡‡] AD: apical dendrites; DB: double bouquet cell axon bundles; MB: myelin bundles

[§§] *Macaca fascicularis*, *M. mulatta*, *M. fuscata*, and *M. nemestrina*.

Note: There is no corresponding relationship between column size and brain volume or size of a cortical region.

A number of researchers have studied species-specific differences among primates, including humans. In an area of the brain associated with human language, several studies have demonstrated differences between nonhuman anthropoids and humans. The posterior portion of Brodmann's area 22, part of the auditory association cortex included within Wernicke's area, was examined in normal human, chimpanzee, and rhesus monkey brains [28]. The study analyzed digitized images from Nissl-stained sections by a computerized imaging program that detected and described minicolumnar morphology. The results indicated that minicolumns in humans are about 1.3 times the width of, and have considerably more neuropil space within them than, those of the nonhuman primates. The increase in peripheral neuropil space in human minicolumns appears closely related to their larger width. Viewing peripheral neuropil space as a ratio of the column width, the proportions are similar for all three species. While the increase in humans may be absolute rather than relative, the result provides more space for dendritic branching, spines, and other features generally found in this part of the column.

An examination of the "core" region of the cell column (where 90 % of the cells are located) revealed a reduction in cellular density in humans. The grey level index of the core area in the human brain was twice that derived for the column as a whole, while the gray level index of the core was 1.8 times and 1.7 times that of the whole minicolumn in the chimpanzee and monkey, respectively. While seemingly small, the differences were highly significant [23]. Because human cell columns are much wider and contain greater neuropil space in the periphery, the concentration of cells in the core area is relatively higher. This means that the core area has not expanded in proportion to the increase in width. This suggests that human neural tissue has an emphasis on increased peripheral neuropil space, or more non-cell rich areas between cell arrays.

A recent study by Letinic and Rakic [67] may offer a glimpse into some of the reasons for this increase in neuropil space. The authors found a pathway between the ganglionic eminence and pulvinar nucleus in the dorsal thalamus in the human brain but not in the monkey or mouse brains. The GABAergic neurons are thought to represent an additional set of neurons in the thalamic association nuclei during fetal development, to "accommodate" the input from the expanding cortex. This might account for some of the increase in neuropil space in human brains in cortex regions served by the dorsal thalamus, which includes the auditory association cortex.

Previous studies [2,3] (also Casanova et al., unpublished data, 2003) report that the smallest minicolumns, outside of area 17 in primates, are found in the brain of the mouse, with columns as small as 20 μm (Table 1). The rat brain has considerably larger cell columns that are typically around 50 μm to 60 μm [4-8.10], so a very significant difference exists between these rodent species. Considering the discrepancies among techniques, the size of minicolumns in the cat, rabbit, and rat appears to be generally similar (Table 3). On the other hand, the size range reported in monkey or chimpanzee cortex appears to be smaller than these other mammals, despite their much larger brain volumes. In studies that measured the width or center-to-center spacing, minicolumns in monkey were 20 μm to 30 μm in V1 and 36 μm in Brodmann area 22. The Kaas study [27] indirectly estimated minicolumn width from i*n vivo* conditions, which lack shrinkage, so it is not a direct comparison. A study of the great apes reveals similar-sized minicolumns. The common chimpanzee has been studied the most, and the minicolumns in Brodmann area 22 are approximately 36.5 μm. Recently, very small samples were obtained of other anthropoid apes, including orangutan, gorilla, and the pygmy chimpanzee. The size for columns ranged from 32 μm to 35 μm. A summary of some parameters shows how the great apes and humans differ. The human columns are wider, typically in mid-forty to mid-fifty microns in width, the neuropil space is typically over 20 μm compared to only 12 μm to 17 μm in the great apes and monkeys. The only non-primate mammal for which these parameters are available is the mouse (Table 4). In this case the mean value of 8.7 μm represents the smallest neuropil space for any adult mammal examined.

Table 4. Cell Columns in Mammals

	Cortical area	Sample size	CW (μm)	MCS (μm)	NS (μm)	CGLI (%)
Apes	22	14	35.4 (5.2)	16.1 (2.8)	15.5 (2.1)	42.3 (7.7)
Human	22	28	47.4 (8.6)	22.2 (3.7)	18.9 (3.6)	34.3 (8.0)
Monkeys	22	7	36.8 (5.7)	17.9 (1.5)	15.4 (2.6)	44.4 (6.0)
Mouse	V1	7	26.3 (4.3)	16.1 (0.8)	8.7 (0.6)	42.2 (5.4)

The evidence presented above suggests that minicolumnar width in primates has decreased compared to most other mammals (except for extremely small brains like that of the mouse). Of course, this needs to be verified by extensive studies with standardized techniques. If true, it demonstrates a trend in primates towards decreased minicolumn size with expanded cortical surface area, resulting in absolutely and relatively more minicolumnar units per area and per unit of tissue.

Minicolumns and White Matter

Hofman [68] relates the constraints on brain size to either blood flow or neuronal processing. In the case of the latter, the basic requirement is to enable quick processing and information integration. As grey matter increases, white matter volume must increase even more if each cell is to be interconnected. The general principle is that the number of connections increases much faster than the number of units (cells or modules). A primate brain with volume 3000 cm^3 would consist of 1470 cm^3 white matter, or nearly half of the entire brain volume [68]. At some upper limit, increasing brain size diminishes efficiency. It has been suggested that the addition of neurons degrades efficiency because of the needed connections and increasingly larger distances between the units [40]. According to Hofman, the disproportionate increase in white matter volume accounts for more of the neocortical expansion of primate brain than does the increase in cortical neurons. Anderson provided a mathematical description for Ringo's model as well as describing the basic thesis: In a randomized system,

> "...any increase in the absolute number of connections is exactly offset by the spatial separation that increases between elements so that the number of communications that occur per a given fixed time interval remains unchanged. The only way this disadvantage can be overcome is to rearrange the increased connections such that the neurons that are spatially proximate have a greater chance of connecting" [58].

As a result, there must be a decrease in the fraction of mass devoted to wiring. This concept provides a rationale for the brain to localize function and to increase the number of cytoarchitectonic areas of the human and primate brain compared to that of other mammals [69,70].

In this context the size of cell columns may be significant. Provided that a similar number of cells per column give rise to myelinated efferent bundles and to the extent that each column in turn receives myelinated afferents, a brain with narrower cell columns (more per unit area) should have an increase in the white matter. However, the number of cells per column, the size of the neurons and their type, and the ratio of long to short distance connections must also be considered. Cell columns, whether large or small, with more pyramidal cells or longer distance ones within them, would have thicker individual axons, more total axons, or both.

Minicolumns and Development

It is a basic model in neuroscience that the developing brain produces many more neurons than is required while a pruning process removes excess neurons over time. The number of synaptic connections also increases far beyond what will be found in the adult cortex, also resulting in death of early connections. The cause may be a combination of genetic programming and Darwinian competitive process. In the latter case, connections strengthened through learning or through exposure survive, while those that fail to connect do not. Studies of cell death have focused on single cells, but these cells occur within individual cell columns. This process affects the adult configuration of cell minicolumns by varying their cell numbers, types, the number of afferent and efferent projections, and both local and horizontal connectivity. During development another source of individuation of the cell minicolumn is the potential effect of inhibition and excitation [71].

There is abundant evidence that the reiterative vertical organization within a given region of the brain is highly variable in a number of anatomical features, such as the thickness of bundles, number of fibers within bundles, column width, amount of neuropil space, and cell density within a minicolumn. Table 5 provides an example of the variation for width, neuropil space, and core grey level index (CGLI). Minicolumns exhibit a high degree of variability even within the same region of interest. In a study that carefully documented variation in the spacing of fiber bundles and their composition, Peters and Sethares [21] reported that the mean number of myelinated axons within a bundle ranged from less than 10 to more than 70, with a mean center-to-center spacing of 34 μm (standard deviation 13 μm). The thickness of the individual axons ranged from 0.4 μm to 2.0 μm. The number of individual dendrites per apical dendrite cluster varied with a mean of about 8 μm (standard deviation 3.2 μm). The mean center-to center spacing between them was 22.2 μm (standard deviation 7.0 μm, range 6 μm to 37 μm). The thickness of the axon bundles varied in a similar manner. Lohmann and Koppen [9] found large differences in the diameters of apical dendrite and axon bundles. The center-to-center spacing for apical dendrite bundles ranged between 25 μm and 90 μm, and for labeled axon bundles it was 20 μm to 100 μm. Schmolke and Kunzle [11] reported the center-to-center spacing distances for apical dendrite bundles ranged from 7 μm to 76 μm. The center-to-center spacing distances for the honeycomb mosaics at the Layer I and II border reported by Ichinohe et al. [72] ranged from 50 μm to 120 μm.

Table 5. Mean Coefficient of Variation in Cell Columns According to Cortical Regions

Cortical area	CW	NS	CGLI
Apes			
22	0.15	0.32	0.27
Human			
22	0.18	0.34	0.31
41	0.17	0.41	0.27
4	0.21	0.34	0.34
17	0.10	0.16	0.21
21	0.15	0.33	0.27
40	0.18	0.33	0.29
9	0.17	0.34	0.23
46	0.17	0.33	0.33
Monkeys			
22	0.16	0.32	0.24
Mouse			
S1	0.16	—	—
V1	0.15	—	—

Schmolke [16] describes how the neuropil space between the dendrite bundles is different from that within the bundles. The space outside contains a larger number of thin unmyelinated axons than are found within the bundles, and irregularly shaped smooth and spiny dendrites are the prevailing postsynaptic structures compared to spines within the apical dendrites. The appearance of the space between dendritic bundles is determined by whether or not there are myelinated axon bundles (most axon bundles cannot be traced beyond the superficial portion of layer IV). On the basis of these findings, there is little doubt that the number of cells per minicolumn and the types of cells within them also vary. Rockel's earlier study [73] purporting to find cell number homogeneity in arbitrary 30 μm vertical slabs has been revised by later findings [74,75], which reported that the number of neurons in different cortical areas is not uniform.

Minicolumns and Macrocolumns

Minicolumns are considered to be subunits of macrocolumns. In the future, one of the more vital and interesting topics will be to understand how these units interface, and it is quite possible that some assumptions about their relationships will need modification. While few dispute the evidence for the larger macrocolumn, their functionality in some areas of the cortex has been disputed [76]. For instance, ocular dominance columns are not found in all mammals and are apparently absent in some primates [77]. A recent study describes a situation in which ocular dominance columns, as indicated by cytochrome oxidase labeling, were present in some squirrel monkey brains but not others. The squirrel monkey is one of those primates that lacks ocular dominance columns. In an examination of 12 squirrel monkeys, cytochrome oxidase-labeled ocular dominance columns were present in varying degrees from clearly obvious in some to completely absent in others, leading the authors to conclude that these columns appeared to lack function that may later have adapted to fulfill a functional role in other species [78]. One implication from this is that it is the minicolumn (in all its varieties), and not the macrocolumn, that is the most generalized functional unit of the mammalian brain. It is possible that the minicolumn will be found to be the building block of cortical modules found throughout the mammalian class.

Conclusions

One of the more fascinating questions about minicolumns concerns their origin. Minicolumns of all types may be derived from non-cortical modules, such as nuclei and neuropil, since modular organization is a common organizing principle of all brains, not just in mammals [37]. There is undoubtedly a common principle shared by modules found in subcortical brain tissue and cortical columns; however, it can be argued that cortical columns are a specialized form that differ from other kinds of modules [79]. The inquiry into columnar organization is still at its most rudimentary level, especially regarding their evolutionary history. Among the questions that have yet to be addressed include when and in what animals did they originate? How ubiquitous are they across different organisms? Are they present in the entire cortex, or do some areas organize differently? What are the different forms of columnar organization among different species? Are they most pronounced in the primate order? Finally, we should ask ourselves whether minicolumns are the basic building block of the neocortex from which specialized macrocolumns later emerged. If the latter is correct, then there will be instances where functioning minicolumns but not macrocolumns will be present.

REFERENCES

[1] Jerison HJ. The study of primate brain evolution: Where do we go from here? In: Falk D, Gibson KR, eds. *Evolutionary Anatomy of the Primate Cerebral Cortex*. Cambridge, UK: Cambridge University Press; 2001:305-337.

[2] Escobar MI, Pimenta H, Caviness VS Jr, Jacobson M, Crandall JE, Kosik KS. Architecture of apical dendrites in the murine neocortex: dual apical dendritic systems. *Neuroscience.* 1986;17:975-989.

[3] White EL, Peters A. Cortical modules in the posteromedial barrel subfield (Sm1) of the mouse. *Journal of Comparative Neurology.* 1993;334:86-96.

[4] Gabbott PL, Bacon SJ. Local circuit neurons in the medial prefrontal cortex (areas 24a,b,c, 25 and 32) in the monkey, II: quantitative areal and laminar distributions. *Journal of Comparative Neurology.* 1996;364:609-636.

[5] Peters A, Walsh TM. A study of the organization of apical dendrites in the somatic sensory cortex of the rat. *Journal of Comparative Neurology.* 1972;144:253-268.

[6] Feldman ML, Peters A. A study of barrels and pyramidal dendritic clusters in the cerebral cortex. *Brain Research.* 1974;77:55-76.

[7] Peters A, Kara D. The neuronal composition of area 17 in rat visual cortex, IV: the organization of pyramidal cells. *Journal of Comparative Neurology.* 1987;260:573-590.

[8] Kohn A, Pinheiro A, Tommerdahl MA, Whitsel BL. Optical imaging *in vitro* provides evidence for the minicolumnar nature of cortical response. *Neuroreport.* 1997;8:3513-3518.

[9] Lohmann H, Köppen H-J. Postnatal development of pyramidal dendritic and axonal bundles in the visual cortex of the rat. *Journal für Hirnforschung.* 1995;36:101-111.

[10] Winkelmann E, Brauer K, Berger U. Zur columnaren Organisation von Pyramidenzellen im visuellen Cortex der Albinoratte. *Zeitschrift für mikroskopisch-anatomische Forschung*. 1975;89:239-256.

[11] Schmolke C, Künzle H. On the presence of dendrite bundles in the cerebral cortex of the Madagascan lesser hedgehog tenrec and the red-eared pond turtle. *Anatomy and Embryology.* 1997;196:195-213.

[12] Peters A, Yilmaz E. Neuronal organization in area 17 of cat visual cortex. *Cerebral Cortex*. 1993;3:49-68.

[13] Tommerdahl M, Favorov O, Whitsel BL, Nakhle B, Gonchar YA. Minicolumnar activation patterns in cat and monkey S1 cortex. *Cerebral Cortex.* 1993;3:399-411.

[14] Favorov OV, Diamond ME. Demonstration of discrete place-defined columns—segregates—in the cat SI. *Journal of Comparative Neurology*. 1990;298:97-112.

[15] Schmolke C, Viebahn C. Dendrite bundles in lamina II/III of the rabbit neocortex. *Anatomy and Embryology*. 1986;173:343-348.

[16] Schmolke C. Morphological organization of the neuropil in laminae II-V of rabbit visual cortex. *Anatomy and Embryology*. 1987;176:203-212.

[17] Viebahn C. Correlation between differences in the structure of dendrite bundles and cytoarchitectonic patterns in the cerebral cortex of the rabbit. *Journal für Hirnforschung*. 1990;31:645-652.

[18] Detzer K. Course and distribution of apical dendrites of layer V pyramids in the barrel field and area parietalis of the mouse. *Anatomy and Embryology*. 1976;149:251-258.

[19] Fleischhauer K, Petsche H, Wittkowski W. Vertical bundles of dendrites in the neocortex. *Zeitschrift für Anatomie und Entwicklungsgeschichte*. 1972;136:213-223.

[20] DeFelipe J, Hendry S, Hashikawa T, Molinari M, Jones EG. A microcolumnar structure of monkey cerebral cortex revealed by immunocytochemical studies of double bouquet cell axons. *Neuroscience*. 1990;37:655-673.

[21] Peters A, Sethares C. Myelinated axons and the pyramidal cell modules in monkey primary visual cortex. *Journal of Comparative Neurology*. 1996;365:232-255.

[22] Peters A, Sethares C. Organization of pyramidal neurons in area 17 of monkey visual cortex. *Journal of Comparative Neurology*. 1991;306:1-23.

[23] Buxhoeveden DP, Switala AE, Roy E, Litaker M, Casanova MF. Morphological differences between minicolumns in human and nonhuman primate cortex. *American Journal of Physical Anthropology*. 2001;115:361-371.

[24] Peters A, Cifuentes JM, Sethares C. The organization of pyramidal cells in area 18 of the rhesus monkey. *Cerebral Cortex*. 1997;7:405-421.

[25] Sakai M. Dendritic bundles formed by layer VI pyramidal cells in the monkey frontal association cortex. *Experimental Brain Research*. 1985;58:609-612.

[26] Peters A, Sethares C. The organization of double bouquet cells in monkey striate cortex. *Journal of Neurocytology*. 1997;26:779-797.

[27] Kaas JH, Nelson RJ, Sur M, Merzenich MM. Organization of somatosensory cortex in primates. In: Schmitt FO, Worden FG, Adelman G, Dennis SG, eds. *The Organization of the Cerebral Cortex*. Cambridge, MA: MIT Press; 1981:237-261.

[28] Buxhoeveden DP, Switala AE, Roy E, Litaker M, Casanova MF. Lateralization in human planum temporale is absent in nonhuman primates. *Brain, Behavior and Evolution*. 2001;57:349-358.

[29] Schlaug G, Schleicher A, Zilles K. Quantitative analysis of the columnar arrangement of neurons in the human cingulate cortex. *Journal of Comparative Neurology*. 1995;351:441-452.

[30] Seldon HL. Structure of human auditory cortex, I: cytoarchitectonics and dendritic distributions. *Brain Research*. 1981;229:277-294.

[31] del Río MR, DeFelipe J. Synaptic connections of calretinin-immunoreactive neurons in the human neocortex. *Journal of Neuroscience*. 1997;17:5143-5154.

[32] Buldyrev SV, Cruz L, Gomez-Isla T, et al. Description of microcolumnar ensembles in association cortex and their disruption in Alzheimer and Lewy body dementias.

Proceedings of the National Academy of Sciences of the United States of America. 2000;97:5039-5043.

[33] Kenan-Vaknin G, Ouaknine GE, Razon N, Malach R. Organization of layers II–III connections in human visual cortex revealed by *in vitro* injections of biocytin. *Brain Research.* 1992;594:339-342.

[34] Morgane PJ, Glezer II, Jacobs MS. Visual cortex of the dolphin: an image analysis study. *Journal of Comparative Neurology.* 1988;273:3-25.

[35] Manger P, Sum M, Szymanski M, Ridgway SH, Krubitzer L. Modular subdivisions of dolphin insular cortex: does evolutionary history repeat itself? *Journal of Cognitive Neuroscience.* 1998;10:153-166.

[36] Buxhoeveden DP, Casanova MF. The minicolumn and evolution of the brain: a review: *Brain, Behavior and Evolution.* 2002;60:125-151.

[37] Leise EM. Modular constructs of nervous systems: a basic principle of design for vertebrates and invertebrates. *Brain Research: Brain Research Reviews.* 1990;15:1-23.

[38] Mountcastle VB. The columnar organization of the neocortex. *Brain.* 1997;120:701-722.

[39] Cherniak C. Component placement optimization in the brain. *Journal of Neuroscience.* 1994;14:2418-2427.

[40] Ringo JL. Neuronal interconnection as a function of brain size. *Brain, Behavior and Evolution.* 1991;38:1-6.

[41] Hubel DH, Wiesel TN. Functional architecture of the macaque monkey visual cortex. *Proceedings of the Royal Society of London, Series B: Containing Papers of a Biological Character.* 1977;198:1-59.

[42] Michael CR. Columnar organization of color cells in monkey's striate cortex. *Journal of Neurophysiology.* 1981;46:587-604.

[43] LeVay S, Hubel DH, Wiesel TN. The pattern of ocular dominance columns in macaque visual cortex revealed by a reduced silver stain. *Journal of Comparative Neurology.* 1975;159:559-576.

[44] Wiesel TN, Hubel DH, Lam DM. Autoradiographic demonstration of ocular-dominance columns in the monkey striate cortex by means of transneuronal transport. *Brain Research.* 1974;79:273-279.

[45] Romanski LM, Bates JF, Goldman-Rakic PS. Auditory belt and parabelt projections to the prefrontal cortex in the rhesus monkey. *Journal of Comparative Neurology.* 1999;403:141-157.

[46] Bourgeois JP. Synaptogenesis, heterochrony and epigenesis in the mammalian neocortex. *Acta Paediatrica (Oslo) Supplement.* 1997;422:27-33.

[47] Amir Y, Harel M, Malach R. Cortical hierarchy reflected in the organization of intrinsic connections in macaque monkey visual cortex. *Journal of Comparative Neurology.* 1993;334:19-46.

[48] Silver MA, Stryker MP. Distributions of synaptic vesicle proteins and GAD65 in deprived and nondeprived ocular dominance columns in layer IV of kitten primary visual cortex are unaffected by monocular deprivation. *Journal of Comparative Neurology.* 2000;422:652-664.

[49] Kornack DR, Rakic P. Radial and horizontal deployment of clonally related cells in the primate neocortex: relationship to distinct mitotic lineages. *Neuron.* 1995;15:311-321.

[50] Rakic, P, Kornack, DR. Neocortical expansion and elaboration during primate evolution: a view from neuroembryology. In: Falk D, Gibson KR, eds. *Evolutionary Anatomy of the Primate Cerebral Cortex.* Cambridge, UK: Cambridge University Press; 2001:30-56.

[51] Creutzfeldt OD. Generality of the functional structure of the neocortex. *Die Naturwissenschaften.* 1977;64:507-517.

[52] Buxhoeveden DP, Lefkowitz W, Loats P, Armstrong E. The linear organization of cell columns in human and nonhuman anthropoid Tpt cortex. *Anatomy and Embryology.* 1996;194:23-36.

[53] Seldon HL. Structure of human auditory cortex, II: axon distributions and morphological correlates of speech perception. *Brain Research.* 1981;229:295-310.

[54] Peters A, Payne BR. Numerical relationships between geniculocortical afferents and pyramidal cell modules in cat primary visual cortex. *Cerebral Cortex.* 1993;3:69-78.

[55] Schmolke C. The ontogeny of dendritic bundles in rabbit visual cortex. *Anatomy and Embryology.* 1989;180:371-381.

[56] Galuske RA, Schlote W, Bratzke H, Singer W. Interhemispheric asymmetries of the modular structure in human temporal cortex. *Science.* 2000;289:1946-1949.

[57] Buxhoeveden DP, Roy E, Switala AE, Casanova MF. Reduced interneuronal space in schizophrenia. *Biological Psychiatry.* 2000;47:681-683.

[58] Anderson B, Southern BD, Powers RE. Anatomic asymmetries of the posterior superior temporal lobes: a postmortem study. *Neuropsychiatry, Neuropsychology, and Behavioral Neurology.* 1999;12:247-254.

[59] Hutsler JJ, Gazzaniga MS. Acetylcholinesterase staining in human auditory and language cortices: regional variation of structural features. *Cerebral Cortex.* 1996;6:260-270.

[60] Buxhoeveden DP, Casanova MF. Comparative lateralisation patterns in the language area of human, chimpanzee, and rhesus monkey brains. *Laterality.* 2000;5:315-330.

[61] LeMay M. Asymmetries of the brains and skulls of nonhuman primates. In: Glick SD, ed. *Cerebral Lateralization in Nonhuman Species.* Orlando, FL: Academic Press; 1985:223-245.

[62] Yeni-Komshian GH, Benson DA. Anatomical study of cerebral asymmetry in the temporal lobe of humans, chimpanzees, and rhesus monkeys. *Science.* 1976;192:387-389.

[63] Gannon P, Holloway RL, Broadfield DC, Braun AR. Asymmetry of chimpanzee planum temporale: humanlike pattern of Wernicke's brain language area homolog. *Science.* 1998;279:220-222.

[64] Hopkins WD, Marino L, Rilling JK, MacGregor LA. Planum temporale asymmetries in great apes as revealed by magnetic resonance imaging (MRI). *Neuroreport.* 1998;9:2913-2918.

[65] Livingstone MS, Hubel DH. Specificity of intrinsic connections in primate connections in primate primary visual cortex. *Journal of Neuroscience.* 1984;4:2830-2835.

[66] Orban GA. *Neuronal Operation in the Visual Cortex.* Berlin, Germany: Springer; 1984.

[67] Letinic K, Rakic P. Telencephalic origin of human thalamic GABAergic neurons. *Nature Neuroscience.* 2001;4:931-936.

[68] Hofman MA. Brain evolution in hominids: Are we at the end of the road? In: Falk D, Gibson KR, eds. *Evolutionary Anatomy of the Primate Cerebral Cortex.* Cambridge, UK: Cambridge University Press; 2001:113-127.

[69] Kaas J. The organization of the neocortex in mammal: implications for theories of brain function. *Annual Review of Psychology.* 1987;38:129-151.

[70] Welker WI. The significance of foliation and fissuration of cerebellar cortex: the cerebellar folium as a fundamental unit of sensorimotor integration. *Archives italiennes de biologie.* 1990;128:87-109.

[71] Favorov OV, Kelly DG. Minicolumnar organization within somatosensory cortical segregates, I: development of afferent connections. *Cerebral Cortex.* 1994;4:408-427.

[72] Ichinohe N, Fujiyama F, Kaneko T, Rockland KS. Honeycomb-like mosaic at the border of layers 1 and 2 in the cerebral cortex. *Journal of Neuroscience.* 2003;23:1372-1382.

[73] Rockel AJ, Hirons RW, Powell TP. The basic uniformity in structure of the neocortex. *Brain.* 1980;103:221-244.

[74] Beaulieu C. Numerical data on neocortical neurons in adult rat, with special reference to the GABA population. *Brain Research.* 1993;609:284-292.

[75] Skoglund TS, Pascher R, Berthold CH. Aspects of the quantitative analysis of neurons in the cerebral cortex. *Journal of Neuroscience Methods.* 1996;70:201-210.

[76] Swindale NV. Is the cerebral cortex modular? *Trends in Neurosciences.* 1990;13:487-492.

[77] Hendrickson AE, Wilson JR, Ogren MP. The neuroanatomical organization of pathways between the dorsal lateral geniculate nucleus and visual cortex in Old World and New World primates. *Journal of Comparative Neurology.* 1978;182:123-136.

[78] Adams DL, Horton JC. The representation of retinal blood vessels in primate striate cortex. *Journal of Neuroscience.* 2003;23:5984-5997.

[79] Buxhoeveden DP, Casanova MF. The minicolumnar hypothesis in neurosciences. *Brain.* 2002;125:935-951.

In: Neocortical Modularity and the Cell Minicolumn
Editor: Manuel F. Casanova, pp. 137-144
ISBN 1-59454-301
© 2005 Nova Science Publishers, Inc.

Chapter VII

The Generation and Migration of Cortical Interneurons

John G. Parnavelas*
University College London, London, UK

Introduction

The cerebral cortex is by far the largest part of the mammalian brain, containing about half of its neurons. Neurons are organized in six layers with each layer containing a complement of the two main neuronal types, the pyramidal and nonpyramidal cells. Pyramidal neurons, which make up approximately 75 % of all neurons of the cortex, are the projection neurons that use the excitatory amino acid glutamate as a neurotransmitter. Nonpyramidal cells, the cortical interneurons, are a much more diverse group of cells that display a range of morphologies and molecular identities. They all contain the inhibitory neurotransmitter GABA as well as one or more neuropeptides and/or calcium-binding proteins [1].

The cerebral cortex develops from the rostral part of the neural tube named the telencephalic pallium. The wall of the pallium is initially formed of neuroepithelial germinal cells whose continued proliferation causes the outward bulging of the pallial walls to form the cerebral vesicles. Neuroepithelial cells close to the ventricular lining of the neural tube, the so-called ventricular zone (VZ), are destined to give rise to neurons and some of the glial cells of the cortex. The radial alignment of the neuroepithelial cells imposes a radial pattern on the histogenesis of the pallium. The conventional scheme of cortical formation [2],[3], described in Figure 1, shows that early postmitotic neurons migrate away from the VZ towards the surface of the cerebral vesicles to form the primordial plexiform layer, or preplate

* Corresponding author: John G. Parnavelas, Department of Anatomy and Developmental Biology, University College London, Gower Street, London WC1E 6BT, UK. Tel +44 20 7679-3366; Fax +44 20 7679-7349; E-mail j.parnavelas@ucl.ac.uk

(PP). The later-generated neurons migrate to form a layer within the PP, the so-called cortical plate (CP), thus splitting it into a superficial marginal zone (MZ; layer I) and a deep subplate (SP). The neurons of the CP assemble into layers II–VI in an "inside-out" sequence, that is, the deepest cellular layers are assembled first and those closest to the surface last. The SP is separated from the VZ by the intermediate zone (IZ), a layer that will eventually contain the afferent and efferent axonal tracts of the cortex (future white matter). As the CP emerges, another layer of proliferating cells appears between the VZ and IZ, the so-called subventricular zone (SVZ). This germinal zone contains cells, produced in the VZ, that give rise to neurons [4] and to most of the glial cells of the cortex [5],[6]. According to this conventional scheme of cortical development, the processes of radial glial cells support and direct the migration of young neurons from the their origin in the VZ to their positions in the CP [7]. However, this view had to be modified recently in light of emerging evidence showing that, in addition to guiding migration, radial glia produce cortical neurons and glia [8]–[11].

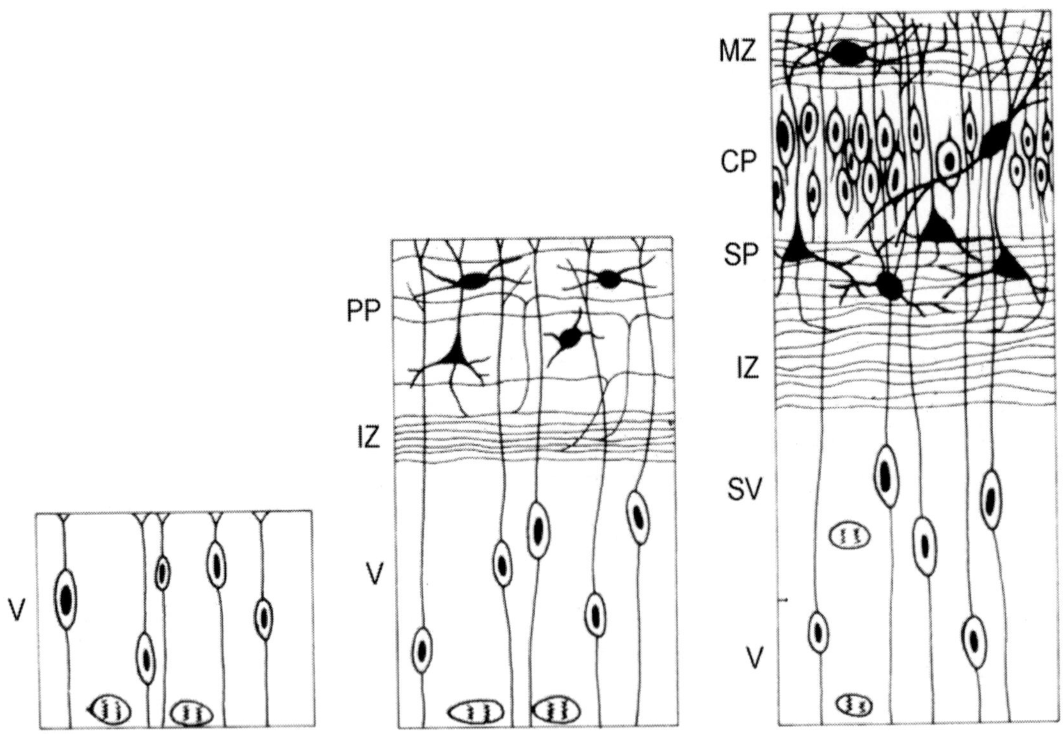

Figure 1. Three panels illustrate the layers of the cerebral wall at different stages of development. VZ, ventricular zone; PP, preplate; IZ, intermediate zone; MZ, marginal zone; CP, cortical plate; SP, subplate; SV, subventricular zone.

Development of Neuronal Lineages

Earlier lineage studies, using defective retroviruses, described single-labeled cells or discrete clusters of two or more neurons in the cerebral cortex of rats and mice following the placement of intraventricular injections at any day of gestation during the period of corticogenesis [12],[13]. The clones of two or more cells contained for the most part either neurons or glial cells. When neuronal clones were examined further by electron microscopy or immunohistochemistry, they were all found to be nearly homogeneous, composed of all pyramidal or all nonpyramidal neurons [14],[15]. These studies suggested that pyramidal and nonpyramidal neurons arise from different progenitors in the VZ. Further examination of clonally related neurons from brains injected with retrovirus at different stages of corticogenesis revealed remarkable differences in the number and laminar distribution of pyramidal and nonpyramidal neurons. Nonpyramidal cells appeared for the most part as single cells and, on very few occasions, as clones of two neurons present in the same or adjacent layers. Clones of pyramidal neurons were larger, and they were either dispersed in one layer or in several layers following earlier injections. Their size and laminar distribution was progressively reduced following later retrovirus injections [15]. This finding suggested the existence of different mechanisms that generate the two main neuronal types of the cerebral cortex. More recent studies have clearly demonstrated that the specification of the pyramidal lineage occurs at the level of the progenitor in the VZ, before the onset of corticogenesis [16]. Further, pyramidal neurons maintain a close spatial relationship with their clonal relatives in the developing cortex, which can be achieved through radial migration [17]. However, nonpyramidal cells have the tendency to be diffusely scattered in the cortex and are likely part of larger clones [16],[17]. This has raised the question of whether the VZ contains progenitors committed to producing only nonpyramidal neurons. The presence in the cortex of a relatively small number of nonpyramidal neurons following intraventricular injections of retrovirus compared to the large pyramidal clones prompted speculation that there are other potential sources of nonpyramidal neurons.

Nonpyramidal Neurons: Origin and Tangential Migration

Sources of neurons destined for the cerebral cortex have been discovered in the ganglionic eminence, the primordium of the basal ganglia in the ventral telencephalon or subpallium. Porteus et al. [18] first reported that cells expressing Dlx2 appear to migrate from the ventral telencephalon to the neocortex. Subsequently, De Carlos et al. [19] and Tamamaki et al. [20] provided strong evidence that cells in the lateral ganglionic eminence (LGE), the primordium of the striatum, migrate into the developing neocortex and are distributed predominantly in the IZ. More recently, a number of studies have confirmed that the cells that migrate from the ventral telencephalon to the cortex are indeed GABAergic (Figure 2) [21]–[25]. Three streams of neurons originating in the ventral telencephalon were observed to round the corticostriatal notch and follow tangentially oriented paths to enter the cortex. An early cohort (E12 in mouse; E14 in rat), originating in the medial ganglionic eminence (MGE), invades mainly the PP. These cells are tangentially oriented and some show features typical of Cajal-Retzius cells. A second and more prominent cohort, composed also of MGE cells, has been observed to migrate predominantly through the IZ slightly later in development (E13-15 mouse; E15-17 rat) (Figure 2A). At the late stages of corticogenesis, cells originating in the LGE and MGE appear in the lower IZ and SVZ [26].

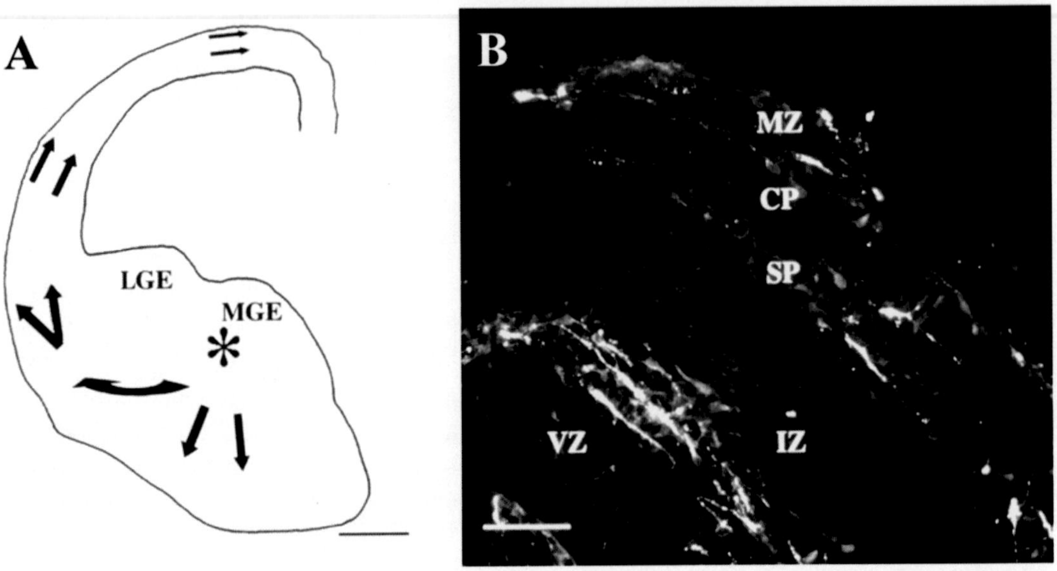

Figure 2. (A) Drawing of a coronal section through part of the rat forebrain after placement of crystals of the fluorescent marker DiI in the medial ganglionic eminence (MGE) at embryonic day 16. Arrows indicate the direction of migration of labeled cells in the cortical primordium 3 days after DiI application. (B) DiI-labeled cells in different layers of the developing cortex and particularly in the lower intermediate zone (IZ), subplate (SP) and marginal zone (MZ). Scale bars: A, 600 μm; B, 100 μm.

Genetic manipulations have provided further evidence for the origin of the cortical GABAergic interneurons in the subpallium. For example, mice lacking transcription factors that regulate regionalization (Nkx2.1) or differentiation (Dlx1/2, Mash1) in the ventral telencephalon have significantly reduced numbers of GABAergic neurons in the cortex [21],[27],[28]. Specifically, Nkx2.1 mutants that lack a functional MGE show approximately a 50 % reduction in GABA-containing neurons in the cortex, but the olfactory bulbs of these mutants contain nearly a normal number of GABAergic cells. In contrast, the Dlx1/2 mutants that lack migration of cells out of the LGE and MGE in slice cultures have about a 75 % reduction of GABA cells in the cortex and virtually no GABAergic cells in the olfactory bulb. These observations suggest that the MGE is the main source of interneurons to the cerebral cortex, while the LGE provides some cells to the cortex and many to the olfactory bulb. In a more recent study, Stühmer et al. [29] have shown that all cortical GABAergic neurons in the adult mouse brain are derived from cells that express the Dlx genes. This finding suggests that the vast majority, if not all, GABA-containing neurons in the rodent cortex are derived from progenitors in the ventral telencephalon.

Little is known about the genes that play a role in the specification and migration of cortical interneurons from the ventral telencephalon. Earlier studies [22] have shown that the origin, migration, and distribution of interneurons in the cortex coincide with the pattern of expression of the LIM-homeobox gene Lhx6 in the developing telencephalon, and indeed, these cells were found to express this transcription factor. The specific expression of Lhx6 in neurons of the MGE, including those destined for the developing cortex, suggested a role for this transcription factor in the neurochemical identity and migration of these neurons. Using RNA interference, recent loss-of-function studies for Lhx6 have found that this transcription factor does not regulate the expression of GABA in MGE neurons, but it does control their migration from the ventral telencephalon [30].

Following their generation, cortical interneurons use the chemorepellent activity provided by Slit1 and other chemotropic signals to move away from the MGE towards the cortex [31]. Their movement is facilitated by hepatocyte growth factor, a known motogen that is produced in the ganglionic eminence [32]. Recent studies have demonstrated that interneurons destined to populate the cortex express neuropilin1 and neuropilin2 receptors, enabling them to respond to chemorepulsive signals provided by class 3 semaphorins in the striatal mantle [33]. Moreover, it seems that the repulsive activity of semaphorins in the developing striatum creates an exclusion zone and channels cortical interneurons into adjacent paths, leading to the formation of the MZ and IZ migratory routes.

Little is known about the substrates used by interneurons to reach the cortex, but their tangential migration appears largely independent of interactions with radial glia. However, a close association has been observed between tangentially oriented cells and corticofugal axons, predominantly in the IZ and MZ of the developing cortex [34], suggesting that interneurons may use this axonal system as a scaffold for their migration into the cortex. Earlier studies had suggested that axons provide a substratum for nonradial migration in the developing CNS including the cerebral cortex [35]. Recent studies have provided evidence that the neural adhesion molecule TAG-1, a member of the immunoglobulin superfamily present on corticofugal fibers, serves as a substrate upon which GABAergic interneurons migrate. Blocking TAG-1 function in cortical slices with anti-TAG-1 antibodies or soluble TAG-1 protein results in marked reduction of migrating GABAergic interneurons [36].

If tangentially migrating neurons use the corticofugal system to enter the neocortex, how do they migrate into specific layers with their pyramidal counterparts? Using time-lapse imaging of cortical slices together with tracer-labeling techniques, Nadarajah et al. [37] have shown that interneurons arising in the ventral telencephalon actively migrate towards the cortical VZ upon reaching the dorsal telencephalon, a mode of movement that has been termed "ventricle-directed migration." After a pause in this proliferative zone, they migrate radially in the direction of the pial surface to take positions in the developing CP.

Earlier birthdating studies [38] and more recent transplantation experiments [23] have demonstrated that, similar to pyramidal cells, cortical interneurons are disposed in an "inside-out" pattern within the CP. How is it that two neuronal types generated in two distinct regions of the developing brain, the pallium and subpallium, and shown to follow different migratory paths can assemble in the cortex in a way that they are linked temporally and spatially? Nadarajah and colleagues [37] have proposed that cortical interneurons follow ventricle-directed migration actively seeking the VZ to obtain the type of positional information that the pyramidal cells acquire prior to becoming postmitotic. These cues may be obtained from the local environment or from the pyramidal cells themselves through neural-neural interactions. The mechanism that guides interneurons to the VZ before they move to the positions in the developing cortex is not known, but a combination of chemoattractant (e.g., semaphorins) and chemorepellent (e.g., Slit) molecules may be involved.

REFERENCES

[1] Parnavelas JG, Dinopoulos A, Davies SW. The central visual pathways. In: Björklund A, Hökfelt T, Swanson LW, eds. *Handbook of Chemical Neuroanatomy*, vol. 7, part II. Amsterdam, Netherlands: Elsevier; 1989:1-164.

[2] Boulder Committee. Embryonic vertebrate central nervous system: revised terminology. *Anatomical Record.* 1970;166:257-261.

[3] Uylings HBM, Van Eden CG, Parnavelas JG, Kalsbeek A. The prenatal and postnatal development of rat cerebral cortex. In Kolb B, Tees RC, eds. *The Cerebral Cortex of the Rat*. Cambridge, MA: MIT Press; 1990:35-76.

[4] Noctor SC, Martínez-Cerdeño V, Ivic L, Kriegstein AR. Cortical neurons arise in symmetric and asymmetric division zones and migrate through specific phases. *Nature Neuroscience.* 2004;7:136-144.

[5] Levison SW, Goldman JE. Both oligodendrocytes and astrocytes develop from progenitors in the subventricular zone of postnatal rat forebrain. *Neuron.* 1993;10:201-212.

[6] Parnavelas JG. Glial cell lineages in the rat cerebral cortex. *Experimental Neurology.* 1999;156:418-429.

[7] Rakic P. Mode of cell migration to the superficial layers of fetal monkey neocortex. *Journal of Comparative Neurology.* 1972;145:61-83.

[8] Miyata T, Kawaguchi A, Okano H, Ogawa M. Asymmetric inheritance of radial glial fibers by cortical neurons. *Neuron.* 2001;31:727-741.

[9] Noctor SC, Flint AC, Weissman TA, Dammerman RS, Kriegstein AR. Neurons derived from radial glial cells establish radial units in neocortex. *Nature.* 2001;409:714-720.

[10] Parnavelas JG, Nadarajah B. Radial glial cells: are they really glia? *Neuron.* 2001;31:881-884.

[11] Heins N, Malatesta P, Cessoni F, et al. Glial cells generate neurons: the role of the transcription factor Pax6. *Nature Neuroscience.* 2002;5:308-315.

[12] Price J, Turner D, Cepko C. Lineage analysis in the vertebrate nervous system by retrovirus mediated gene transfer. *Proceedings of the National Academy of Sciences.* 1987;84:156-160.

[13] Luskin MB, Pearlman AL, Sanes JR. Cell lineage in the cerebral cortex of the mouse studied *in vivo* and *in vitro* with a recombinant retrovirus. *Neuron.* 1988;1:635-647.

[14] Parnavelas JG, Barfield JA, Franke E, Luskin MB. Separate progenitor cells give rise to pyramidal and nonpyramidal neurons in the rat telencephalon. *Cerebral Cortex.* 1991;1:463-468.

[15] Luskin MB, Parnavelas JG, Barfield JA. Neurons, astrocytes, and oligodendrocytes of the rat cerebral cortex originate from separate progenitor cells: an ultrastructural analysis of clonally related cells. *Journal of Neuroscience.* 1993;13:1750-1770.

[16] Tan SS, Kalloniatis M, Sturm K, Tam PP, Reese BE, Faulkner-Jones B. Separate progenitors for radial and tangential cell dispersion during development of the cerebral cortex. *Neuron.* 1998;21:295-304.

[17] Mione MC, Cavanagh JFR, Harris B, Parnavelas JG. Cell fate specification and symmetrical/asymmetrical divisions in the developing cerebral cortex. *Journal of Neuroscience.* 1997;17:2018-2029.

[18] Porteus MH, Bulfone A, Liu JK, Puelles L, Lo LC, Rubenstein JLR. DLX-2, MASH-1, and MAP-2 expression and bromodeoxyuridine incorporation define molecularly distinct cell populations in the embryonic mouse forebrain. *Journal of Neuroscience.* 1994;14:6370-6383.

[19] De Carlos JA, Lopez-Mascaraque L, Valverde F. Dynamics of cell migration from the lateral ganglionic eminence in the rat. *Journal of Neuroscience.* 1996;16:6146-6156.

[20] Tamamaki N, Fugimori KE, Takauji R. Origin and route of tangentially migrating neurons in the developing neocortical intermediate zone. *Journal of Neuroscience.* 1997;17:8313-8323.

[21] Anderson SA, Eisenstat DD, Shi L, Rubensteinn JLR. Interneuron migration from the basal forebrain to neocortex: dependence on *Dlx* genes. *Science.* 1997;278:474-476.

[22] Lavdas AA, Grigoriou M, Pachnis V, Parnavelas JG. The medial ganglionic eminence gives rise to a population of early neurons in the developing cerebral cortex. *Journal of Neuroscience.* 1999;19;7881-7888.

[23] Wichterle H, Turnbull DH, Nery S, Fishell G, Alvarez-Buylla A. In utero fate mapping reveals distinct migratory pathways and fates of neurons born in the mammalian basal forebrain. *Development.* 2001;128:3759-3771.

[24] Anderson SA, Kaznowski CE, Horn C, Rubenstein JLR, McConnell SK. Distinct origins of neocortical projection neurons and interneurons *in vivo*. *Cerebral Cortex.* 2002;12:702-709.

[25] Valcanis H, Tan SS. Layer specification of transplanted interneurons in the developing mouse neocortex. *Journal of Neuroscience.* 2003;23:5113-5122.

[26] Anderson SA, Marin O, Horn C, Jennings K, Rubenstein JLR. Distinct cortical migrations from the medial and lateral ganglionic eminences. *Development.* 2001;128:353-363.

[27] Casarosa S, Fode C, Guillemot F. *Mash1* regulates neurogenesis in the ventral telencephalon. *Development.* 1999;126:525-534.

[28] Sussel L, Marin O, Kimura S, Rubenstein JLR. Loss of *Nkx2.1* homeobox gene function results in a ventral to dorsal molecular respecification within the basal telencephalon: evidence for a transformation of the pallidum into the striatum. *Development.* 1999;126:3359-3370.

[29] Stühmer T, Puelles L, Ekker M, Rubenstein JLR. Expression of a *Dlx* gene enhancer marks adult mouse cortical GABAergic neurons. *Cerebral Cortex.* 2002;12:75-85.

[30] Alifragis P, Liapi A, Parnavelas JG. Lhx6 regulates the migration of cortical interneurons from the ventral telencephalon but does not specify their GABA phenotype. *Journal of Neuroscience*. 2004;24:5643-5648.

[31] Zhu Y, Li H, Zhou L, Wu JY, Rao Y. Cellular and molecular guidance of GABAergic neuronal migration from an extracortical origin to the neocortex. *Neuron.* 1999;23:473-485.

[32] Powell EM, Mars WM, Levitt P. Hepatocyte growth factor/scatter factor is a motogen for interneurons migrating from the ventral to dorsal telencephalon. *Neuron.* 2001;30:79-89.

[33] Marin O, Yaron A, Bagri A, Tessier-Lavigne M, Rubenstein JLR. Sorting of striatal and cortical interneurons regulated by semaphorin-neuropilin interactions. *Science.* 2001;293:872-875.

[34] Metin C, Godement P. The ganglionic eminence may be an intermediate target for corticofugal and thalamocortical axons. *Journal of Neuroscience.* 1996;16:3219-3235.

[35] Rakic P. Contact regulation of neuronal migration. In: Edelman GM, Thiery JP, eds. *The Cell in Contact*. New York, NY: Wiley; 1985:67-91.

[36] Denaxa M, Chan CH, Schachner M, Parnavelas JG, Karagogeos D. The adhesion molecule TAG-1 mediates the migration of cortical interneurons from the ganglionic eminence along the corticofugal fiber system. *Development.* 2001;128:4635-4644.

[37] Nadarajah B, Alifragis P, Wong ROL, Parnavelas JG. Ventricle-directed migration in the developing cerebral cortex. *Nature Neuroscience.* 2002;5:218-224.

[38] Miller MW. Cogeneration of retrogradely labeled corticocortical projection and GABA-immunoreactive local circuit neurons in cerebral cortex. *Developmental Brain Research.* 1985;23:187-192.

ACKNOWLEDGEMENTS

Research in our laboratory was supported by the Wellcome Trust.

In: Neocortical Modularity and the Cell Minicolumn
Editor: Manuel F. Casanova, pp. 145-160
ISBN 1-59454-301
© 2005 Nova Science Publishers, Inc.

Chapter VIII

MINICOLUMNAR PATTERNS IN THE GLOBAL CORTICAL RESPONSE TO SENSORY STIMULATION

Mark Tommerdahl,* Joannellyn Chiu and Oleg V. Favorov
Department of Biomedical Engineering,
University of North Carolina School of Medicine, Chapel Hill, North Carolina
Barry L. Whitsel
Department of Cellular and Molecular Physiology,
University of North Carolina at Chapel Hill

INTRODUCTION

In 1978 Mountcastle [1] hypothesized that the smallest functional unit of neocortical organization (the "minicolumn") is a radial cord of cells about 30–50 μm in diameter, and that sensory stimuli activate local groupings of minicolumns (called "macrocolumns"). This hypothesis subsequently received support from multiple lines of experimental evidence, leading to its substantial elaboration.

Structurally, minicolumns are attributable to the radially-oriented cords of neuronal cell bodies evident in Nissl-stained sections of cerebral cortex. It is likely that they also are related to ontogenetic columns [2] and to the radially-oriented modules defined by the clustering of the apical dendrites of pyramidal neurons [3]. Among the various elements of neocortical microarchitecture, *spiny-stellate* cells and *double-bouquet* cells [4–6] are most directly relevant to Mountcastle's concept of the minicolumn. Spiny-stellates are excitatory intrinsic cells that are especially prominent in layer 4 of primary sensory cortex. They are the

* Corresponding author: Mark Tommerdahl, Associate Professor, Department of Biomedical Engineering, 434 MacNider Hall, CB #7575, University of North Carolina School of Medicine, Chapel Hill, North Carolina 27599-7575; Telephone: (919)966-8985; E-mail: Mark_Tommerdahl@med.unc.edu

major recipients of thalamocortical connections and, in turn, they (especially the star pyramid subclass of spiny-stellates) distribute afferent input radially to cells in other layers. Double-bouquet cells are GABAergic cells whose somas and dendritic trees are confined to the superficial layers. The axons of double-bouquet cells descend in tight 50 μm diameter bundles across layers 3 and 4 and into layer 5, making synapses along the way on the distal dendrites of pyramidal and spiny-stellate cells, but avoiding the main shaft of apical dendrites [4,5,7,8]. Because the double-bouquet cells are more likely to inhibit cells in adjacent minicolumns rather than in their own, they offer a mechanism by which a minicolumn can inhibit its immediate neighbors.

Overall, the detailed features of primary sensory cortical microarchitecture are clearly suggestive of a *structural* substrate for the minicolumns hypothesized by Mountcastle. But it remains unproven that these structurally-defined units act as *functional* entities—that is, that there is a minicolumnar dimension to primary sensory cortical information processing and representation. In this paper we review some of the experimental evidence that supports the proposal that primary sensory cortical information processing and representation exhibits a minicolumnar nature, and consider the possible functional utility of this dimension of the primary sensory cortical response to natural stimulation of peripheral receptors.

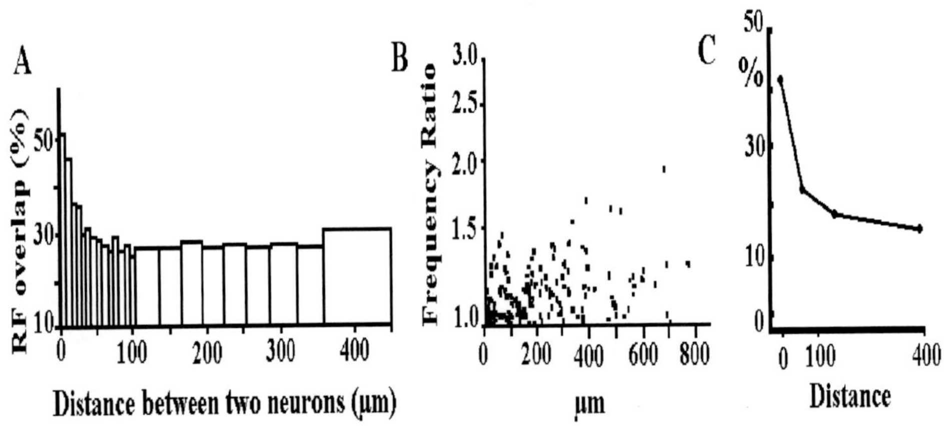

Figure 1. RF similarity as a function of the tangential distance separating neurons in primary sensory cortex. The plots show that neurons that are near neighbors in the tangential plane of the cortex have very similar RF properties, and that similarity declines with increasing distance. The decline in RF similarity with increasing tangential separation has two distinct phases: In the first phase, at separations less than 50 μm, average RF similarity declines very quickly with distance; in the second phase, at separations greater than 50 μm the rate of decline is much slower. In contrast, neurons with very similar RFs are found at much greater separations in the radial dimesion of sensory cortex—a finding that suggests the presence of radially-oriented strands of cells, <50 μm in diameter, within each there is relatively limited RF diversity (see refs. 9 and 10 for in-depth discussion). (A) Ordinate indicates the average degree of RF overlap of pairs of neurons in somatosensory cortex (reproduced, with modifications, from Favorov and Whitsel [9]). (B) Ordinate indicates the ratio of optimal stimulus frequencies of pairs of cells in auditory cortex (higher frequency/lower frequency; reproduced with permission from Abeles and Goldstein [11]). (C) The ordinate is the frequency of encountering 2 visual cortical neurons with optimal stimulus orientations differing by less than 7.5° (reproduced, with modifications, from Albus [13]).

MINICOLUMNAR RECEPTIVE FIELD ORGANIZATION

Receptive field (RF) mapping studies carried out in primary somatosensory cortex (SI) of cats and monkeys obtained experimental evidence that strongly supports Mountcastle's minicolumnar hypothesis [9,10]. These studies found that the receptive fields (RFs) of neurons within fine (~50 μm in diameter) radial cords are very similar in size, shape, and position on the skin. In contrast, the same studies found that neurons located in adjacent minicolumns typically have RFs that differ significantly in size and shape, and frequently overlap only minimally on the skin (on average, RFs of neurons in adjacent minicolumns overlap by only 22 % in cat, and 28 % in macaque monkey). Comparable results have been reported in the primary auditory and visual cortical areas of cat and monkey [11–13]. These findings are schematically summarized in Figure 1.

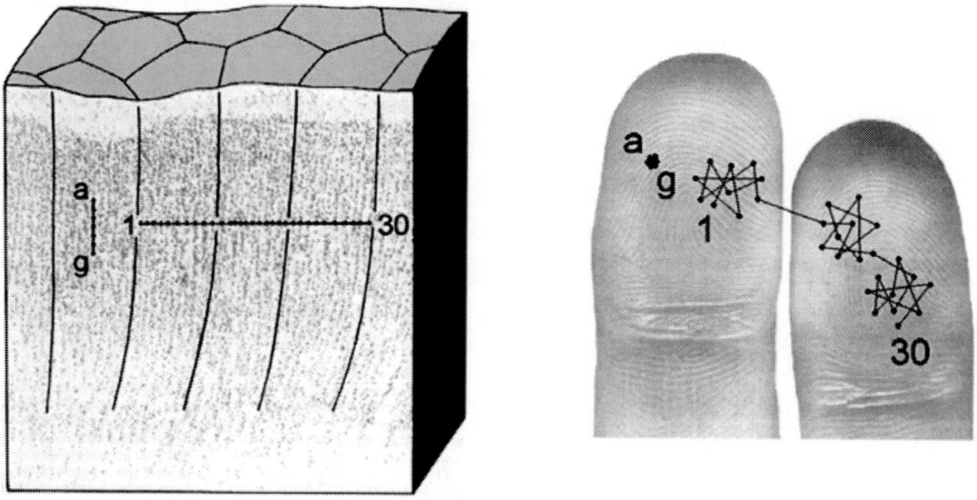

Figure 2. Summary of minicolumnar RF organization in SI somatosensory cortex. Left: Drawing of cross-section of Nissl-stained cortical tissue showing darkly-stained cell bodies organized in radially oriented cords, interpreted as minicolumns. Filled circles labeled *a–g*—sequence of neurons located within a single minicolumn; *1–30*—sequence of neurons located in series of adjacent minicolumns. Right: Sequences of RF centers (connected dots) mapped by neuron sequences *a–g* and *1–30*. Note that RF centers for SI neurons that occupy the same minicolumn stay close together, whereas the RF centers for pairs of neurons located in neighboring minicolumns shift back and forth over large distances, and occupy totally non-overlapping skin regions when the pair of neurons occupies different SI macrocolumns. Based on Favorov and Whitsel [9], and Favorov and Diamond [10].

Most of the experimental literature that has addressed the topographical organization within the primary somatosensory, visual, auditory, and motor cortical areas (and association cortex as well) at high resolution shows that while neighboring neurons exhibit a remarkable uniformity from the standpoint of some RF property (e.g., stimulus orientation in visual cortex), they tend to differ prominently in other properties (for review see ref. [14]). In fact, when sensory cortical neuron RF dimensions are considered *in toto*, neighboring neurons typically have little in common—that is, a stimulus optimal for one cell frequently activates its neighbor much less effectively. The studies reviewed above [9–13,15] suggest, however, that this prominent diversity in the receptive field properties of neurons located in the same locale in sensory cortex is constrained substantially in the radial dimension—that is, cells that occupy the same radially-oriented minicolumn have very similar RF properties. In other words, the tendency for the RF properties among neighboring sensory cortical neurons to be different is mainly attributable to the diverse RF properties of neurons that occupy neighboring minicolumns. Figure 2 illustrates the minicolumnar organization of single neuron RF properties that published studies have identified within cat and monkey primary sensory cortex.

Model of Minicolumnar RF Formation

The predominance of radially-oriented intrinsic connectivity within cerebral cortex clearly predicts that cells lying in a particular minicolumn will have very similar RFs. But why are the RFs of neurons in adjacent minicolumns so different? Favorov and Kelly [16,17] suggested in a modeling study that during perinatal development minicolumns might actively drive their neighbors to establish afferent connections with different, only partially overlapping sets of thalamic neurons. This might be accomplished via the lateral inhibitory interactions among adjacent minicolumns expressed via the connectivity attributable to double-bouquet cells. In the model of Favorov and Kelly [16,17] (shown schematically in Figure 3) each minicolumn is driven during self-organization of the network by inhibitory interactions with adjacent minicolumns (mediated by double-bouquet cells) to acquire a set of afferent (thalamic) connections *different* from those of its immediate neighbors. On the other hand, each minicolumn also is driven by excitatory interactions with neurons in a larger circle of neighboring minicolumns (mediated by spiny-stellate cells) to make its set of afferent connections *similar* to theirs. According to this model these opposing pressures are satisfied by the achievement (during early development) of a permuted arrangement of the minicolumns in the macrocolumn. To achieve this arrangement the RFs of adjacent minicolumns in the macrocolumn move farther apart, and at the same time the RFs of the entire macrocolumn are prevented from diverging too widely. In this way the model of Favorov and Kelly [16,17] generates complex patterns of RFs across the macrocolumn similar to those observed experimentally in microelectrode penetrations through SI cortex in adult subjects [10,16,17].

In Vivo Stimulus-evoked Minicolumnar Activity Patterns

Because of the prominent differences in RF properties that exist among neighboring minicolumns in sensory cortex in adults, even the simplest sensory stimulus should evoke a spatially complex minicolumnar pattern of activity in the engaged cortical region—such a pattern consisting of a patchwork of active and inactive minicolumns [17]. This expectation is in accord with experimental observations obtained in high-resolution 2-deoxyglucose (2-

DG) metabolic studies of mouse (barrel field) and monkey SI [18–20]. Those studies revealed not only that the distribution of stimulus-evoked 2-DG labeling in somatosensory cortex is modular on a macrocolumnar scale, but is highly non-uniform within such a macrocolumnar module. Analysis of the spatial distribution of activity within the characteristic column-shaped patches of 2-DG label evoked in primary somatosensory cortex by natural skin stimuli suggested that such patches are made up of groupings of highly active minicolumns interdigitated with less active minicolumns. The experimental evidence that led the authors to propose this concept is summarized in Figure 4.

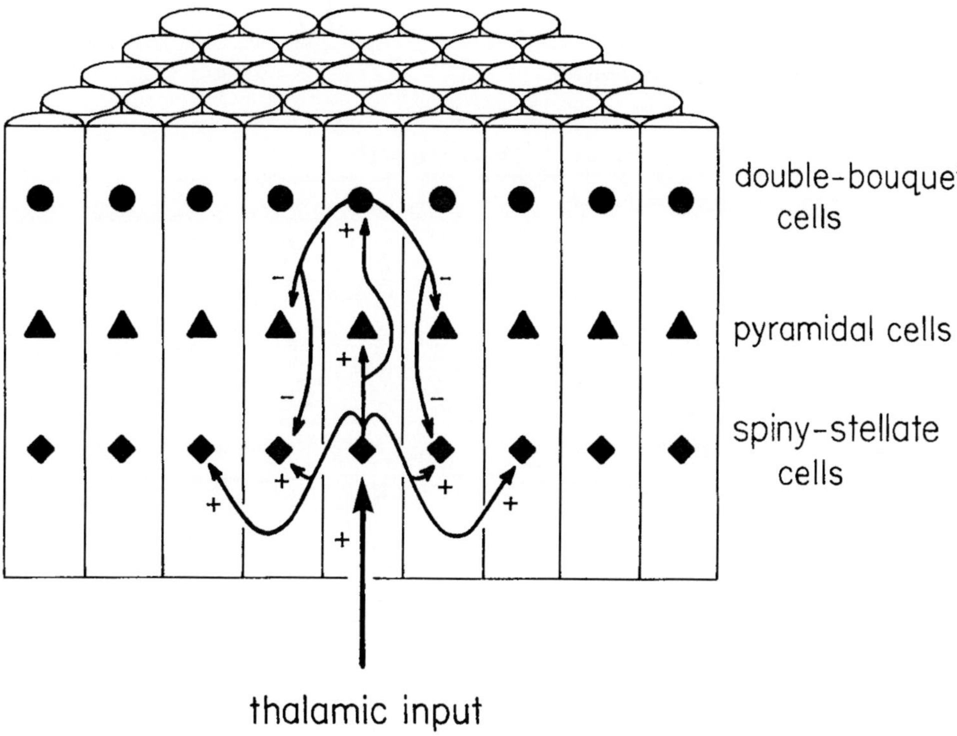

Figure 3. Pattern of minicolumnar connections (modified from Favorov and Kelly [16]). Shown is a section across an idealized cortical region, represented as a tightly packed field of cylinder-shaped minicolumns, each containing one representative spiny stellate, pyramidal, and double bouquet cells. Afferent, intra-minicolumnar, and local inter-minicolumnar connections are shown for one minicolumn.

More recently our laboratory has employed a very different imaging modality to continue our investigation of the response of primary somatosensory cortex at the minicolumnar level of resolution—in these studies we used near-infrared (830 nm) imaging of the optical intrinsic signal (OIS) evoked by mechanical stimulation of the skin [21,22]. The spatial resolution of this imaging method is fine enough to enable direct visualization of stimulus-evoked patterns of active/inactive minicolumns in local cortical territories viewed from above. An example of such a minicolumnar activity pattern within SI cortex of the cat is shown in Figure 5.

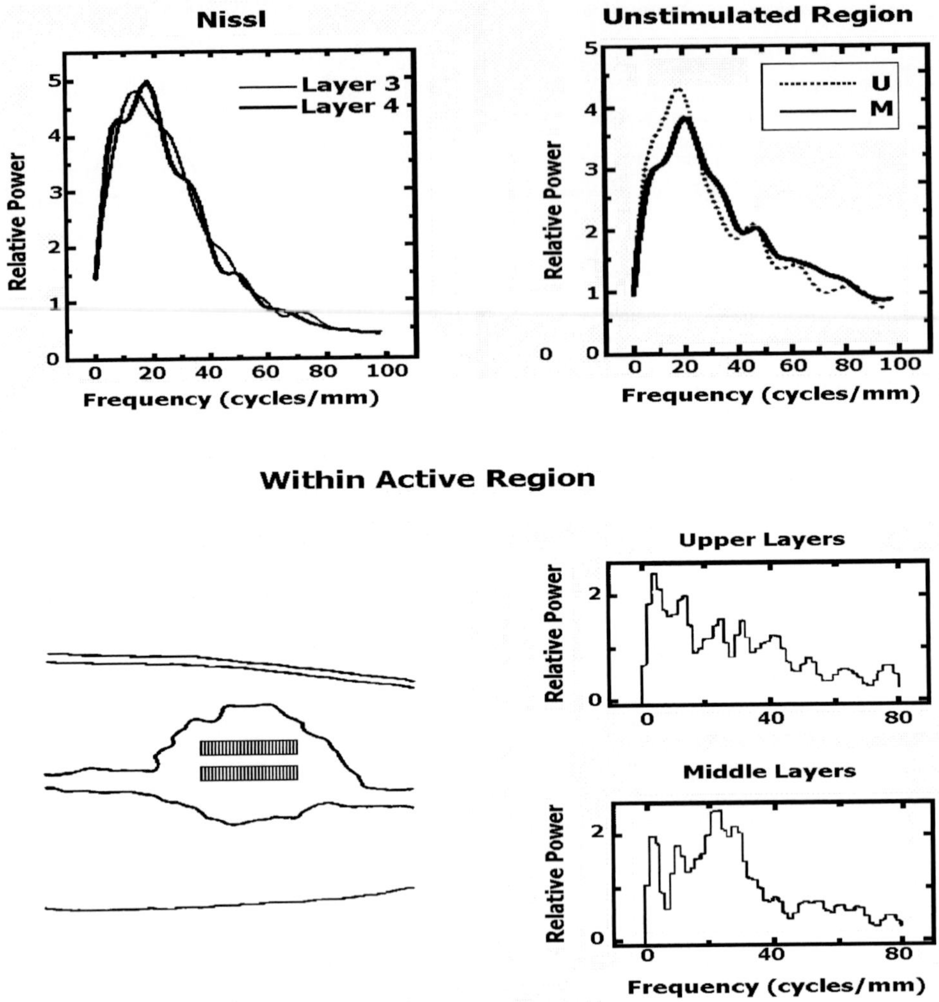

Figure 4. Minicolumnar pattern of stimulus-evoked activation in monkey SI cortex: Spatial frequency analysis of stimulus-evoked 2-DG labeling (modified from Tommerdahl *et al.* [20]). Discrete Fourier transforms were computed across linear, tangentially-oriented sectors of middle and upper cortical layers, and plotted as periodograms. *Top-left:* Average periodograms for optical density data sampled from Nissl-stained sections of SI cortex. Note that distribution of spatial frequencies is the same in the upper and middle layers, and that the radial striation of Nissl-stained sections is reflected by the prominent peak near the minicolumnar frequency of 20 cycles/mm. *Top-right:* Average periodograms of 2-DG labeling in an unstimulated region of SI. Note close similarity of periodograms for 2-DG labeling to those obtained from Nissl-stained sections: both demonstrate prominent minicolumnar periodicity of 20 cycles/mm. *Bottom:* Outline of a patch of above-background 2-DG labeling in a section through stimulus-activated SI region. Fourier transforms were computed across the two rectangular regions and plotted as periodograms on the right. Note that the periodogram of the middle layers is similar to those obtained from both the unstimulated region and the Nissl-stained sections, in that its peak is near to the minicolumnar frequency. In contrast, in the upper-layer periodogram the peak is prominently shifted to lower spatial frequencies, indicating that in the upper layers the activated SI column consists of interdigitated radial strands of elevated and near-background 2-DG labeling. This outcome suggests that neighboring minicolumns were differentially activated by the stimuli that were used.

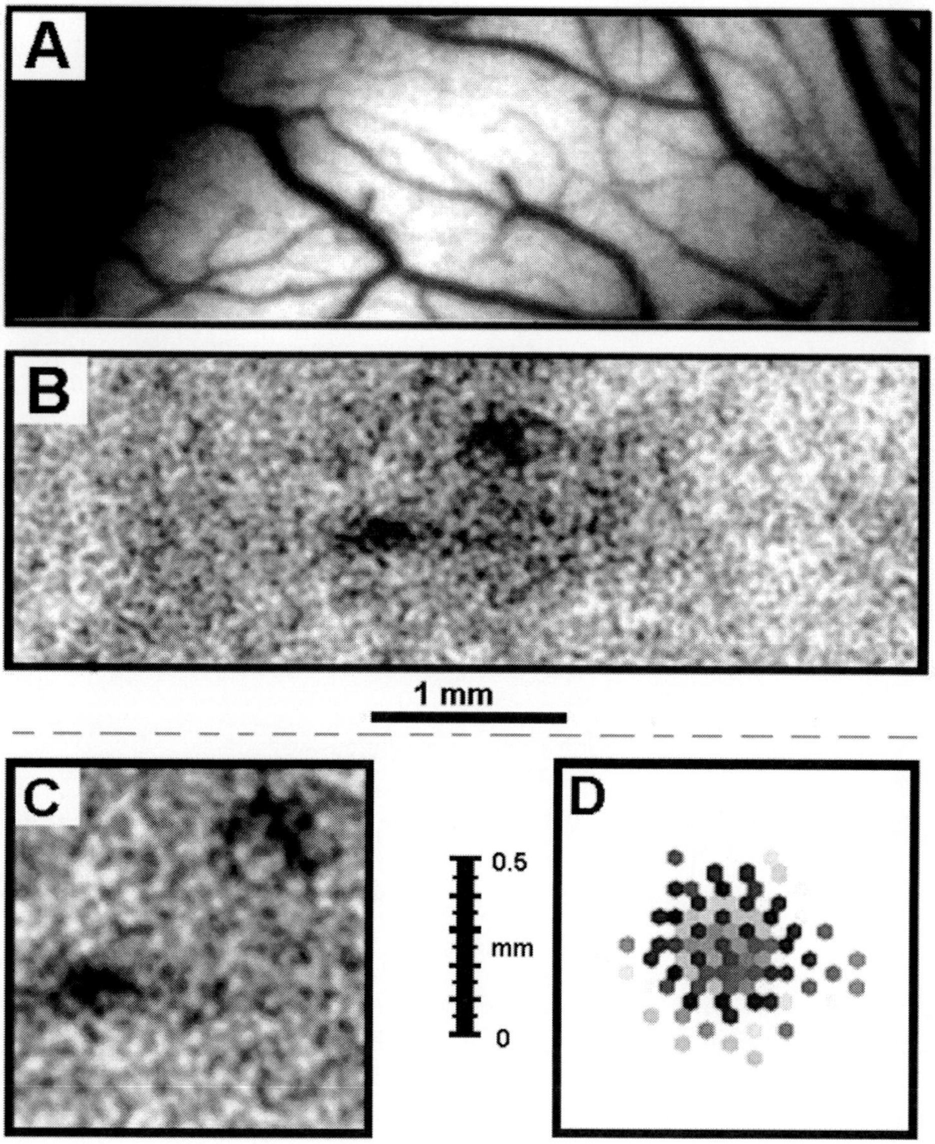

Figure 5. Minicolumnar pattern of activation in cat SI cortex: OIS imaging of the stimulus-evoked intrinsic signal (*B & C*) and modeling prediction (*D*). The response in B and C was evoked by 400 μm amplitude 25 Hz vibrotactile stimulation of the ulnar eminence on a contralateral foreleg. Image in B shows two activated cortical regions, the bottom one in area 3b, top one in area 3a. Upon closer inspection shown in C, each active region appears to consist of a patchwork of minicolumn-sized spots. Note that the spots tend to be organized in short parallel strings, and that orientation of the strings varies across the activated region. Image in D was generated by the minicolumnar model of Favorov and Kelly. [16,17] It shows a spatial pattern of active minicolumns, driven by a punctate stimulus. This model-generated pattern is similar to the one on the left in that minicolumns activated by the stimulus are also organized in short parallel strings which run in different directions in different parts of the pattern.

The optical intrinsic signal (OIS) is an activity-dependent change in the light scattering properties of neural tissue. Although both the OIS evoked in cortical tissue by natural stimulation and the OIS evoked in a cortical slice by electrical stimulation co-localize with stimulus-evoked neuronal activity, and increase in magnitude with increasing stimulus intensity, the OIS recorded *in vivo* or *in vitro* is primarily non-neuronal in origin. That is, the OIS mainly reflects the changes in the extracellular space and cell swelling attributable to glia and neurons. Specifically, repetitive activity in a neuronal population leads to a local excess of potassium and glutamate in the extracellular space that, after a brief delay, is restored to normal by the surrounding glia. The movement of potassium from the extracellular space into glial cells (via ion pumps, transporters and channels), is accompanied by glial uptake of water and swelling. The resultant decrease in extracellular space causes the stimulus-activated region in a brain slice to increase its light transmittance, and the stimulus-activated region in the cortex of an intact subject to undergo an increase in light absorbance. Since the glial swelling that results from uptake of the activity-related excesses in extracellular potassium and glutamate are highly correlated with the degree and spatial extent of neuronal activity, the change in light transmittance *in vitro* can be used to characterize the spatial characteristics of the distributed response of the neocortical slice to controlled afferent drive, and the increase in absorbance observed *in vivo* can be used to evaluate the spatially distributed response of the intact sensory cortex to natural skin stimulation.

In Vitro Stimulus-evoked Minicolumnar Activity Patterns

Optical imaging has been used extensively to study the global patterns of response to natural tactile stimulation [21–24]. However, only a few studies have evaluated the minicolumnar patterns of activity evoked by skin stimulation (e.g., Figure 5). *In vitro* studies of the sensory cortical response to controlled afferent drive at the minicolumnar level of resolution are also relatively rare, but the few studied of this type that have been carried out have provided observations that make it evident that the column-shaped SI response evoked by stimulation at layer VI/WM border is not spatially homogenous (Figure 6). Instead, spatial frequency analysis revealed that although all minicolumns are activated at the level of the cortex at which most direct thalamocortical afferents terminate (i.e., layer IV), at more superficial levels (in layers II-III) activated groupings of minicolumns in the responding macrocolumn are separated from one another by less active minicolumns [25].

The above-described spatial variations in OIS intensity indicate the presence of a repeating radially-oriented structure within layer IV of the responding column with a center-to-center spacing equal to that of the cortical minicolumn. That these spatial variations correspond to activated minicolumns is supported by the observation that no change in spatial frequency occurred in the radial direction. More recently, we have investigated the patterns of SI minicolumnar activation detected under different stimulus conditions *in vitro*. Figure 7 exemplifies the influence of increasing stimulus intensity of electrical stimulation in the sensorimotor cortical slice on the spectral content of the stimulus evoked OIS.

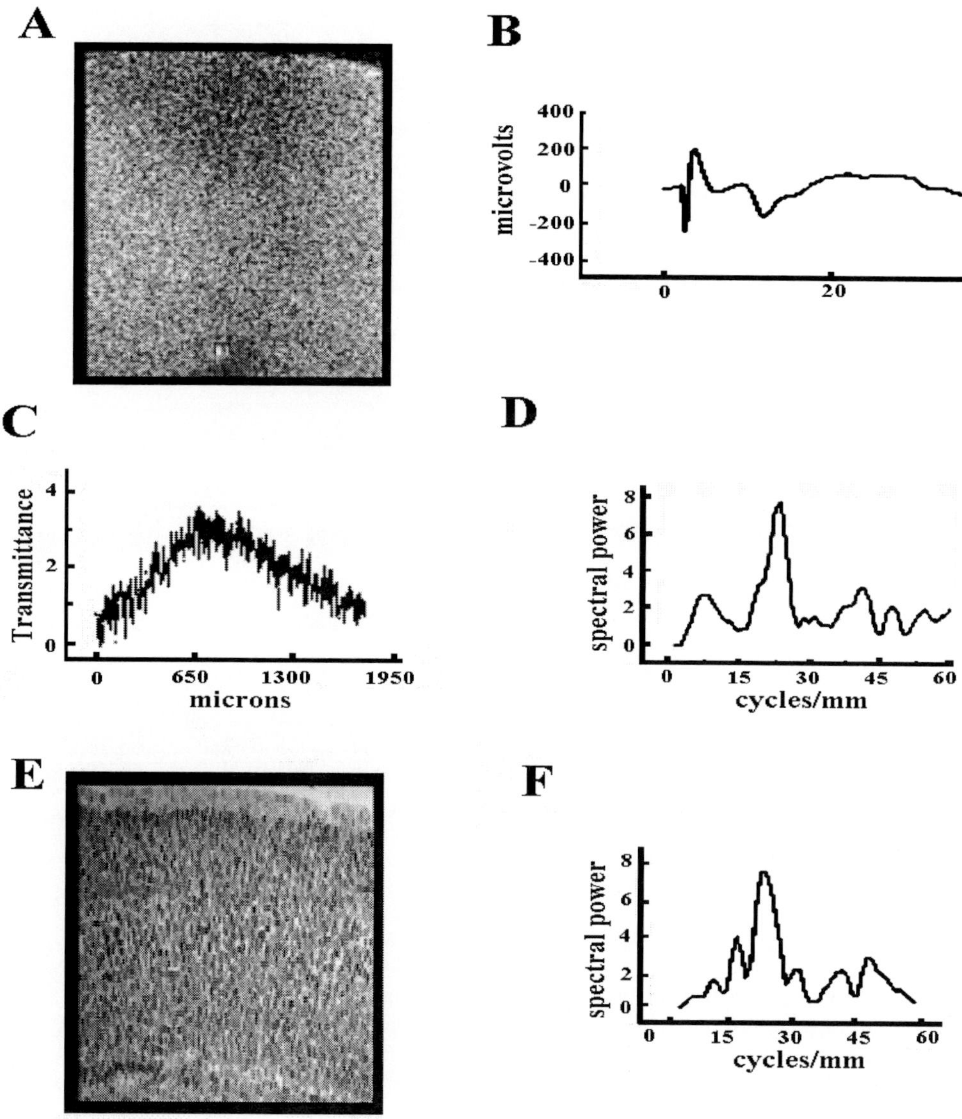

Figure 6. Measures of OIS minicolumnar SI activity patterns *in vitro* in rat somatosensory cortical slice preparation. *(A)* Image of column-shaped OIS evoked by a threshold pulse stimulus delivered to the layer VI/WM junction. *(B)* Evoked potential evoked from the same layer VI/WM locus by single pulse at same intensity. *(C)* Spatial intensity histogram obtained by averaging all pixel values sampled radially across middle layers. *(D)* Power spectrum of the spatial intensity histogram in C. Note a prominent peak at approximately minicolumnar frequency of 24 cycles/mm, or 42 μm period, as well as a second peak at ~8 cycles/mm. *(E)* Image of a Nissl-stained section from the same slice that yielded the OIS response in A. *(F)* Power spectrum of the distribution of optical densities in layer IV of the Nissl-stained section. Note the presence of a peak at the minicolumnar frequency, but not at the frequency of ~8 cycles/mm. This difference in power spectra of OIS and Nissl images suggests that the stimulus activated the cortical macrocolumn non-uniformly, preferentially driving on average every third minicolumn.

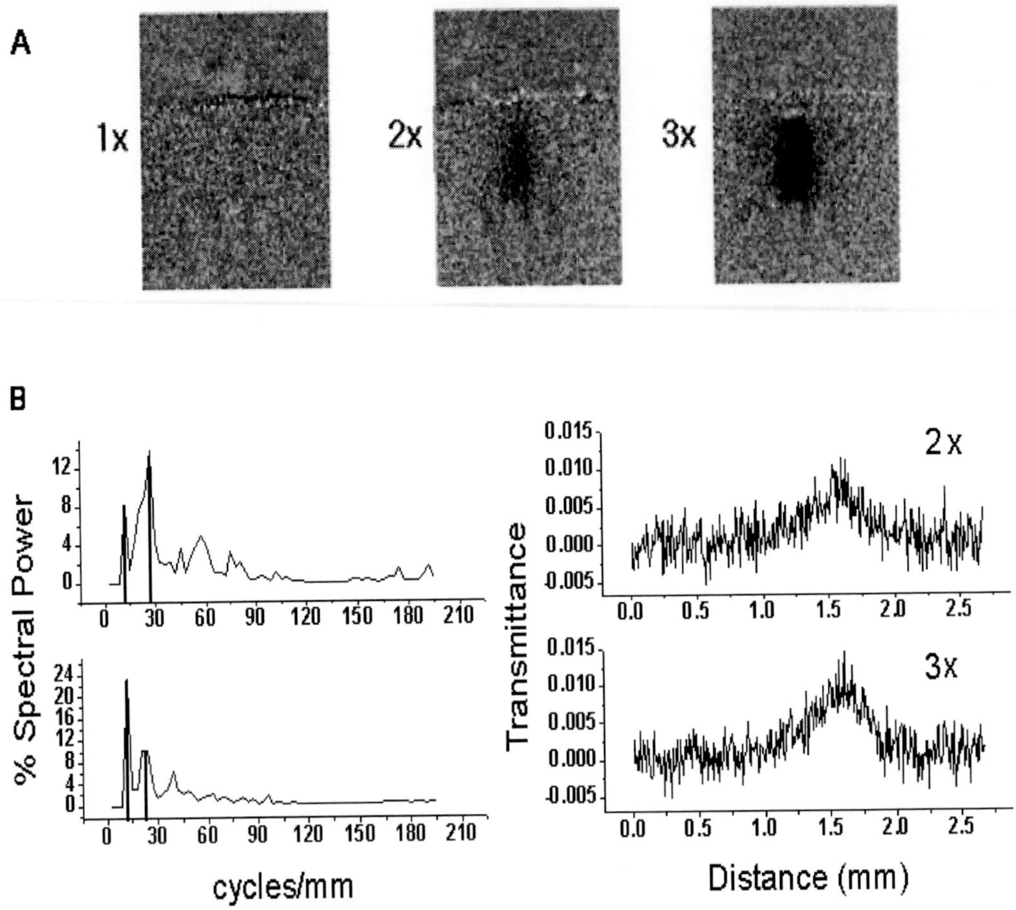

Figure 7. Stimulus intensity influences the pattern of minicolumnar activity within the responding SI macrocolumn. *A*: 3 OIS images obtained in response to 3 different intensities of stimulation (1×, 2×, and 3× threshold) delivered to the layer VI/WM junction. *B: Left column:* Power spectra of OIS activity across the columnar response evoked by stimuli of two different intensities (2× and 3× threshold). *Right Column:* Histograms showing spatial distribution of the response at each stimulus intensity. Note that at both stimulus intensities the spectrum contains two peaks—one at the minicolumnar frequency of 25 cycles/mm, or 40 μm period, the other at 13 cycles/mm, or 80 μm period. However, the relative powers of these two peaks change with stimulus intensity, with 13 cycles/mm frequency growing in power at stronger stimulus.

While prominent power is observed at the minicolumnar spatial frequency (~25 cycles/mm) when using relatively low intensities of layer VI/WM stimulation, a consistent leftward shift in the power spectrum occurs when higher intensities of stimulation are used. We interpret this enhanced low-frequency component at higher intensities of stimulation to be a result of increased local lateral interactions among minicolumns, resulting in significant numbers of minicolumns becoming inhibited, or "turned off," by their neighbors.

We also have initiated an examination of the patterns of SI minicolumnar activity evoked by multi-site afferent drive more representative of the spatially distributed input patterns evoked *in vivo* by natural skin stimuli. Figure 8 demonstrates a method which provides detailed information about this more complex, but probably much more realistic pattern of afferent drive. Arrays consisting of 3–5 electrodes placed at the layer VI/WM junction were used to deliver input to the SI slice. In the example shown in Figure 8, the stimulus intensity in the central electrode was maintained at threshold while the intensity at the 2 electrodes positioned to either side of the central electrode were systematically modified.

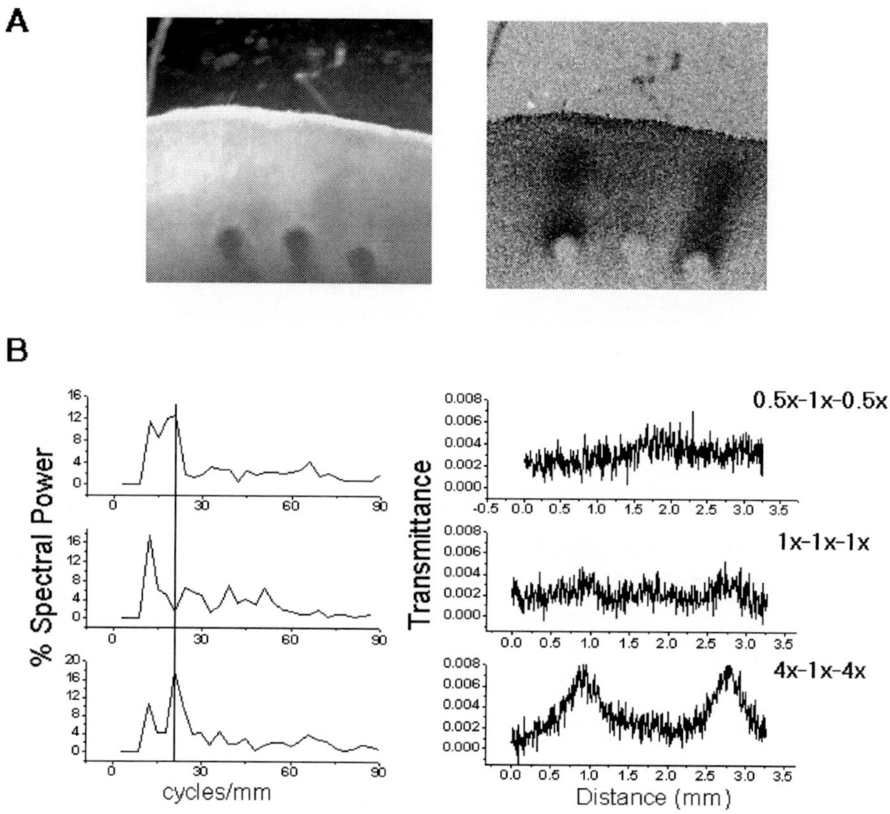

Figure 8. Lateral influence of adjacent cortical territories on stimulus-evoked minicolumnar activity patterns. In this experiment, threshold for each stimulating electrode was set independently. Responses shown in this figure were those obtained when stimuli of the indicated intensities (1× = threshold) were delivered at each of the electrodes simultaneously. *(A) Left panel:* Image of a neocortical slice with 3 stimulating bipolar electrodes located at layer VI/white matter border. *Right panel:* OIS image evoked by all three stimulating electrodes simultaneously. For this particular response the stimulus condition used was 4× threshold intensity at the left electrode, 1× threshold at the central electrode, and 4× threshold at the right electrode (denoted by 4×-1×-4×). *(B)* Stimulus conditions are denoted at far right. *Right column:* Spatial intensity histograms obtained by sampling OIS data tangentially across the region of slice activated by the three electrodes. *Left column:* Power spectra of the spatial intensity histograms sampled above the central stimulating electrode. Note the presence of a peak at the minicolumnar frequency of ~21 cycles/mm (48 μm period) under 0.5×-1×-0.5× and 4×-1×-4× stimulus conditions, and another peak at lower spatial frequency of 12 cycles/mm (83 μm period) under all three stimulus conditions. The relative magnitudes of these two peaks vary depending on the stimulus conditions. In particular, the minicolumnar frequency peak completely disappears when a larger cortical region is driven by the stimulus (1×-1×-1×), even though the stimulus intensity here is near threshold, which in the case of single-electrode stimulation produces a prominent peak at the minicolumnar frequency (see for example Figure 7).

While the observations obtained to date in our *in vitro* studies are preliminary, they clearly indicate that competitive (inhibitory) minicolumnar interactions leading to a "checkerboard-like" interleaved pattern of local groupings of activated and non-activated minicolumns occurs under 2 conditions: (1) when the afferent drive evoked by a single electrode placed at VI/WM border is strong; and (2) when the minicolumns within a large cortical territory receive simultaneous, equal-intensity (suprathreshold) afferent drives from a linear array of layer VI/WM sites. On the other hand, when the afferent drive provided at the same multiple layer VI/WM sites is unequal (for example, the 4×-1×-4× condition in Figure 8) activity in the minicolumns within the weakly-driven macrocolumn is suppressed by lateral inhibitory influences arising in the neighboring, more strongly activated macrocolumns.

Discussion

What picture of sensory information processing in somatosensory cortex has emerged from the studies reviewed in this paper? Most fundamentally, it is apparent that cortical processing is modular on at least two different scales, macrocolumnar and minicolumnar.

With regard to macrocolumns, according to Favorov et al. [9,10,18], the mystacial vibrissa region of rodent somatosensory cortex is not unique in being organized as a mosaic of discrete macrocolumns; i.e., barrel-based columns. Favorov and colleagues demonstrated a similar honeycomb-like pattern made up of discrete place-defined macrocolumns—"segregates"—in the region of cat and monkey somatosensory cortex that receives input from forelimb skin, and proposed that discrete place-defined macrocolumns are a common mode of topographic organization throughout somatosensory cortex. Within such discrete macrocolumns, as one moves from one minicolumn to the next, the RFs of neurons shift back and forth on the skin, displaying local RF diversity without yielding any overall RF shift across the entire macrocolumn. Only at a border separating adjacent macrocolumns do RFs shift en masse in a single step to a new skin position (see Figure 2 for a graphic illustration).

The studies of Pearson et al. [26], Montague et al. [27], Senft and Woolsey [28], and Xing and Gerstein [29] suggest that such discrete macrocolumns—either barrels or segregates—emerge during perinatal development when small (0.3-0.5 mm diameter) cortical regions become innervated each by a selected group of thalamic neurons, sharing similar RFs, whose axons all terminate extensively throughout the territory of that macrocolumn. Within a macrocolumn, according to Favorov and Kelly [16], thalamocortical axons do not connect to all the minicolumns uniformly, but connect selectively so that each minicolumn receives afferent connections from a unique subset of the thalamic neurons projecting to that macrocolumn. The differences in afferent inputs to neighboring minicolumns in a macrocolumn are further amplified by lateral inhibitory interactions among adjacent minicolumns. As a result, in response to a tactile stimulus (even a simple punctate stimulus), an activated macrocolumn generates a complex, spatially heterogeneous pattern of activity that consists of active minicolumns interdigitated throughout the macrocolumn with much less active minicolumns. Furthermore, tactile stimuli, even the most spatially restricted ones, usually activate not a single macrocolumn but a local group of macrocolumns [20]. Each macrocolumn in such an active group generates its own pattern of minicolumnar activation. Thus, the SI response to a skin stimulus takes the form of a patchwork of active minicolumns that extends across multiple macrocolumns (as illustrated in Figure 5). The Favorov and Kelly model predicts that the richly-detailed spatiointensive minicolumnar patterns evoked by tactile stimuli should be very stimulus-specific, exhibiting exquisite sensitivity to stimulus location, shape, and temporal characteristics (such as direction of motion for moving stimuli). One demonstration of such sensitivity is provided in Figure 9.

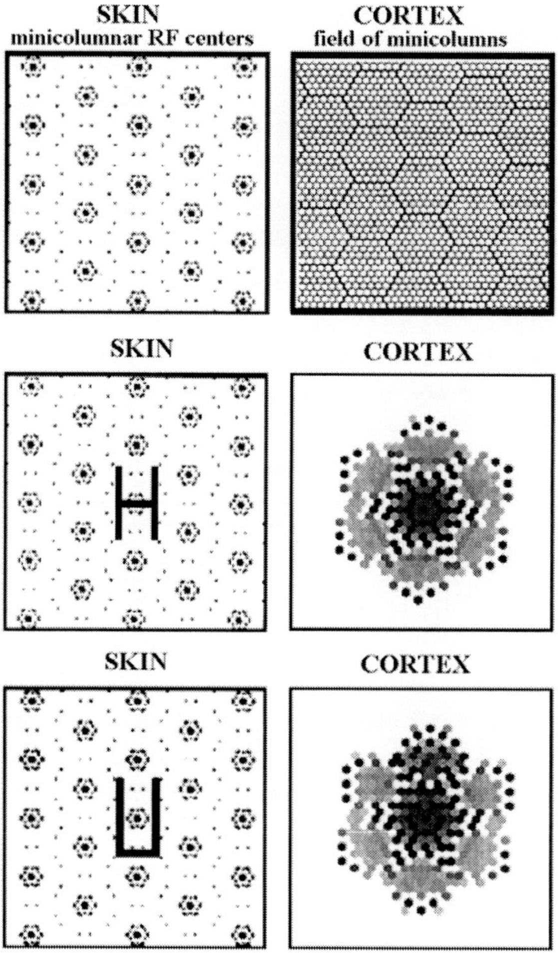

Figure 9. Minicolumnar activity patterns generated by Favorov and Kelly [16,17] model in response to spatially detailed stimulus patterns in a shape of letters H and U. *Top row:* on the right, the field of minicolumns (small hexagons) organized into larger groups, macrocolumns (large hexagons). On the left, locations on the model skin of the RF centers (dots) of the minicolumns shown in the right panel. *Middle row:* on the left, the shape and location on the skin of the stimulus pattern. On the right, the pattern of activities evoked by the stimulus in the minicolumns (activity level is grayscale-coded from white—no activity—to black—maximal activity). *Bottom row:* minicolumnar response pattern evoked by another stimulus. Note the prominent differences in spatial details of the two minicolumnar activity patterns *throughout* the activated cortical field, despite the fact that the two stimuli were quite similar to each other (the change from H to U is merely a small downward shift of the horizontal bar).

In conclusion, while the subject of the existence and functional significance of minicolumns has received relatively little experimental exploration, primarily due to profound technological difficulties associated with addressing it, the combination of experimental and modeling studies reviewed in this paper suggest that cortical networks respond to sensory stimulation with spatially complex patterns of differentially activated minicolumns. An intriguing possibility is that such spatial patterns of activities among minicolumns in an activated cortical field might function to encode highly detailed information about stimulus properties such as, for example, its location, motion, and various spatiotemporal features.

REFERENCES

[1] Edelman GM. Group selection and phasic reentrant signaling: A theory of higher brain function. In: Edelman GM, Mountcastle VB. *The Mindful Brain: Cortical Organization and the Group-Selective Theory of Higher Brain Function*. Cambridge, MA: MIT press; 1978:51-100.

[2] Rakic P. Specification of cerebral cortical areas. *Science*. 1988;241:170-176.

[3] Peters A, Yilmaz E. Neuronal organization in area 17 of cat visual cortex. *Cerebral Cortex*. 1993;3:49-68.

[4] Jones EG. Varieties and distribution of non-pyramidal cells in the somatic sensory cortex of the squirrel monkey. *Journal of Computational Neurology*. 1975;160:205-267.

[5] Jones EG. Anatomy of cerebral cortex: columnar input-output organization. In: Schmitt FO, Worden FG, Adelman G, Dennis SG, eds. *The Organization of the Cerebral Cortex*, Cambridge, MA: MIT Press; 1981:199-235.

[6] Lund JS. Spiny stellate neurons. In: Jones EG, ed. *Cellular Components of the Cerebral Cortex*. New York: Plenum Press; 1984:255-308. *Cerebral Cortex*, vol 1.

[7] DeFelipe J, Hendry MC, Jones EG. Synapses of double bouquet cells in monkey cerebral cortex visualized by calbindin immunoreactivity. *Brain Research*. 1989;503:49-54.

[8] DeFelipe J, Farinas I. The pyramidal neuron of the cerebral cortex: morphological and chemical characteristics of the synaptic inputs. *Progress in Neurobiology*. 1992;39:563-607.

[9] Favorov OV, Whitsel BL. Spatial organization of the peripheral input to area 1 cell columns, I: the detection of "segregates." *Brain Research Reviews*. 1988;13:25-42.

[10] Favorov OV, Diamond ME. Demonstration of discrete place-defined columns—segregates—in the cat SI. *Journal of Computational Neurology*. 1990;298:97-112.

[11] Abeles M, Goldstein MH Jr. Functional architecture in cat primary auditory cortex: columnar organization and organization according to depth. *Journal of Neurophysiology*. 1970;33:172-187.

[12] Hubel DH, Wiesel TN. Sequence regularity and geometry of orientation columns in the monkey striate cortex. *Journal of Computational Neurology*. 1974;158:267-294.

[13] Albus K. A quantitative study of the projection area of the central and the paracentral visual field in area 17 of the cat, I: the spatial organization of the orientation domain. *Experimental Brain Research*. 1975;24:181-202.

[14] Favorov OV, Kelly DG. Local receptive field diversity within cortical neuronal populations. In: Franzén O, Johansson R, Terenius L, eds. *Somesthesis and the Neurobiology of the Somatosensory Cortex*. Basel: Birkhäuser-Verlag; 1996:395-408.

[15] Merzenich MM, Sur M, Nelson RJ, Kaas JH. Organization of the SI cortex: multiple cutaneous representations in areas 3b and 1 of the owl monkey. In: Woolsey CN, ed. *Cortical Sensory Organization*, vol 1. Clifton, NJ: Humana Press; 1981:47-66.

[16] Favorov OV, Kelly DG. Minicolumnar organization within somatosensory cortical segregates, I: development of afferent connections. *Cerebral Cortex*. 1994;4:408-427.

[17] Favorov OV, Kelly DG. Minicolumnar organization within somatosensory cortical segregates, II: emergent functional properties. *Cerebral Cortex*. 1994;4:428-442.

[18] Tommerdahl M, Whitsel BL, Cox EG, Diamond M, Kelly DG. Analysis of the periodicities in somatosensory cortical activity patterns. *Abstracts: Society for Neuroscience*. 1987;13:470.

[19] McCasland JS, Woolsey TA. High-resolution 2-deoxyglucose mapping of functional cortical columns in mouse barrel cortex. *Journal of Comparative Neurology*. 1988;278:555-569.

[20] Tommerdahl M, Whitsel BL, Nakhle B, Favorov O. Minicolumnar activation patterns in cat and monkey SI cortex. *Cerebral Cortex*. 1993;3:399-411.

[21] Tommerdahl M, Delemos KA, Whitsel BL, Favorov OV, Metz CB. Response of anterior parietal cortex to cutaneous flutter versus vibration. *Journal of Neurophysiology*. 1999;82:16-33.

[22] Tommerdahl M, Favorov OV, Whitsel BL. Optical imaging of intrinsic signals in somatosensory cortex. *Behavioral Brain Research*. 2002;135:83-91.

[23] Chen LM, Friedman RM, Roe AW. Optical imaging of a tactile illusion in area 3b of the primary somatosensory cortex. *Science*. 2003;302:881-885.

[24] Shoham D, Grinvald A. The cortical representation of the hand in macaque and human area S-I: high resolution optical imaging. *Journal of Neuroscience*. 2001;21:6820-6825.

[25] Kohn A, Pinheiro A, Tommerdahl MA, Whitsel BL. Optical imaging *in vitro* provides evidence for the minicolumnar nature of cortical response. *Neuroreport*. 1997;8:3513-3518.

[26] Pearson JC, Finkel LM, Edelman GM. Plasticity in the organization of adult cerebral cortical maps: a computer simulation based on neuronal group selection. *Journal of Neuroscience*. 1987;7:4209-4223.

[27] Montague PR, Gally JA, Edelman GM. Spatial signaling in the development and function of neural connections. *Cerebral Cortex*. 1991;1:199-220.

[28] Senft SL, Woolsey TA. Mouse barrel cortex viewed as Dirichlet domains. *Cerebral Cortex*. 1991;1:348-363.

[29] Xing J, Gerstein GL. Networks with lateral connectivity, II: development of neuronal grouping and corresponding receptive field changes. *Journal of Neurophysiology*. 1996;75:200-216.

ACKNOWLEDGEMENTS

This work was supported, in part, by US Army Research Office grant P43077-LS (M. Tommerdahl, P.I.), NIH NS050587 (M. Tommerdahl, P.I.) and NIH NS35222 (B. Whitsel, P.I.). A special thanks goes to Ms. Sharlini Sankaran for technical support and assistance with manuscript preparation.

In: Neocortical Modularity and the Cell Minicolumn
Editor: Manuel F. Casanova, pp. 161-179
ISBN 1-59454-301
© 2005 Nova Science Publishers, Inc.

Chapter IX

MINICOLUMNAR MORPHOMETRY: COMPUTERIZED IMAGE ANALYSIS

Manuel F. Casanova* and Andrew E. Switala
Department of Psychiatry, University of Louisville, Louisville, KY

INTRODUCTION

Notwithstanding marked cytoarchitectural variability, most neuroimaging and postmortem studies select brain regions based on gross anatomical landmarks. Brodmann's areas [1], for example, were defined in terms, not of their location within particular gyri, but of their particular cellular characteristics revealed by the Nissl stains. Unfortunately, Nissl stains provide fragmentary knowledge regarding the structure of neurons. These stains render visible the types and arrangements of cell somata, but they fail to describe the rich dendritic and axonal arborizations as well as synaptic endings. It is reasonable to presume that conventional stains reveal at most 20 % or less of the surface area of most neurons. Understanding the intricate relationships of intracortical circuits and the relationship between neurons is one of the premier objectives of neurosciences. Unsurprisingly, researchers have used different methods in their quest for this understanding. Brain parcellation techniques have included, among others, the use of pigment, pathoclisis (selective vulnerability to certain insults), neurochemistry, and myelin. Regardless of their different approaches and techniques, all of these studies agree in the use of serial sections, special stains, generous sampling, and avoidance of artifacts.

This chapter will provide a mechanistic understanding of how to use computerized imaging in the analysis of cell minicolumns. The minicolumn is an anatomically identifiable structure that constitutes part of the larger macrocolumn. Reasons for focusing study on the

* Corresponding author: Manuel F. Casanova, MD, Gottfried and Gisela Kolb Endowed Chair in Psychiatry, University of Louisville, Department of Psychiatry, 500 South Preston St., A Bldg., Rm. 217; Louisville, KY 40292. Tel: (502)852-4077; Fax: (502)852-4078; E-mail: M0CASA02@louisville.edu

minicolumn include the following: It is the basic anatomical unit of neuronal aggregation in the neocortex when considering the radial direction from the white matter border to the pial surface. Conceptually as well as geometrically, the minicolumn is orthogonal to the tangential unit of aggregation, *viz.* the cortical lamina. Long-range afferent and efferent fiber systems are all arranged about this radial unit of cells. All neuronal types save one, the Cajal-Retzius cell, can be found within the minicolumn. It is a readily identifiable, fixed anatomical structure that is generalized throughout the neocortex. Lastly, the ontogenetic cell column, precursor to the minicolumn, is the earliest organization of neurons in the developing cortex.

Quantifying Radial Organization

Researchers have used at least four major features to detect and describe the radial organization of the cortex:

1. Arrays of pyramidal cell somata (e.g. Kohn et al. [8]),
2. Apical dendrite bundles (e.g. Lohmann and Köppen [9]),
3. Myelinated fiber bundles (e.g. Peters and Sethares [50]), and
4. Double bouquet cell axon bundles (e.g. DeFelipe et al. [20]).

Of these four objects, pyramidal cell arrays are probably the most difficult to work with. Cell somata are rarely as obviously oriented as fibers, and they do not aggregate so tightly into distinct bundles. These problems are offset by several advantages: The soma is more amenable to quantitative analysis than a structure that is detectable only with immunocytochemistry, such as the apical dendrite. Tissue to be stained for cell somata may be embedded in celloidin, where the durable nature of the material allows for long-term archival of the tissue, which in turn increases the reproducibility of results. Furthermore, cell somata are the sources and sinks of signal transmission along the apical dendrites and bundles of myelinated fibers, and have been linked directly to physiological units. The radial array of cells is also the first discernible structure in the neocortex *in utero*, [49] allowing researchers trace cortical development from the prenatal period to advanced age.

Of the major characteristics (1–4, above) used to identify minicolumns, the cell soma array provides the most information. However, because cell column study alone has other shortcomings, multiple approaches should always be favored. Fiber bundles, which provide information on the horizontal spacing between columns and the thickness of the bundles, are more easily defined than cell arrays. On the other hand, cell soma arrays, unlike fiber bundles, extend from lamina II to lamina VI, nearly the full depth of the cortex. They also allow columns to be measured on a lamina-by-lamina basis since laminar boundaries are readily apparent in a field of cell somata. Other important measurements, such as unbiased cell counts, can be made using precisely the same Nissl-stained tissue used for image analysis of cell soma arrays, facilitating studies of the relationships between these measurements and minicolumnar morphology.

Despite all the potential problems with postmortem tissue, strong arguments exist for the overall accuracy of cell column measurements. Measurements reported by multiple researchers—using different brains, preparation techniques, and methods—have achieved great consistency (Table 1). [5] At least two other studies [30],[29] used pyramidal cell arrays to estimate minicolumn size. Seldon [30] used celloidin-embedded, Nissl-stained, thick sections of auditory cortex. The study of Schlaug and associates [29] was confined to the cingulate and pericingulate cortex. The number of brains used to obtain these measures is not specifically given. The approach taken by Buldyrev et al. [36] is very different, and the relationship between its output and anatomy is not clear. However, it demonstrates that radially oriented structure can be observed within a field of neurons. Overall, the similarities of different studies' results (Table 1) are striking, considering they employed different protocols for both tissue processing and image analysis.

Table 1. Comparison of Cell Column Arrays in Different Studies

Cortical area	Number of brains	Mean CW (µm)	Tissue processing	Investigator
4	1	51.7	Celloidin-imbedded; sectioned at 35 µm	Casanova et al. (2003)
9	16	48.0		
17	13	31.6		
21	14	48.0		
22	30	46.6		
40	14	49.7		
41	3	38.5		
46	2	52.4		
22	*	46.7	Celloidin-imbedded; sectioned at 50–80 µm	Seldon [30],[53]
41	*	46.1		
42	*	44.8		
7	1	39.5	Paraffin-imbedded; sectioned at 30 µm	Schlaug et al.[29]
19	1	40.1		
23b	1	39.5		
24b	1	45.0		
31	1	40.8		
STS	11	80.0	Frozen; sectioned at 50 µm	Buldyrev et al.[36]

* The number of brains in which cell arrays were measured was listed as "a few"; the exact number is unknown.

Note: In cases where measurements were provided for both left and right hemispheres, the mean minicolumnar width (CW) is the average of both. Seldon [30] reported individually the width of cell soma arrays and the width of neuropil between them. The CW given here here is the sum of these two values.

[5] See also table 1 of Buxhoeveden and Casanova, "Encephalization, minicolumns, and hominid evolution," this volume.

Methodology

Image Acquisition

Methods in this chapter operate on digital images of cerebral cortex. Since the first step is to binarize the image, classifying each pixel as belonging to the foreground phase (stained cell somata) or background phase (unstained neuropil), it makes little difference whether the original images are in color or grayscale. Unless the chosen segmentation algorithm uses color information, storing such might be a waste of space. More important is striking the right balance between image resolution and field of view. Profiles of individual cell somata, some very small (on the order of 10 μm^2 in area), must be identifiable, whereas the structure of interest, the pyramidal cell array, is about 50 μm wide and can be traced across the full width of the cortex excluding lamina I. In our experience a resolution in the neighborhood of 1 μm per pixel works well.

Either a CCD or a traditional film camera can be used. Suppose for concreteness that one would like to photograph section of cerebral cortex 3 mm thick, which spans the entire microscopic field of view, with resolution at least 1 μm per pixel. The digital image must be 3000 pixels or more in at least one dimension. High-end digital cameras can produce images larger than that already, and they are bound to improve in future. At the time this chapter was written, Kodak T-MAX 100 film [11] had a resolving power of 63 lines per millimeter at "low" contrast, i.e. a factor of 1.6 separating bright from dark. The resolving power of a digital image is half the sampling frequency, so the film corresponds to a resolution of 126 "pixels" per millimeter. One 35 mm frame is then equivalent to a 4410 line digital image. Digital and film photography today both produce images more than adequate for the image analysis routines to follow.

Segmentation

Image foreground, i.e. stained objects, is distinguished from image background via thresholding. The problem of uneven illumination demands that the threshold be selected adaptively. One simple, effective method is to partition the image into blocks then use Otsu's method [12] in each block to compute a threshold value for the pixel at the block's center. These values are interpolated to obtain the threshold gray level for every pixel in the full image. Otsu's venerable algorithm is widely used and known to produce good results when the foreground and background phases don't differ greatly in size [13]. This is the case for images of Nissl-stained cerebral cortex outside of lamina I. For alternative thresholding techniques readers are directed to the extensive review by Sezgin and Sankur [13]. It omits some particular algorithms, but provides good coverage of all approaches to threshold determination.

Thresholding by itself is sufficient to preprocess images for methods, such as the verticality index (Schleicher and Zilles, this volume), which study the spatial distribution of stained material. A connected region of foreground pixels in the thresholded image often comprises several overlapping cell profiles, however. Further image processing is required before applying methods, such as that described in the next section, which study the spatial distribution of cell somata. The watershed transformation of mathematical morphology produces images more suitable for such purposes. The input to this transform consists of the inverse distance map of the thresholded image, where every pixel is replaced by the additive inverse of the distance to the nearest background pixel. Foreground objects appear as negative "basins" in a plain of zeros, and the watershed transform locates "ridges" by conceptually filling these basins with water, keeping track of where two pools merge when the water reaches a certain level. Ridges emanate from concavities in the foreground objects' boundaries, thus segmenting the foreground into non-overlapping, convex regions. If cell somata, or rather their profiles, are not convex, the watershed transformation may produce too many objects where thresholding alone produced too few.

Buldyrev and colleagues [36] avoid the problems with automated image segmentation by identifying cells visually and marking their locations for subsequent analysis. Identifying biological structures by eye is, of course, *the* accepted procedure in cell counting or other stereological investigations. There is little need, however, for such a labor-intensive step in image analysis, where the results are not unbiased, stereological estimates of three-dimensional quantities at any rate.

Feature Extraction: Minicolumn Fragments

We have developed software to quantify minicolumnar structure with minimal human interaction. It operates orthogonally to the image segmentation step, taking for input the (x,y) coordinates of the centroids of foreground objects, as well as their areas. Each point must also be labeled according to whether it is from one of the laminas III, V, or VI. The software assumes that columnar structure is present and that the Y-axis is parallel to the image radial direction r', being the two-dimensional projection of the direction r along which minicolumns extend from the white matter boundary to the pial surface. Minicolumn orientation varies with location in general; r' is consequently a vector field, assumed to be constant or nearly so across the region of interest within an image. The software does not check these assumptions, which must be independently verified (see below). The vector field t' is the local tangential direction, everywhere perpendicular to r'.

Objects are partitioned into three classes based on size: Anything with an area less than 15 μm^2 is simply discarded as "noise." Objects larger than 30 μm^2 are grouped into clusters that we call *minicolumn fragments*. Objects of intermediate size (between 15 μm^2 and 30 μm^2 in area) are allocated after the fact to the nearest minicolumn fragment. These object size thresholds are more-or-less arbitrary and can be changed, but they must be kept fixed for any particular data set to ensure that data from different images are comparable. In ascending order of size, the classes are meant to represent glia or image/segmentation artifacts, possible neuron soma profiles, and likely neuron soma profiles. Our lab has consistently used the above values. Apart from these two thresholds provided by the user, the software operates automatically.

Since minicolumns in laminas III, V, and VI are about one neuron wide [14], the typical distance between Δ adjacent columns should be of the same order of magnitude as the distance between adjacent pyramidal cell somata. Adjacency for a point set in any number of dimensions (two in our case) may be rigorously defined in terms of the Dirichlet tessellation. The region that the points occupy is divided into cells (polygons in two dimensions), where each cell contains one point of the given point set, and everywhere in the interior of a cell is closer to the enclosed point than to any other point in the set (Figure 1). Two points are considered adjacent if the corresponding cells in the Dirichlet tessellation share a side. There is a graph dual to the Dirichlet tesselation called the Delaunay triangulation, where each pair of adjacent points in the set is joined by an edge (line segment). Our software takes the median length of these edges for an estimate of the distance Δ. Efficient algorithms for constructing the Delaunay triangulation [15] of N points take $O(N \log N)$ time, allowing for the analysis of large images capturing many thousands of neurons.

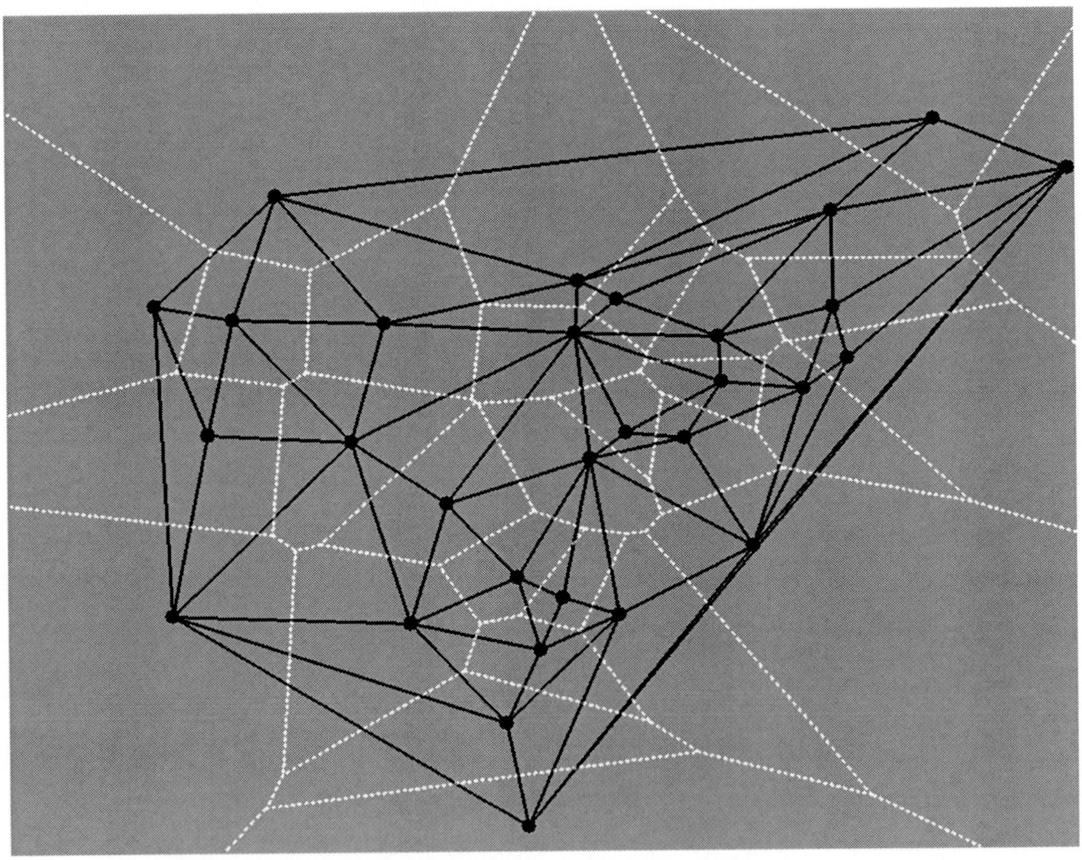

Figure 1. The Dirichlet tesselation (dotted white lines), also called a Voronoi diagram, portions space into neighborhoods of the points of a given point set (black dots). Its dual construct, the Delaunay triangulation (solid black lines), joins each pair of points whose neighborhoods share a boundary in the Dirichlet tesselation. Both structures exist not only for planar point sets but for point sets in any number of dimensions. In three dimensions the Delaunay "triangulation" is actually made up of tetrahedra, and in general comprises $n + 1$ point simplices in n dimensions.

The reason for labeling points according to lamina becomes clear. Seldon's description of minicolumn width [14], the heuristic basis for estimating Δ, does not apply to laminas II and IV. Edges of the Delaunay triangulation with either endpoint in one of these laminas are discarded before the median edge length is obtained.

Now the cell somata are grouped into clusters. The image is divided vertically into rectangles with height 2Δ. (Recall the Y-axis is parallel to r'.) Each rectangle overlaps the bottom half of the rectangle immediately below, and the top half of the rectangle immediately above. Let $k(x)$ be a bell-shaped kernel function, symmetric about the origin, with unit width in the sense that the greatest value of ε such that $k(x) + k(\varepsilon - x)$ is unimodal is $\varepsilon = 1$. The gaussian $k(x) = \exp(-x^2/2)$ and the centered cubic B-spline

$$k(x) = \begin{cases} \frac{3}{8} - x^2 + \frac{2}{3}x^3, & |x| < 0.75 \\ \frac{3}{4} - \frac{3}{2}x + x^2 - \frac{2}{9}x^3, & 0.75 \le |x| < 1.5 \\ 0, & |x| \ge 1.5 \end{cases}$$

are examples of suitable kernel functions. Let x_j be the X-coordinate of the centroid of image object j, and for each rectangle compute

$$f(x) = \sum_j k\left(\frac{x_j - x}{\Delta/2}\right),$$

where the sum is over all object centroids within the given rectangle. Some constant multiple of $f(x)$ is an estimate of the local numeric density of cell somata along the local tangential direction t' (Figure 2). Fluctuations in $f(x)$ occur on the scale taken from Seldon [14]: Rectangle height multiplied by kernel width, $(2\Delta) \times (\Delta / 2) = \Delta^2$, is the area of a square containing about one cell soma profile in the image. Local maxima of f(x) are taken as clustering centers, and each object in the rectangle is associated with the nearest clustering center.

The final stage of the routine links clusters in overlapping rectangles into minicolumn fragments. For each pair of overlapping rectangles, if two clustering centers, one from each rectangle, are mutually nearest neighbors, the corresponding clusters are combined. That is to say, given cluster C1 in a rectangle R1 and cluster C2 in an adjacent rectangle R2, if the center of C1 is nearer than any other cluster center in R1 to the center of C2 *and* the center of C2 is nearer than any other cluster center in R2 to the center of C1, then C1 and C2 are part of the same minicolumn fragment. It is easy to see that this criterion ensures one cluster center cannot belong to more than one minicolumn fragments, i.e. the minicolumn fragments do not branch. Note, however, that an individual image object may become part of more than one minicolumn fragment, so the result is a "fuzzy" clustering.

After the minicolumns are identified, the program computes several parameters to describe the distribution of neurons and interneuronal space (neuropil) in each fragment. When these parameters are subsequently averaged to estimate, e.g., the mean minicolumnar width in a particular cortical area of a particular brain, minicolumn fragments comprising ten or fewer image objects are given a weight of zero. Small fragments might occupy relatively little image area, while being numerous enough to exert undue influence on the mean parameter values if included in the average.

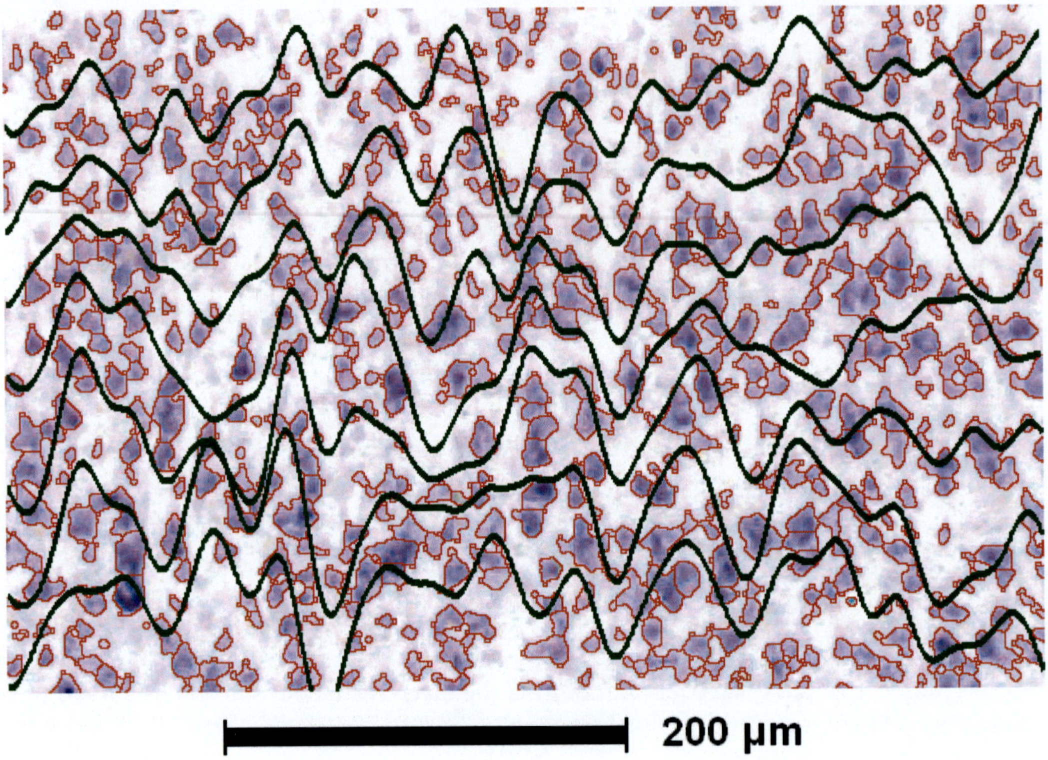

Figure 2. Superposed on an image of cortical layer III are the boundaries of cells (dark outlines) as determined using an automatic segmentation algorithm including a watershed transformation step. The cell density profiles $f(x)$ are shown at several positions along the local radial direction (Y-axis). Peak-to-peak distances on these profiles provide an estimate of minicolumnar width CW.

Three descriptive parameters are of general interest. First among them is minicolumnar width or CW, [6] the horizontal distance from the clustering center of one minicolumn fragment to the clustering center of its neighbor. CW resembles the notion of minicolumn size in the fiber bundle literature, where it refers almost universally to the bundles' center-to-center spacing [50],[33],[40].

Interneuronal distance or MCS is the mean edge length of a graph, the minimum spanning tree, itself a subgraph of the Delaunay triangulation described above. The minimun spanning tree of a point set is connected (meaning there is a sequence of edges joining any one point to any other point), acyclic (meaning there are no closed loops), and among all such graphs it is the one with the least total edge length. Given the Delaunay triangulation of a minicolumn fragment, constructing its minimum spanning tree takes little time using the

---

[6] Symbols for descriptive parameters are CW for "columnar width," MCS for "mean cell spacing," and NS for "neuropil space." These symbols, which we've used since the earliest version of the methodology,[57] have been retained for consistency even as the parameter names have been replaced by more precise terms.

Kruskal or Prim algorithms [19] even without optimization. The Delaunay triangulations are themselves constructed using the quickhull algorithm [15] so the entire procedure is computationally efficient.

Estimation of peripheral neuropil space—NS—makes use of the local *minima* of the density $f(x)$. The minima to either side of the chain of clustering centers defining a minicolumn fragment define a kind of boundary, or shape, for the fragment. Imagine squeezing this shape by scaling the distances between clustering center and the neighboring local minima by some factor $k < 1$. Let k be made as small as possible with the constraint that the squeezes shape encloses at least 90% of the objects in the minicolumn fragment. The mean width of the resulting shape, subtracted from the fragment's CW, yields NS.

Texture Analysis: Local Radial Orientation

The feature extraction method constructs, then measures, vertical clusters of neuron profiles. Prior to input to the routine, an image must be oriented so that its Y-axis is parallel to r'. This cannot be achieved in general since r' can vary appreciably over distances on the order of 1 mm in regions where the cerebral cortex folds sharply, and also near the white matter border where minicolumns themselves take on a curved shape [20].

Columnar structure in an image can be seen in the image's Fourier transform. Consider, for example, a grayscale image of alternating light and dark, vertical bands. At any given position on the x-axis the image, I, is constant for all y: $I(x,y) = I(x)$. All the nonzero components of its Fourier transform $J(f,g)$ then are localized at zero vertical frequency $g = 0$. Let I' be the original image rotated clockwise by an angle θ,

$$I'(x,y) = I(x',y') = I(x\cos\theta - y\sin\theta, x\sin\theta + y\cos\theta).$$

Then the Fourier transform of the rotated image is

$$\begin{aligned} J'(f,g) &= \iint \exp(2\pi i f x)\exp(2\pi i g y) I'(x,y)\,dxdy \\ &= \iint \exp(2\pi i f(x'\cos\theta + y'\sin\theta))\exp(2\pi i g(-x'\sin\theta + y'\cos\theta)) \cdot \\ &\quad I(x',y')\tfrac{\partial(x,y)}{\partial(x',y')}\,dx'dy'. \end{aligned}$$

The Jacobian of a rotation is just unity, so rearranging terms one obtains

$$J'(f,g) = J(f\cos\theta - g\sin\theta, f\sin\theta + g\cos\theta).$$

Thus the Fourier transform is rotated through the same plane angle as the image, and its nonzero components lie on the line $g = f\tan\theta$.

Now let I be an image of Nissl-stained cerebral cortex, with Fourier transform J. Pyramidal cell arrays give rise to a striped appearance, or texture, while the individual cell somata produce a blotchy texture. Superposition of these textures is reflected in J, where minicolumnar structure stands out as a strongly directional signal against an isotropic background (Figure 3). The dominant orientation θ of the signal is found using the formula [21]

$$\theta = \tfrac{1}{2}\tan^{-1}\frac{\sum_k |J_k|^2 \sin 2\theta_k}{\sum_k |J_k|^2 \cos 2\theta_k},$$

where $|J_k|$ is the amplitude of component k of the discrete Fourier transform, and the sum is over all two-dimensional frequencies $f_k = (f_k, g_k)$. The angle θ_k is not the phase of J_k, but the direction of the signal giving rise to the Fourier component at that frequency, i.e. $\tan\theta_k = g_k / f_k$. The directionality, or strength of the directed texture, is given by [21]

$$D^2 = \frac{\sum_k |J_k|^2 \cos 2(\theta_k - \theta)}{\sum_k |J_k|^2},$$

which is normalized to lie between zero and one.

A local estimate of r' (Figure 4) is produced by computing the above quantities in small (about 0.20 mm^2) regions of an image:

$$r'_{\text{region}} = (\cos\theta_{region}, \sin\theta_{region}).$$

Two modifications to this basic method ensure that the estimates of r' do not vary unrealistically across the image: Neighboring regions are made to overlap substantially so that the respective estimates therein are not independent. In addition, the final result is smoothed by a three-by-three weighted median filter. Local directionalities D^2 are used for weights, and the median filter is applied to the components of r' individually. Once r', and consequently t', are known, it is possible to segment the image, transform each image object's (x,y) coordinates to (r',t') coordinates, and input these to the minicolumn fragment routine. Descriptive parameters are computed using the untransformed (x,y) coordinates after fragments have been identified. Subsequent statistical analyses and interpretation must account for the fact that, in the presence of curvature, parameters will in general be a function of r' even within a given lamina.

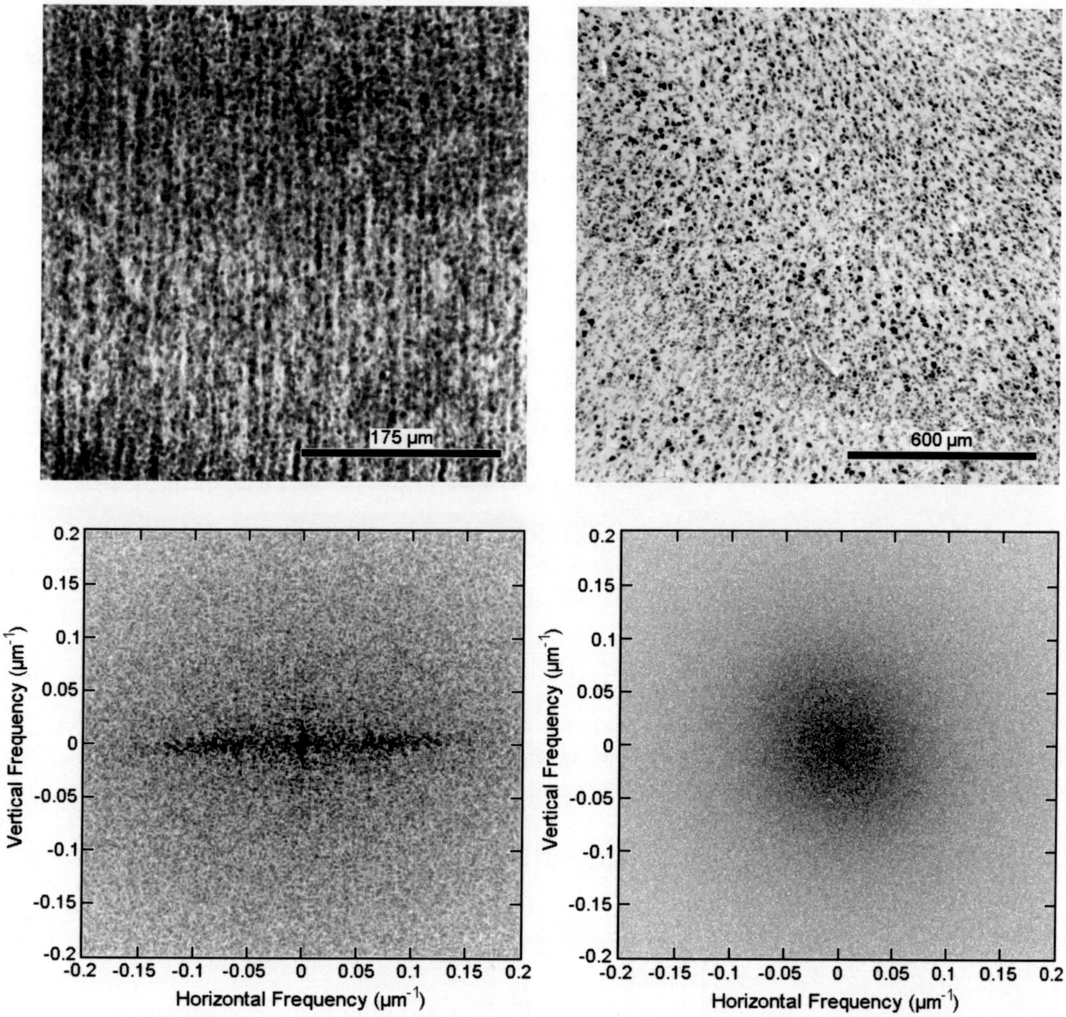

Figure 3. Top left: Ontogenetic cell columns in the fetal cerebral cortex at 28 weeks of gestation have a strikingly linear appearance. Bottom left: The previous image has been transformed into the frequency domain. The power spectrum, or magnitude of the Fourier transform, is shown as grayscale, with darker patches indicating more signal—image structure—at the corresponding frequency. Since the ontogenetic columns are oriented vertically in the image, most of the power is concentrated in a horizontal band. Top right: In this low-magnification image of Brodmann area 4 from an adult human, there is a large amount folding so that the local radial direction changes appreciably across the region. Moreover, the minicolumns are not nearly so visible as the ontogenetic columns. Consequently, the power spectrum (bottom right) is practically isotropic.

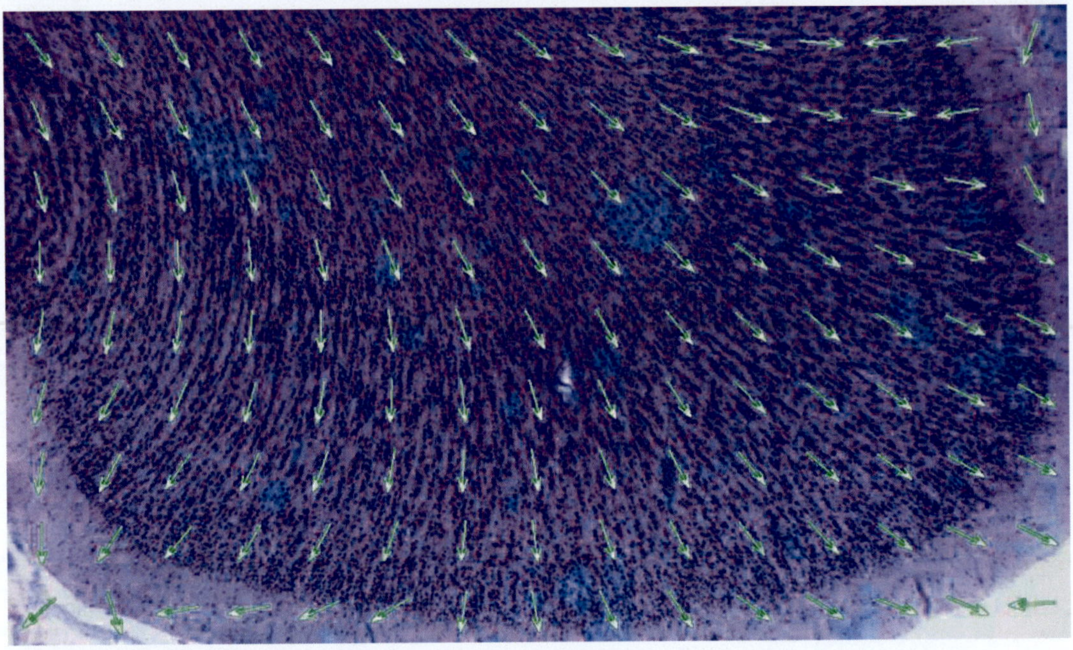

Figure 4. A 35 μm thick section through human cortex (Brodmann area 22) is shown, spanning a region 4.5 mm by 2.7 mm in size. Arrows represent the local radial direction r' computed automatically using the Fourier transform to detect anisotropy. The routine fails in lamina I, where there is no columnar structure present in a Nissl stain, but otherwise performs adequately.

Examples

Relationship of Minicolumn Fragments to Physiological Minicolumns

We compared the output of our method against an experiment to discern physiological minicolumns via optical intrinsic signal, which obtained evidence of metabolic activity after stimulation of the lamina VI/white matter border (Tommerdahl et al., this volume). The experiment was performed in the primary sensory cortex of a monkey (*Macaca fascicularis*) [59]. To determine whether the columns detected by OIS correspond to anatomical minicolumns, the authors measured optical density values from the same material. The resolution was very low (828 pixels/mm), which the authors stated was done intentionally for clarity [59]. The result was strongly in accord with the values attained through OIS. Our measurements of minicolumn fragments in lamina III of *Macaca* primary sensory cortex yielded a mean CW of 33.6 μm, within the range of 29 μm to 56 μm reported by Tommerdahl et al. [59]

Minicolumnar Architecture of Cortical Areas and Laminas

In the context of a study of lamination abnormalities in schizophrenia [23], we recently analyzed columns from laminas III and V in area 9 of Brodmann, and in the primary motor, sensory, and visual cortices from thirteen *post mortem* human brains. The sample consisted entirely of men, with a mean age at death 51.9 years (standard deviation 11.1 years) and a mean interval between death and autopsy 23.7 hours (standard deviation 13.6 hours). All patients were free from any psychopathology, and had in their history neither neurological problems requiring intervention or interfering with cognitive assessment, epilepsy, severe head injury with loss of consciousness, nor diabetes mellitus with poor glycemic control. The cerebral hemispheres were cryoprotected in a mixture of glycerol-dimethylsulfoxide-formalin (after careful removal of the meninges and the pial vessels), embedded in gelatin, deeply frozen at –60 °C, and serially sectioned using a cryomicrotome. Heinsen and Heinsen [24] describe the procedure in detail.

Digital images of the four cortical areas were analyzed with the methods just described. Full factorial linear models were fit to the measurements of CW and MCS, including cortical area, hemisphere, and lamina as fixed factors. Multivariate dependencies on cortical area, on lamina, and on their interaction were statistically significant ($p < 0.05$); there was no significant laterality. Univariate tests revealed no significant variation of CW with lamina, exactly as expected. Joint confidence regions on the mean CW and MCS, estimated using the basic bootstrap method [25], are shown (Figure 5).

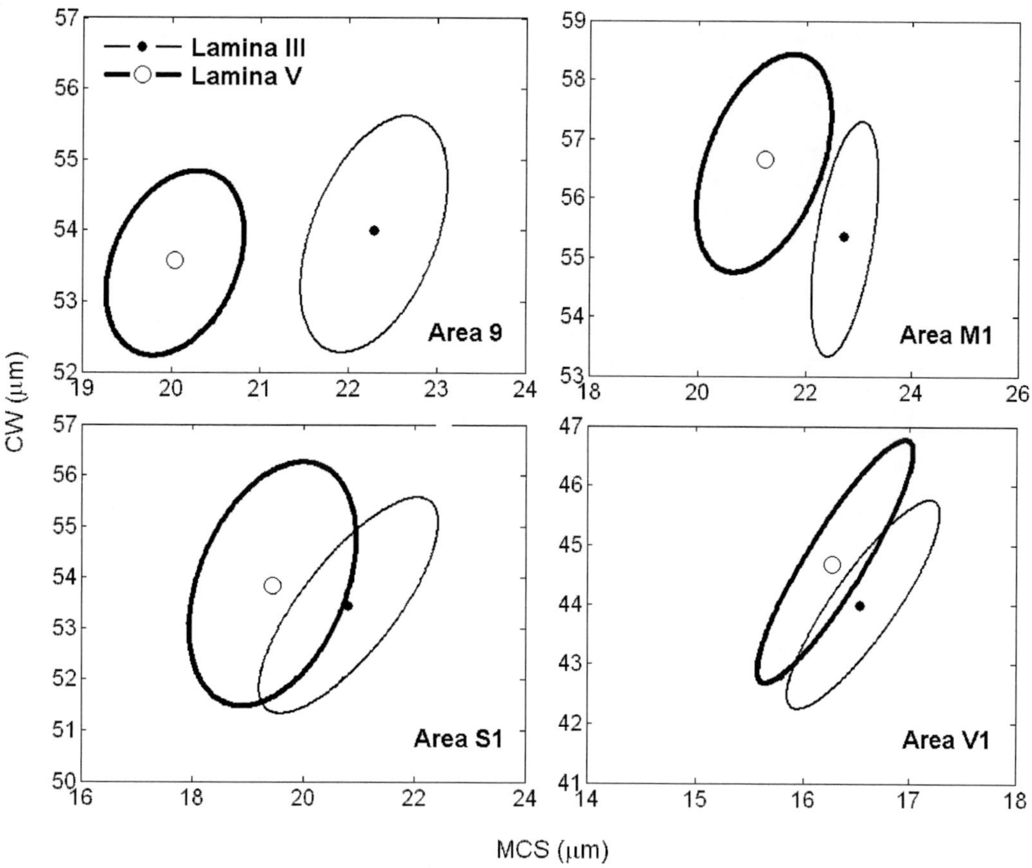

Figure 5. Confidence ellipses for the joint mean CW and MCS were estimated from a sample of normal, adult, male human brains. Points near the ellipses' centers are the maximum likelihood estimates.

Stereological Considerations

Shrinkage

Tissue shrinkage during processing can acquire enormous proportions. Pakkenberg [26] and Robins et al. [27] found shrinkage of approximately 40 % in fixed, paraffin-embedded tissue. Numerical values for shrinkage in this section refer to *linear* shrinkage:

$$\lambda = (l_0 - l) / l_0,$$

where l is the observed straight line distance between two points in processed tissue, and l_0 is the distance between the same two points prior to tissue processing. Measured areas will be reduced by $1 - (1 - \lambda)^2$, and measured volumes will be reduced by a factor of $1 - (1 - \lambda)^3$.

It is implicit in the preceding that λ is constant. Robins and co-workers [27] examined the shrinkage of fixed, stained tissue relative to freeze-dried, unstained tissue from the motor cortex. They found little difference in the relative shrinkage of the distance from the pial surface to the lamina I/II boundary, of the distance from the pial surface to lamina Va (identified by the presence of Betz cells), and of the full cortical thickness. They conclude, "It is, therefore, probable that the shrinkage of the stained vertical sections affected all layers of the cortex approximately equally" [27].

Measurements with units of length—including CW, MCS, and NS—should be multiplied by the correction factor $(1 - \lambda)^{-1}$ to obtain their proper values prior to tissue processing. This might appear a gratuitous nicety when the "proper" values are no more stereologically unbiased than the measured values. If, however, brains from different subpopulations are to be compared, e.g. the brains of schizophrenic patients *versus* those exhibiting no psychopathology, systematic differences in shrinkage between normal and pathological cases would confound the results. Tissue processing, moreover, increases variance as well as introducing a systematic bias. Pakkenberg [26] reported shrinkage as low as $\lambda = 17$ % and as great as $\lambda = 49$ % in different blocks of tissue (eight in all) from three different brains. Variation in λ was observed even between different blocks from the same brain.

For some studies shrinkage may be safely ignored. Suppose, for example, one is interested in laterality in a parameter x (CW, MCS, or NS). If whole-brain coronal sections are available, measurements from the left (x_L) and right (x_R) hemispheres in any given section will be equally reduced by tissue processing. The feature of interest is captured by the dimensionless quantity $(x_L - x_R) / (x_L + x_R)$, invariant with respect to λ. Also among invariant parameters, possibly of interest for testing certain hypotheses, is the relative width of peripheral neuropil space NS / CW, an indicator of the compactness of a pyramidal cell array.

Adaptation to 3-D Proportions

Consider an idealized minicolumn in three dimensions, cylindrical in shape. Its minicolumnar width CW_{true} is the diameter of its circular cross section, and its peripheral neuropil space NS_{true} is twice the thickness of the tube containing at most 10% of the column's cells. The interneuronal distance MCS_{true} is just the mean edge length of the minimum spanning tree in three dimensions. The subscript "true" indicates that these are three-dimensional quantities, of which CW, MCS, and NS are biased estimates. An artificial array of just such idealized minicolumns, packed hexagonally [71],[29] in a 1 mm [2] patch of cortex 1 mm deep. Spherical "neurons" were randomly distributed throughout each minicolumn with a radial distribution peaking at the column core and tapering off toward the edge. Two parallel planes 35 μm apart define a virtual slice of the artificial cortex. Every neuron, or fragment thereof, falling between the planes is collapsed along one dimension, and the result is output as an image suitable for input to the minicolumn fragment routine (Figure 6).

Figure 6. Virtual slices through a computer generated, columnar arrangement of neurons were used to examine the relationship between the dimensions of minicolumns in 3-D and the dimensions of minicolumn fragments extracted from an image.

A total of 140 artificial images were generated and analyzed by the column method. CW_{true} was allowed to range from 40 μm to 80 μm. Comparison of the minicolumn fragment measurements with the known three-dimensional quantities, CW, NS, and MCS are found to consistently underestimate CW_{true}, NS_{true}, and MCS_{true}, respectively (Figure 7). Nevertheless, the measurements are strongly correlated with the true column parameters. The intent of this simulation is not to derive model-based stereological "correction" factors, with all their inherent problems. Rather, it is to show that fragment measurements are suitable for hypothesis testing in that differences in anatomical characteristics between two tissue samples will manifest as differences in the same sense in the measured parameters.

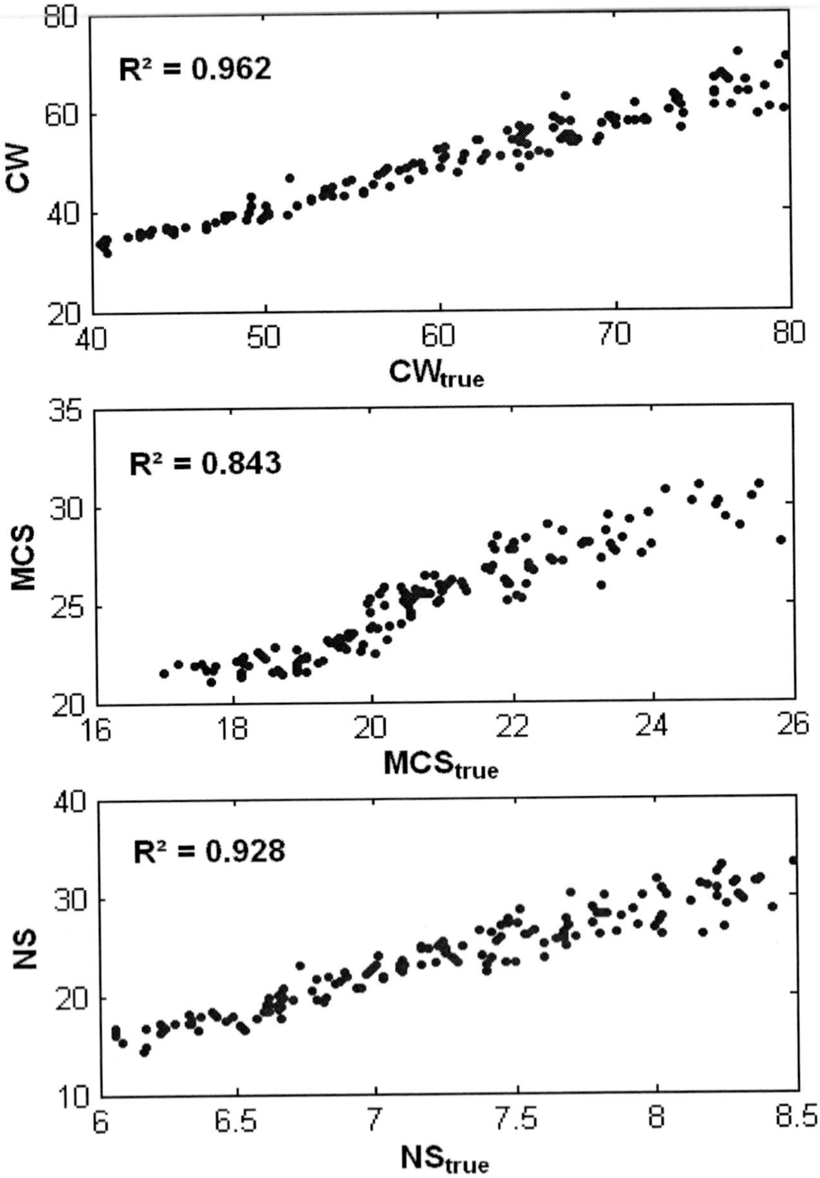

Figure 7. Correlation coefficients R [2] near unity indicate that trends in minicolumn fragment measurements (unsubscripted) are indicative of similar trends in minicolumnar architecture (subscripted "true"). Values are in μm.

Concluding Remarks

Thus far classical neuropathology has primarily concerned itself with neuronal lesions such as cell loss, homogenization of cytoplasm or nucleoplasm, eosinophilia, and so forth. These examples of cellular pathology offer only limited clues as to a causal agent. In essence, trauma, hypoxia, and hypoglycemia may all offer a similar exposition under microscopic examination. After many decades of investigation it is now abundantly clear that the majority of psychiatric conditions do not exhibit changes typical of classical pathology. This conclusion has made some psychiatric researchers retreat to the molecular realm in search of possible causative explanations. Although the molecular approach has yielded many findings, few have been replicated, and most have been marred by methodological issues. If psychiatric conditions are reflections of brain abnormalities, how then should we best approach its pathological investigation?

It appears that a reductionist neuropathological approach has failed to provide any answers to major psychiatric conditions. By looking at the neuron, classical methods may have focused on the tree and lost sight of the forest. Neurons are particulates of canonical circuits. Taken as a whole, these circuits provide the microprocessing capability of the cortex. Neurons along with their afferent and efferent projections are integrated into arrangements called minicolumns. Although the study of these arrangements escaped the processing power of the human eye, their morphological features are readily defined with modern computer methods.

It is within the neocortex that a modular organization is most readily discernible within the central nervous system. A hierarchical organization provides the neocortex with emergent properties subsumed under the term "higher cortical functions." It is these properties that fall under the purview of psychiatry. Cortical lesions provide explanatory power when invoked as pathological explanations to psychiatric conditions. Cellular arrays suggestive of minicolumns have been found in all areas of neocortex from all mammalian species examined. In marked contrast to its ubiquity, few pathological studies have concerned themselves with this structure. Thus far, a failure to explore higher orders of cellular arrangements may have been the result of a failure to implement proper computer algorithms.

In this chapter we have concerned ourselves with the analysis of the cell minicolumn as portrayed by cell arrays. We have focused on cellular arrays because they are fixed units that can be measured by image analysis techniques. A similar approach can be taken using myelinated fiber bundles. The resultant information, although more limited, offers complementary information to that obtained by cellular arrays.

References

[1] Brodmann K. *Vergleichende Lokalisationslehre der Grosshirnrinde in ihren Prinzipien dargestellt auf Grund des Zellenbaues*. Leipzig, Germany: Johann Ambrosius Barth Verlag; 1909. Translated as: Brodmann's "*Localisation in the Cerebral Cortex*." Garey LJ, tr. London, England: Smith-Gordon; 1994.

[2] Kohn A, Pinheiro A, Tommerdahl MA, Whitsel BL. Optical imaging *in vitro* provides evidence for the minicolumnar nature of cortical response. *Neuroreport.* 1997;8:3513-3518.

[3] Lohmann H, Köppen H-J. Postnatal development of pyramidal dendritic and axonal bundles in the visual cortex of the rat. *Journal für Hirnforschung*. 1995;36:101-111.

[4] Peters A, Sethares C. Myelinated axons and the pyramidal cell modules in monkey primary visual cortex. *Journal of Comparative Neurology.* 1996;365:232-255.

[5] DeFelipe J, Hendry S, Hashikawa T, Molinari M, Jones EG. A microcolumnar structure of monkey cerebral cortex revealed by immunocytochemical studies of double bouquet cell axons. *Neuroscience*. 1990;37:655-673.

[6] Kornack DR, Rakic P. Radial and horizontal deployment of clonally related cells in the primate neocortex: relationship to distinct mitotic lineages. *Neuron*. 1995;15:311-321.

[7] Seldon HL. Structure of human auditory cortex, I: cytoarchitectonics and dendritic distributions. *Brain Research.* 1981;229:277-294.

[8] Seldon HL. Structure of human auditory cortex, II: axon distributions and morphological correlates of speech perception. *Brain Research.* 1981;229:295-310.

[9] Schlaug G, Schleicher A, Zilles K. Quantitative analysis of the columnar arrangement of neurons in the human cingulated cortex. *Journal of Comparative Neurology.* 1995;351:441-452.

[10] Buldyrev SV, Cruz L, Gomez-Isla T, et al. Description of microcolumnar ensembles in association cortex and their disruption in Alzheimer and Lewy body dementias. *Proceedings of the National Academy of Sciences of the United States of America.* 2000;97:5039-5043.

[11] Eastman Kodak Company. KODAK PROFESSIONAL T-MAX Films. Technical publication F-4016. February, 2004. Available at: *<http://www.kodak.com/global/en/professional/support/techPubs/f4016/f4016.jhtml>*.

[12] Otsu N. A threshold selection method from grey-level histograms. *IEEE Transactions on Systems, Man, and Cybernetics*. 1979;9:377-393.

[13] Sezgin M, Sankur B. Survey over image thresholding techniques and quantitative performance evaluation. *Journal of Electronic Imaging*. 2004;13:146-165.

[14] Seldon HL. Structure of human auditory cortex, III: statistical analysis of dendritic trees. *Brain Research*. 1982;249:211-221.

[15] Barber CB, Dobkin DP, Huhdanpaa H. The quickhull algorithm for convex hulls. *ACM Transactions on Mathematical Software*. 1996;22:469-483.

[16] Buxhoeveden DP, Switala AE, Roy E, Casanova MF. Quantitative analysis of cell columns in the cerebral cortex. *Journal of Neuroscience Methods*. 2000;97:7-17.

[17] Kenan-Vaknin G, Ouaknine GE, Razon N, Malach R. Organization of layers II–III connections in human visual cortex revealed by *in vitro* injections of biocytin. *Brain Research.* 1992;594:339-342.

[18] Peters A, Kara D. The neuronal composition of area 17 in rat visual cortex, IV: the organization of pyramidal cells. *Journal of Comparative Neurology.* 1987;260:573-590.

[19] Preparata FP, Shamos MI. *Computational Geometry: An Introduction*. New York, NY: Springer-Verlag; 1985.

[20] Galaburda AM, Sanides F. Cytoarchitectonic organization of the human auditory cortex. Journal of Comparative. *Neurology*. 1980;190:597-610.

[21] Pourdeyhimi B, Xu B, Nayernouri A. Evaluating carpet appearance loss: pile lay orientation. *Textile Research Journal* 1994;64:130-135.

[22] Tommerdahl M, Favorov O, Whitsel BL, Nakhle B, Gonchar YA. Minicolumnar activation patterns in cat and monkey S1 cortex. *Cerebral Cortex*. 1993;3:399-411.

[23] Casanova MF, de Zeeuw L, Switala AE, et al. Lamination abnormalities in the prefrontal cortex of patients with schizophrenia. *Biological Psychiatry*. 2004;55:214S.

[24] Heinsen H, Heinsen YL. Serial thick, frozen, gallocyanin stained sections of human central nervous system. *Journal of Histotechnology*. 1991;14:167-173.

[25] Davison AC, Hinkley DV. *Bootstrap Methods and Their Application*. Cambridge, England: Cambridge University Press; 1997.

[26] Pakkenberg H. The number of nerve cells in the cerebral cortex of man. *Journal of Comparative Neurology*. 1966;128:17-20.

[27] Robins E, Smith DE, Eydt KM. The quantitative histochemistry of the cerebral cortex, I: architectonic distribution of ten chemical constituents in the motor and visual cortices. *Journal of Neurochemistry*. 1956;1:54-67.

[28] Favorov OV, Kelly G. Minicolumnar organization within somatosensory cortical segregates, I: development of afferent connections. *Cerebral Cortex*. 1994;4:408-427.

[29] Favorov OV, Kelly G. Minicolumnar organization within somatosensory cortical segregates, II: emergent functional properties. *Cerebral Cortex*. 1994;4:428-442.

In: Neocortical Modularity and the Cell Minicolumn
Editor: Manuel F. Casanova, pp. 181-185
ISBN 1-59454-301
© 2005 Nova Science Publishers, Inc.

Chapter X

THE VERTICALITY INDEX: A QUANTITATIVE APPROACH TO THE ANALYSIS OF THE COLUMNAR ARRANGEMENT OF NEURONS IN THE PRIMATE NEOCORTEX

Axel Schleicher*
Heinrich-Heine University Duesseldorf, Duesseldorf, Germany
Karl Zilles
Heinrich-Heine University Duesseldorf;
Institute of Medicine, Research Center Juelich, Juelich, Germany

INTRODUCTION

The grey level index (GLI) is a stereological approach to quantitative cytoarchitecture. In contrast to the classical stereological method of Haug [1], which estimates mean and standard deviation of the volume density of neurons by sampling and point counting in a bounded 3D volume, the GLI estimates this parameter using an automated image analyzing system with a defined spatial resolution. At the light microscopic level, whole histological brain sections or selected regions of interest (ROI) are scanned at a spatial resolution defined by a grid of measuring fields. This image transformation converts the gray value image of the histological specimen into a GLI-image with pixel values indicating the local volume density of neurons.

GLI-images were used in a variety of applications, e.g., enhanced visualization of the cortical laminar pattern [2], analysis of this pattern using GLI-profiles defined perpendicularly to the cortical [3], and detection of boundaries between neighboring cortical areas using an observer-independent procedure [4].

* Corresponding author: Axel Schleicher, C. and O. Vogt Institute of Brain Research, Heinrich-Heine University Duesseldorf, P.O. Box 101007, 40001 Duesseldorf, Germany. E-mail: axel@hirn.uni-duesseldorf.de

METHODS

GLI-transformation

For a detailed description of the GLI-transformation, see Schleicher et al. [7] In short, GLI is defined as the proportion of a measuring field covered by the projected transects of all stained cell bodies. It provides an estimate of the volume density of neuronal somata versus neuropil since glial and endothelial cell nuclei contribute only a small proportion, which does not vary across layers [8].

In histological sections (formalin fixed, paraffin embedded, section thickness 30 μm, cut in the coronal plane approximately parallel to the cell columns, silver stained for cell bodies), rectangular regions of interest (ROI) were interactively defined and completely covered by a continuous, mosaic-like pattern of video frames using an image analyzing system (KS400, Zeiss, Germany). From each video frame, a binary image was generated by adaptive thresholding [5] and subdivided into a grid of square measuring fields. Field size and, thus, spatial resolution was set to 10 μm to resolve vertical structures of a width not smaller than 30 μm. In each field, the area fraction of cellular transects was measured and assigned to pixel values of the resulting data matrix (GLI-image).

Verticality Index

Within GLI-images, frames were interactively centered in the layer being investigated and perpendicular to the cell columns (Figure 1A–B). Frame width was about 2000 μm, frame height was adjusted to the height of the layer. From the GLI-values covered by the frame, GLI-profiles were extracted as column averages describing the course of GLI-values along the cortical layer, i.e., at right angles to the vertically oriented cell columns. GLI-profiles were reduced in noise by applying a median filter (3×1 kernel). As a result, peaks of only one pixel in width were eliminated.

The degree of columnar organization was quantified by extracting five features (Figure 1C) from each GLI-profile: the mean amplitude of profile peaks (A), the mean and standard deviation of the widths of the profiles peaks (W, SD_W), and the mean and standard deviation of the distances between the profile peaks (D, SD_D). These parameters were used for statistical evaluation and comparison of columnar organization among areas.

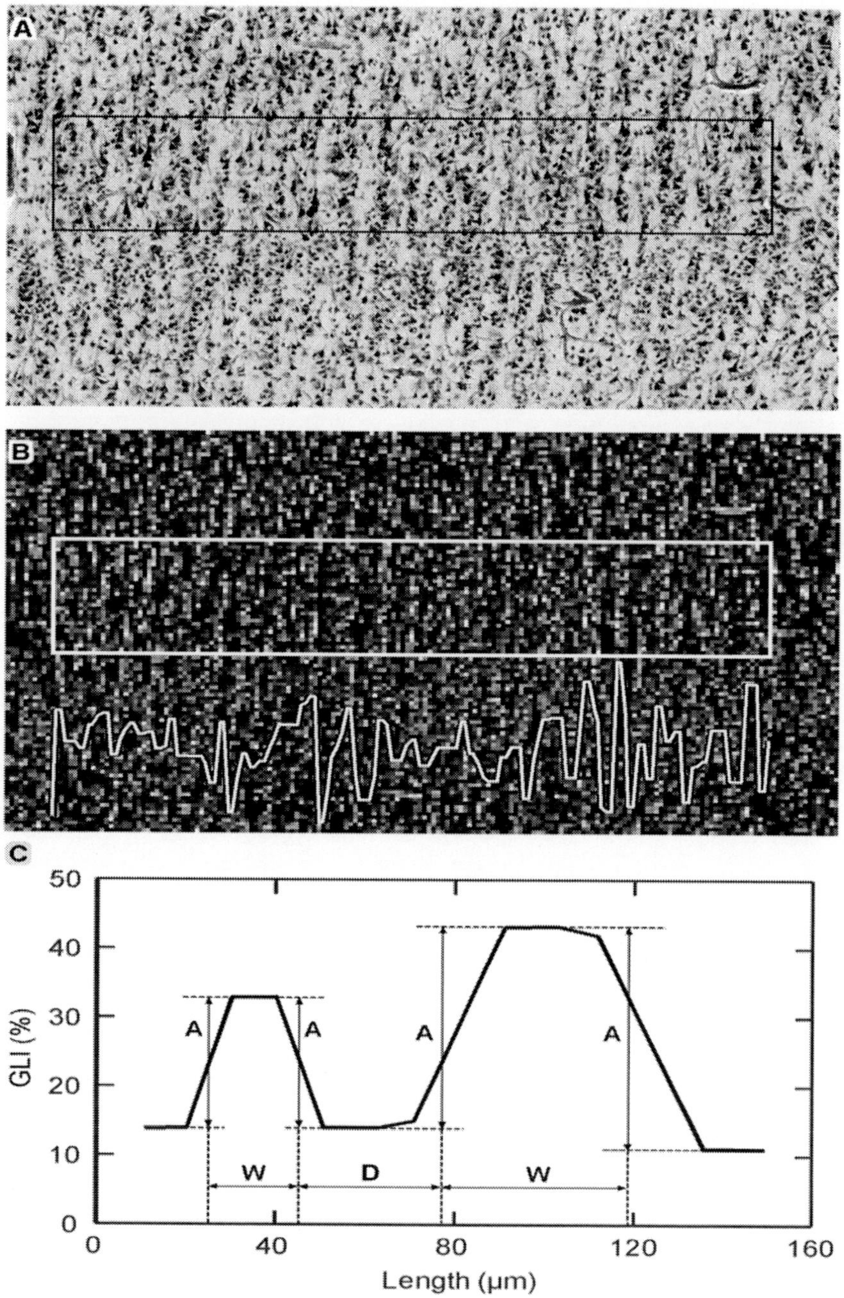

Figure 1. Quantitative evaluation of the degree of columnar organization. (A) Silver-stained histological section from the human temporal area 42. A rectangular frame (width 1600 µm, height 300 µm) is centered over layer IIIb. (B) GLI-image (184×109 pixels) of the grey value image in (A). Each pixel represents a square measuring field 10 µm in size. GLI-values are coded in grey values ranging from 0 % (black) to 100 % (white). The frame corresponds to the frame shown in (A). The respective GLI-profile is shown below (not drawn to scale). (C) Definition of the peak's amplitude A, its width W, and the intercolumnar distance D between two profile peaks.

To facilitate extended, univariate statistics and visualization of data, the degree of columnarity was subsequently expressed by means of the verticality index (VI), which results from a linear combination of three features (A, SD_W, SD_D). To achieve a unified scaling, z-scores for each of the parameters were calculated based on means and standard deviations calculated from all GLI-profiles in all layers and areas. The laminar VI for a specific area and layer was determined as follows:

$$VI = A' - SD'_W - SD'_D$$

The VI indicates the relative degree of columnar organization in a distinct area and layer compared to the overall mean of all areas and layers evaluated in a distinct brain. It increases with increasing mean amplitude and decreases with increasing inhomogeneity of the columnar arrangement, i.e., with increasing standard deviations of the columnar width and the intercolumnar distance. A negative value indicates a degree of columnar organization below the overall average VI across all layers and areas; a positive value indicates a more pronounced columnar pattern.

Application and Results

The verticality index was used as a criteria to characterize the spatial organization of the cingulate (areas 24b, 23b, and 31) and pericingulate (areas 7 and 19) cortex in the human brain [29]. Ten sections per area were analyzed. The average width W of cell columns was about 40 μm, separated by a neuropil rich fascicle (D) of the same dimension (values not corrected for shrinkage).

Differences in the degree of columniation were found among areas and layers, with the maximum value in area 19, layer IIIb (2.44) and the minimum value in area 31, layer IV (-2.03). Multivariate statistics comprising all layers into area VI indicated the lowest value in area 31, which differed significantly from higher values in areas 19, 23b, and 24b. Area 7 was more similar to area 31 than to the other areas.

Discussion

The VI-approach has some advantages over procedures based on single cell analysis. 1) It is robust since it is founded on the basic stereological field parameter "volume density," which is not biased by the high degree of anisotropy in the cortex. This is important when serial sections from highly convoluted brains are analyzed and the plane of the section being investigated is cut in such a way that the columns cannot be detected in full length. 2) No detection of individual columns is required. This allows inclusion of regions with less pronounced or visually unrecognizable columnar organization into an analysis. Even in such areas, regular changes in columnar cell density could be demonstrated by applying the described procedure. 3) It is fast since time-consuming image analyzing procedures, such as deagglomeration, are not required. This facilitates the analysis of large samples. In addition, several ROI can be analyzed within a single GLI-image.

On the other hand, there is one obvious limitation. The VI is a global measure, which supplies no information concerning the internal structure of individual columns, i.e., their spatial cellular organization such as intercellular distance and cell size. It is not an absolute measure but describes the degree of columnar organization, which is defined as the relative deviation from a mean index of all areas and layers included in an analysis.

REFERENCES

[1] Haug H. Remarks on the determination and significance of the gray cell coefficient. *Journal of Comparative Neurology.* 1956;104:473-492.

[2] Schleicher A, Zilles K. A quantitative approach to cytoarchitectonics: analysis of structural inhomogeneities in nervous tissue using an image analyser. *Journal of Microscopy.* 1990;157:367-381.

[3] Amunts K, Schleicher A, Ditterich A, Zilles K. Broca's region: cytoarchitectonic asymmetry and developmental changes. *Journal of Comparative Neurology.* 2003;465:72-89.

[4] Zilles K, Schleicher A, Palomero-Gallagher N, Amunts K. Quantitative analysis of cyto- and receptor architecture of the human brain. In: Toga AW, Maziotta JC, eds. *Brain Mapping: The Methods*, 2nd ed. Amsterdam, Netherlands: Academic Press; 2002:573-602.

[5] Castleman KR. *Digital Image Processing*. Englewood Cliffs, NJ: Prentice Hall; 1979.

[6] Schlaug G, Schleicher A, Zilles K. Quantitative analysis of the columnar arrangement of neurons in the human cingulate cortex. *Journal of Comparative Neurology.* 1995;351:441-452.

[7] Schleicher A, Amunts K, Geyer S, et al. A stereological approach to human cortical architecture: identification and delineation of cortical areas. *Journal of Chemical Neuroanatomyt.* 2000;20:31-47.

[8] Wree A, Schleicher A, Zilles K. Estimation of volume fractions in nervous tissue with an image analyzer. *Journal of Neuroscience Methods.* 1982;6:29-43.

In: Neocortical Modularity and the Cell Minicolumn
Editor: Manuel F. Casanova, pp. 187-203

ISBN 1-59454-301
© 2005 Nova Science Publishers, Inc.

Chapter IX

MOUNTCASTLE PRINCIPLE OF COLUMNAR CORTEX AS BASIS FOR THEORY OF HIGHER BRAIN FUNCTION CLINICAL RELEVANCE

Gordon L. Shaw* and Mark Bodner
M.I.N.D. Institute, Costa Mesa, CA

INTRODUCTION

The understanding of how we think, reason, and create is one of the most important and challenging areas of science. The crucial breakthrough that allows us to investigate this is the Mountcastle Principle of columnar mammalian cortex structure and function. The trion model is a mathematical realization of the Mountcastle Principle. This chapter presents a review of the trion model and its predictions along with the many diverse behavioral, brain imaging, educational, and neurophysiological studies, all of which give strong support for the model and its Mountcastle Principle underpinnings. Perhaps the most well-known set of these studies is the generalized Mozart effect (gMe): defined as enhanced higher brain function in response to music. Proposed tests of the model with large clinical relevance in neuropathologies are outlined.

The cortex is the part of the brain responsible for highest-level thinking. As put forward by Vernon Mountcastle [1] in his groundbreaking columnar principle of mammalian cortex, it is made up of columns forming the fundamental neuronal network and is comprised of small irreducible processing units called minicolumns. (The columnar cortex is now mainstream neuroscience [39]–[4].) Mountcastle proposed that the column has the capability of being excited into complex spatial-temporal firing patterns. The assumption is that higher mammalian brain functions involve the creation and transformation of such spatial-temporal

* Corresponding author: Gordon L. Shaw, M.I.N.D. Institute, 1503 South Coast Drive, Suite 202, Costa Mesa, 92626 CA, USA. Tel: (714)751-5443; Fax: (714)751-5915; E-mail: gshaw@mindinstitute.net

firing patterns as the code for its internal neural language. (This is in contrast to a cortical language or code, which involves sets of neurons firing with high frequency that might be used in emergencies such as when you see a big shark swimming toward you.)

The trion model [5]–[10] is a highly idealized symmetric mathematical realization of Mountcastle's Principle. The trion model has led to several profound predictions. 1) Built into the structured brain is the *innate* ability to do spatial-temporal (ST) reasoning – thinking in pictures as in chess, music and math – involving patterns and symmetries developing in space and time [8]. 2) There is a *causal* connection between music and enhanced ST reasoning [6], as well as the learning of abstract math concepts through an ST approach [10]. 3) There is an innate common ST brain *language* and *grammar* [6],[9],[10], as parts of the brain "talk" with each other, and this is the basis for human language. Predictions 1 and 2 have motivated seminal behavioral, educational and neurophysiological studies supporting and dramatically furthering these concepts; prediction 3 has yet to be tested. Here, we summarize the trion model and its predictions, then give the results from these studies. *We suggest further tests of the model with large potential clinical relevance to neuropathologies.*

TRION MODEL

The trion model [5]–[10] represents a mathematical realization of Mountcastle's Principle of columnar organization and cortex function [1],[39] (Figure 1). The model was developed starting from William Little's seminal neural network analogy [11],[12] to physical spin systems [13]. The trion represents the minicolumn and has three levels of firing activity.

The interactions among the trions are believed be localized, *competing* (between excitation and inhibition), and highly structured, and the firing state of the network (cortical column) of the *distinguishable* trions is updated in a probabilistic way related to the states of the two previous discrete time steps τ. We expect these time steps τ to be roughly 25–100 ms.

Studies of the trion model for learning and memory and higher brain function have been reported. Basically, the success of these studies is based on the localized, competing (between excitation and inhibition), highly symmetric interactions, yielding a huge repertoire of inherent quasi-stable, periodic firing patterns. *Defined as Memory Patterns or MPs*, any of them can be readily learned or enhanced with only small changes in the interaction strengths using the Hebb learning algorithm [7],[12],[14]. An arbitrary spatial-temporal pattern cannot be readily learned. Only an MP can be learned in a "rapid and natural" *selective* manner[7]. The MPs evolve in natural sequences from one to another in probabilistic calculations, as in Figure 2.

A dramatic result of the trion model is that there are families of MPs related by symmetries. Consider an MP enhanced through the Hebb learning rule; the trion network can recognize other members of the symmetry family of this MP in time evolutions [8],[9]. We proposed that perhaps this built-in ability of the structured cortex to recognize MPs related by symmetries was the elemental operation for higher brain functions involved in ST reasoning and processing of music.

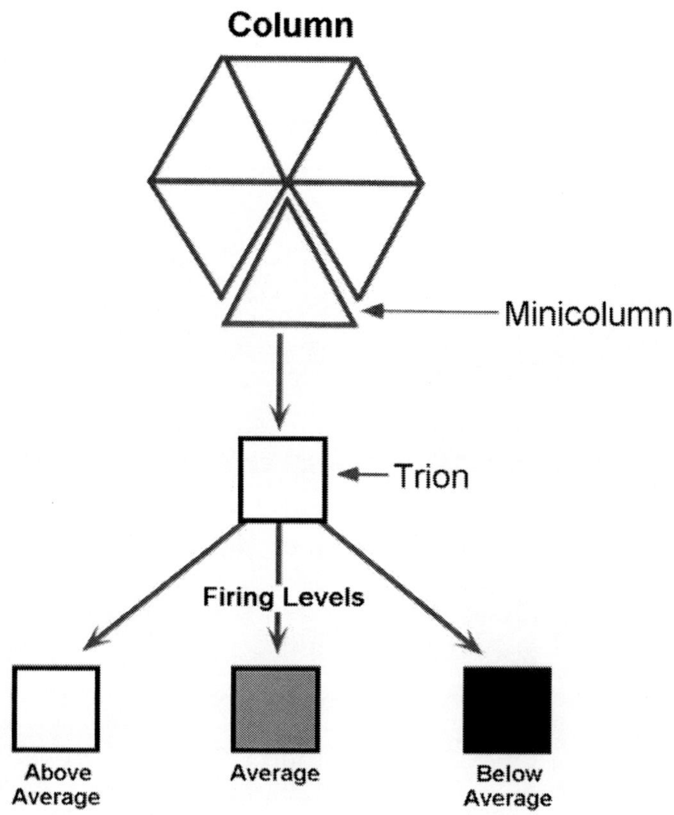

Figure 1. Highly schematic representation of the Mountcastle Principle of cortical organization: a cortical column (horizontal dimension roughly 700 μm, comprising the vertical layers of dimension about 2000 μm) where each triangle is a distinguishable minicolumn (forming irreducible processing units), which encodes the relevant modality or parameter in the stimuli (such as line orientation in the visual cortex). We identify a minicolumn with the idealized trion, and the basic network is the column. The trion has three levels of firing: above average (white), average (gray), and below average (black).

INNATE CORTICAL LANGUAGE AND GRAMMAR

A higher level architecture of cortical columns led to the startling realization that the inherent trion model language had an innate cortical grammar [10]. We calculated the enhancements of global firing of the coupled trion model columns through a Hebb learning rule. Only certain combinations and positions of MPs could be learned, with symmetry properties playing a major role. This then is a cortical grammar.

We suggest that these trion model results represent a glimpse of an inherent internal cortical language with a built-in grammar. We may view the temporal patterns for the individual trion as "letters" in an alphabet, and the resultant MPs as cortical "words," dependent on the connectivity among the trions in a column. Now for cortical columns coupled through a Hebb learning rule, we are able to build reliable short-term memory patterns with different words in each column for specific temporal phases and spatial rotations, but not for all combinations of such words. *This is precisely an inherent internal cortical grammar resulting from the structured Mountcastle columnar principle.*

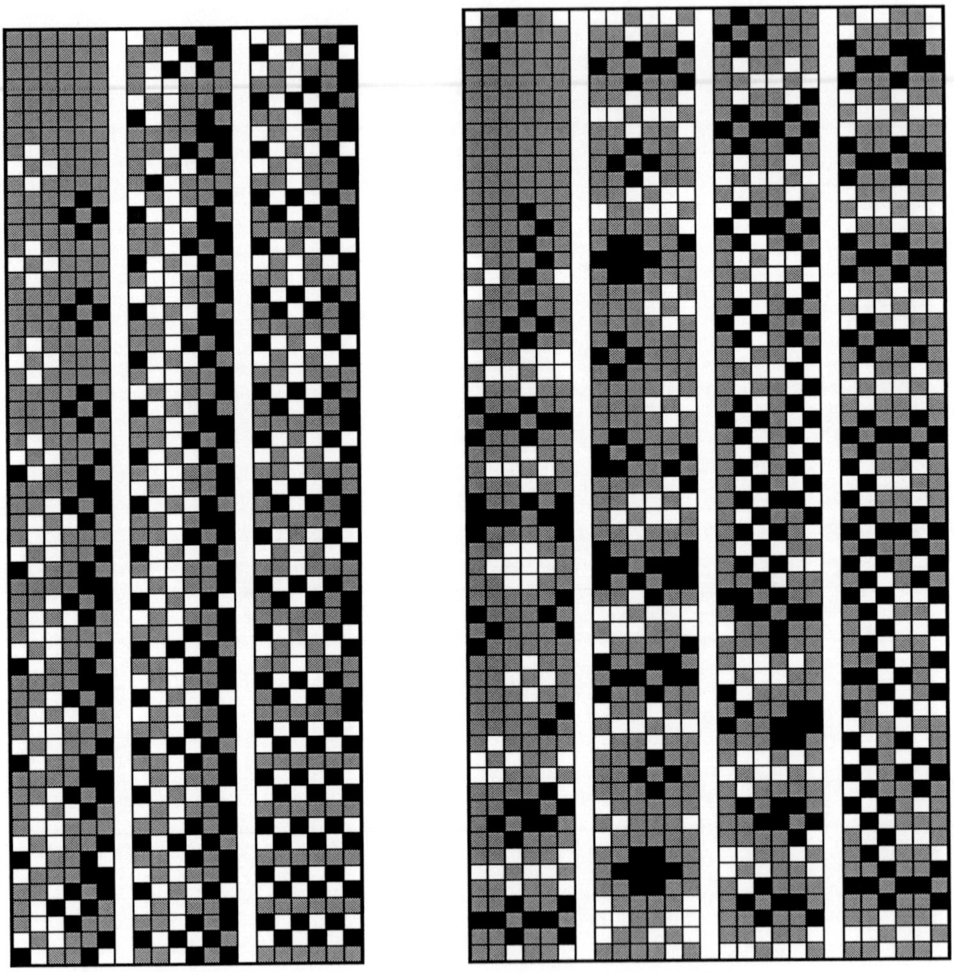

A B

Figure 2. Time evolutions of the firing activity of a columnar network of six trions, as generated by a computer, giving examples of the sequential mode (A) and the creative mode (B). Each square in a given row represents the trion firing level: white is above average, gray is average, and black is below average. Time runs from top left to bottom right. Each horizontal row represents a ring of interconnected trions, as in Figure 1, so that the sixth square wraps around to meet the first. (A) There are seven different memory patterns (MPs) that cycle two or more times. This sequential evolution has low synaptic fluctuations. (B) This time evolution has larger synaptic fluctuations than in (A). This is an example of a creative evolution in that specific MPs appear and reappear. It is these creative evolutions that, when mapped onto music, give the striking results of producing recognizable human type music [6],[9]. (Changes in neuromodulators in the model take one back and forth between evolutions of type A and B as in Figure 5.)

Much further work on the higher columnar trion architectures is necessary before more detailed features of the proposed cortical language and grammar can be discerned. However, already, testable neurophysiological predictions can be made. We suggest searching for a temporal "alphabet" at the minicolumn (or columnar level, as will be discussed later), which is common throughout the cortex. This involves not only the appropriate behavioral experiments but also the appropriate analyses of the resultant cortical data exploiting symmetry.

EXPERIMENTAL TESTS OF THE TRION MODEL

The connection between math and music extends to the ancient Greeks who considered music as one of the four branches of math. The correlation between music training for children and their high math performance has been noted for some time. However, this could simply be due to parents giving music lessons to smart children. The predictive theory of music training *causally* enhancing math abilities began with Leng and Shaw [6].

The brain's innate ability to relate (through symmetry operations) the MPs is the unifying physiological mechanism of higher brain function. The finding that the structure of these MPs and their symmetry relationships, as shown in Figure 2, were that of recognizable human styles of music by Leng and Shaw led to the realization [6] that "music could be used as a window into higher brain function" and the *prediction that specific music and music training could act as exercise for cortical ST function, thus enhancing ST reasoning.* Children can more readily understand math concepts through the ST approach, allowing them to solve standard quantitative equations and word problems.

The trion model [5]–[10] motivated and guided these innovative, collaborative behavioral and neurophysiological experiments, all with *major* results.

Generalized Mozart Effect - gMe (Enhanced Higher Brain Function in Response to Music)

Mozart effect causal experiments [9],[15],[16]: College students, after listening to the first 10 minutes of Mozart's *Sonata for Two Pianos in D Major* (K.448), showed subsequent short-term (10–15 min) enhancement of spatial-temporal reasoning. These results received an *enormous* amount of attention in 1993 and were called the Mozart effect by the media. The following experimental studies generalize these initial Mozart effect studies and should be considered in their entirety along with the motivating trion model as the gMe.

Alzheimer patients [17],[18], after listening to Mozart's sonata, had enhanced short-term spatial-temporal reasoning.

Exposure in epileptic patients (*even those in a coma*) to Mozart's sonata reduced neuropathological spiking activity [19],[20].

Long-term exposure to Mozart's sonata enhanced maze learning by rats; the enhanced performance lasted more than 4 h after the last exposure to music [21]. A recent study with mice [22] has extended this enhancement time to more than 6 h. These animal studies clear the possibility of some long-term enhancement from considerable exposure to Mozart's sonata. Such results may be clinically relevant to the treatment of epilepsy, for example.

An EEG (surface brain wave) coherence study [23] gave evidence for a carryover of listening to Mozart's sonata to subsequent spatial-temporal task in specific cortical regions. This gave the first neurophysiological evidence for the Mozart effect. The idea is that Mozart's sonata "resonates" [9] with the innate columnar structure of the cortex.

Functional magnetic resonance imaging (fMRI) studies comparing cortical blood flow activation by Mozart's sonata versus other music gave striking results [24],[25]. In addition to the expected fMRI activation in cortical regions associated with music, substantial activation was found in cortical regions important for spatial-temporal reasoning. Further fMRI studies (along with EEG studies) should not only be extremely valuable in determining the neurophysiological basis for the Mozart effect but also in determining which other music might give similar enhancements in ST reasoning: a gMe [9], e.g., music of J.S. Bach.

Direct Tests of the Trion Model of Higher Brain Function

A consistency test of the trion model and the Mountcastle columnar ST code for higher brain function came with the demonstration of highly accurate mental rehearsals. The temporal durations of mental rehearsals of pieces of music lasting up to a few minutes were extraordinarily reproducible [26].

Neurophysiological studies confirmed, as predicted, the presence of families of spatial-temporal firing patterns related by symmetries during higher brain function [27].

Music Training Enhances Spatial-temporal Reasoning and Learning Math for Children

Preschool children [28] who received piano keyboard lessons for six months improved dramatically on an age standardized spatial-temporal reasoning task, with the effect lasting for several days.

STAR (ST Animation Reasoning) is ingenious math software developed by Matthew Peterson. We contend that these non-verbal math games utilize innate ST abilities built into our structured cortex. Inner city 2nd graders given piano keyboard training along with STAR training scored significantly higher [29] on proportional math and fractions than children given control training along with STAR. A special interactive version of STAR by Peterson may be found on the CD-ROM enclosed in *Keeping Mozart in Mind*, 2nd ed. [9]

Second graders given piano keyboard training, STAR lessons, and lessons bringing this ST approach into their regular language based math curriculum did as well on advanced math concepts as 4th graders from a higher socioeconomic school lacking our training [9]. They also greatly enhanced their performance on nationwide standardized math tests (Martinez et al., unpublished findings).

A particularly demanding STAR game, Big Seed, was used to train middle and elementary school children. This study [30] gave strong evidence that ST reasoning is not only innate but far exceeds optimistic expectations. This is based on the percentage of children achieving exceptional ST performance in less than 7 h of training and retention of ability when tested 7 months later. We propose that the Mountcastle Principle provided the neurophysiological basis for these striking results.

These 12 highly successful and fundamentally distinct experiments are all extremely relevant to the general theme [6] of "music as a window into higher brain function." *They are all supportive of the basic underlying trion model predictions that motivated them and must be considered as an entire coherent body of knowledge.* This fundamental scientific research continues as we are just at the very beginning. It is as if we have found a vein of gold leading to the gold mine of understanding higher brain function. The trion model [5]–[10] provides a road map to our understanding of higher brain function. We all know that the connections in a young child's brain are rapidly being modified as a result of experience and learning. The crucial distinguishing concept of the trion model (as derived from the Mountcastle columnar principle of cortex) is that the infant's brain starts with an innate, well-defined, and common internal neural language and grammar.

Spatial-Temporal Language of Music

Taking seriously the idea that Mozart's sonata (K.448) could tell us something major about the symmetries of the brain, we mapped [31] the standard music score of this sonata, Figure 3A, onto ST patterns as in the trion brain model and onto actual brain patterns. The result (defined as trion music, Figure 3B) showed symmetries in amazing clarity. This and other similar mappings of music onto trion music patterns are being examined qualitatively and quantitatively for insights into the neural language of higher brain function.

We now have begun to define ST language and grammar [32] for such trion music as in Figure 3B, exploiting symmetry and patterns. For example, we define music ST contours A, B, C, an D (in Figs. 4A–D, respectively) and identify them as "words." Then the trion music of Mozart in measures 55 and 56 shown in Figure 3B (repeated in Figure 4E for clarity) can be expressed simply as a "phrase" in Figure 4E. The entire first movement of Mozart's sonata can be similarly expressed in terms of a fairly small set of analogous contours or words.

We might identify these music contours, Fig 4A–D, as ST music words. We are in the process of analyzing the Mozart trion music (along with other music translated into trion music) for a music language and grammar to be compared with the trion brain model language and grammar presented above. Analysis of real cortical activity data [9],[27],[33] has shown similar trion-like patterns, symmetries, and contours. *These three "languages," (trion brain model language, trion music language, and cortical activity trion-like data language), along with the constraints of innate human language and grammar, will be used to decipher the cortical ST code of higher brain function.*

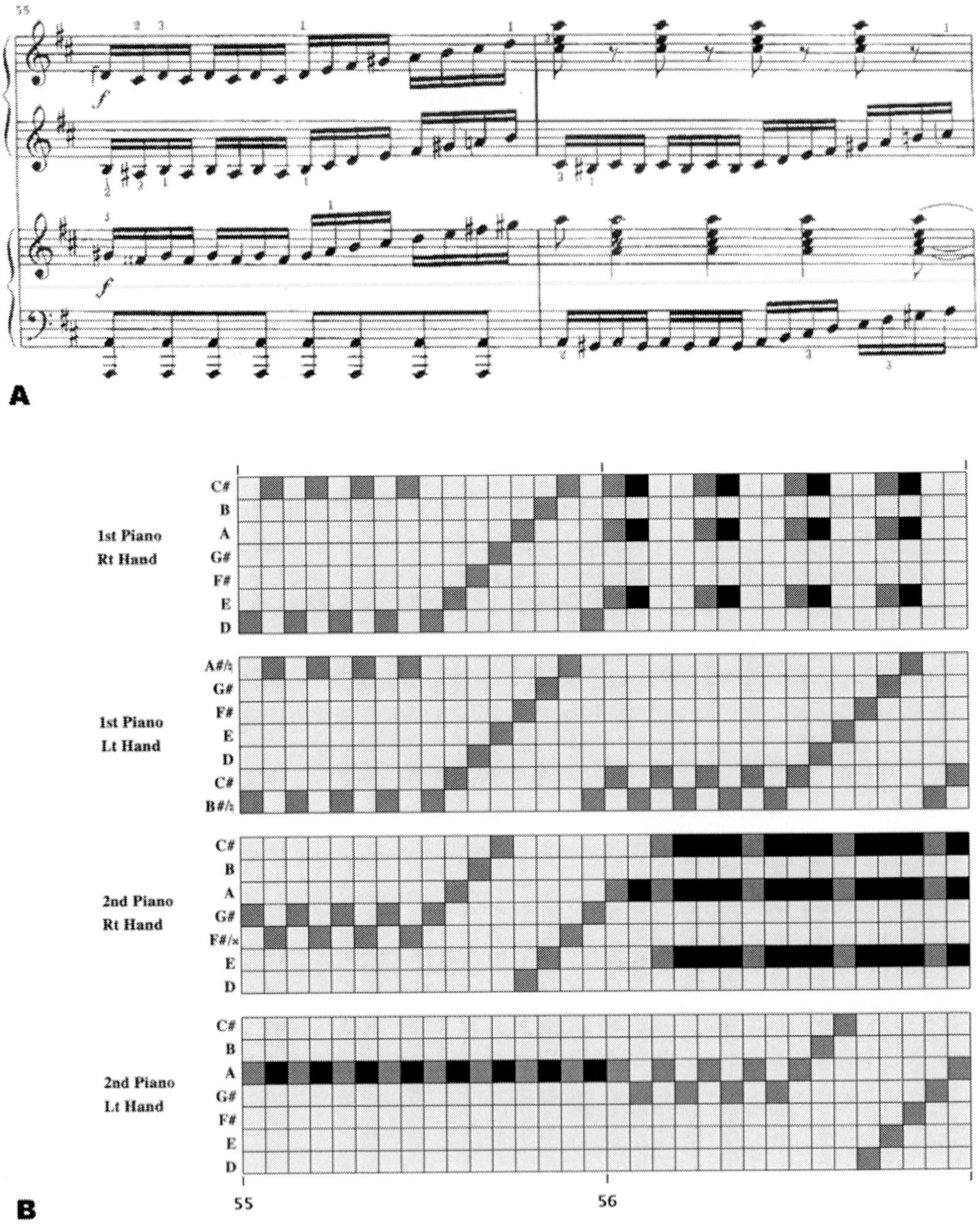

Figure 3. (A) Mozart's *Sonata for Two Pianos in D Major* (K.448) music score for measures 55 and 56 (1781). (B) "Translation" or mapping of the two Mozart music scores measured in (A) onto trion-like patterns [31]. Each square represents a sixteenth note. Dark gray denotes played and black denotes held. The pitches wrap around, octaves are not shown nor are grace notes or thirty-second notes. The visual display of symmetries is striking and dramatic (to the non-musician). This is especially evident when viewed in color on a computer, and the movement of the displayed patterns is synched to the actual music performance (Available at: http://www.MindInstitute.net).

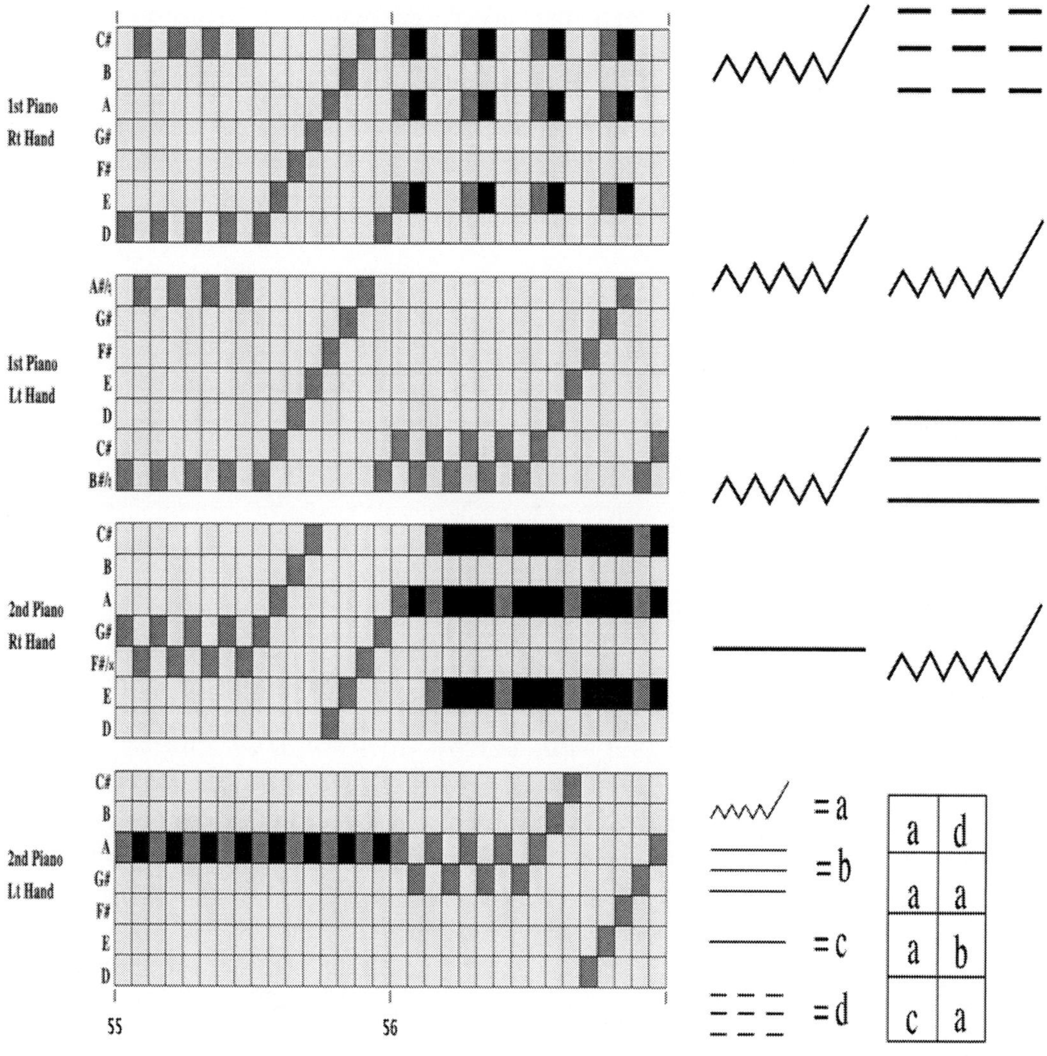

Figure 4. Search for a potential music language and grammar to be compared to the innate brain language and grammar [32]. Define the music contours A, B, C, and D, which include related symmetry family members in A, B, C, and D, respectively. We consider contours A–D as words E. Then measures 55 and 56 of the Mozart's *Sonata* in trion music form, Figure 3B, which we repeat for ease in comparison, are written in terms of A–D and become a "phrase" with possible rules, leading to the Mozart effect.

Formal Human Language and Grammar

It is as yet unclear whether human language systems [34]–[36] in the cortex are the result of a qualitative departure from the general mammalian cortical design or a less radical specialization with origins present in lower mammals. Our finding of the presence of an inherent mammalian cortical language with a built-in grammar strongly supports the second hypothesis, which is further supported by the very clever cross-species experiment of Ramus et al. [37] They showed that newborn infants and tamarin monkeys could discriminate sentences from Dutch and Japanese but not if they were played backward. These experimental results are consistent with the trion model calculations presented here showing that the ordering of the cortical "words" can be crucial.

We see that a cortical language and grammar arises naturally from the trion model realization of the Mountcastle columnar principle of mammalian cortex. In conclusion, there are new tools from the present trion model results, from new neurophysiological analyses, and from cross-species behavioral experiments to explore and examine the possibility of an innate cortical language and grammar. Clearly, one of the most ambitious and important goals in science is to identify and then decode this innate mammalian cortical language of higher brain function.

Tests of Trion Model with Clinical Relevance

There are three features of the trion model we identify, allowing us to suggest tests with significant clinical relevance:

The detailed trion cortical language, as illustrated in Figure 2, led to the landmark prediction [6] that *specific music and music training could act as exercise for cortical ST function and thus enhance ST reasoning*. These predictions led to the seminal studies above of the Mozart effect, the much more inclusive gMe, and the piano keyboard training-causal enhancements. As discussed in Chapter 21 of Shaw [9], these studies have large potential relevance for clinical treatments in Alzheimer's disease [17],[18], autism [38], Down's syndrome, epilepsy [19],[20], stroke recovery, and William's syndrome.

The possibility of inherent ultradian time scales in the brain between one second and one day, as manifested and expressed in neuromodulators, led to discussion [9] concerning clinical treatment of several neuropathologies. In particular, let's consider Parkinson's disease, which involves the regulation of dopamine. The clinical treatment of Parkinson's disease is generally to keep the dopamine levels constant (for example, by giving the dopamine precursor L-DOPA). In rats, a large inherent circadian dopamine rhythm exists [39]. *If this inherent dopamine rhythm is present in humans (with a change in light-dark phase similar to when rats are active), one would presumably want to simulate the magnitude and phase of the natural levels of dopamine in the Parkinson patient.* Further, shorter inherent ultradian rhythms on the order of an hour or less might exist for dopamine or other neuromodulators [9]. These inherent rhythms then should be taken into account in relevant clinical treatments.

The concept illustrated in Figure 2 is that in the trion model contains two major modes of higher cortical thinking, *sequential* and *creative*, and the natural flow between them is regulated by neuromodulators [6],[9], as shown in Figure 5. For example, consider a master chess player evaluating the middle game position. Out of the huge number of possible sequences of moves involved in thinking 5 or 6 steps ahead, the player quickly focuses on a few possibilities while in the creative mode. Then in the sequential mode, the player evaluates them to settle on the move.

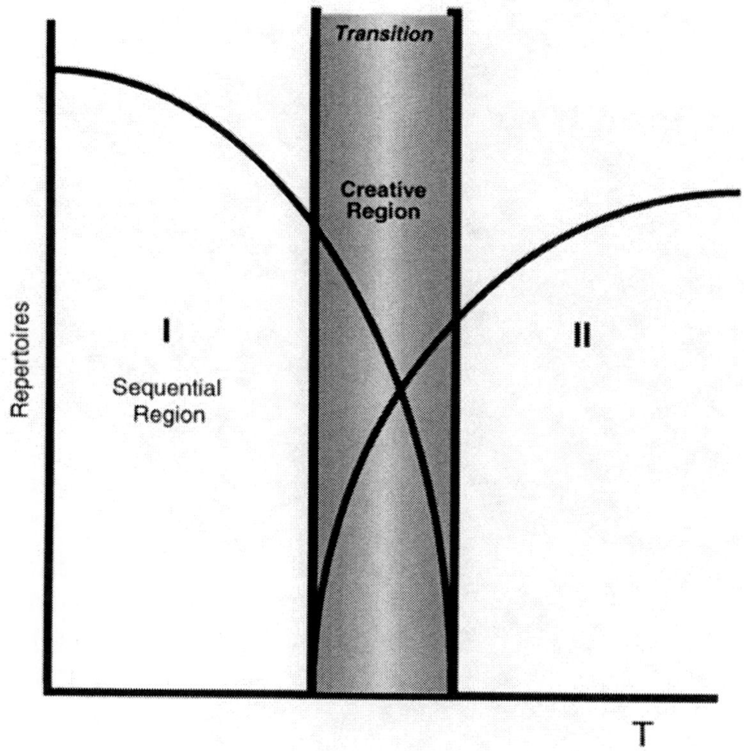

Figure 5. Sequential and creative function regions as a function of fluctuation parameter T in the trion columnar model of cortex [6],[9]. Repertoires of the families of MPs in sequential regions I and II switch and transition into the creative region as T is varied [40]. We proposed that neuromodulators change T and move the cortical function naturally back and forth between sequential and creative modes. We suggest here that getting "stuck" in a sequential mode region might correspond to the neuropathology of autism, and the creative mode region might correspond to schizophrenia.

In the trion model, as the synaptic fluctuation parameter T is varied [40], the cortex oscillates between sequential regions (modes) I and II and the creative region (mode). We suggest [6] that certain neuromodulators can induce this crucial change. Here we will focus on the potential resulting neuropathologies if this oscillating flow, between sequential and creative modes, is faulty. For example, serotonin has been implicated in synaptic fluctuations [41], and a pathology in serotonin release or uptake may cause the cortex to be "stuck." *Being stuck in a sequential mode region might correspond to the neuropathology of autism, while being stuck in the creative mode region might correspond to schizophrenia.*

Other candidate neuromodulators might be involved in these pathologies instead of or in addition to serotonin. In addition to considerations testing these ideas at the neuromodulator level, we refer to a potentially powerful test at the cortical network level. As described in the Appendix, we use our new symmetric method of analysis [33] on EEG data to attempt to understand and diagnose certain neuropathologies, as well as to assess efficacy of clinical treatment.

Conclusion

The trion model of cortex is a specific mathematical realization of the Mountcastle Columnar Principle of mammalian cortex. We have illustrated the wide range of powerful predictions on higher brain function that follow from the trion model and the landmark studies that support and elaborate on these predictions. Due to the robustness of the trion model as far as varying its parameters, we conclude that the Mountcastle Principle directs us to the powerful, qualitative insights presented here on the nature of how we think, reason, and create, as well as insights into how particular neuropathologies might be treated in a non-invasive clinical manner.

Appendix
Clinical Applications of Symmetry Analysis

A potentially powerful new symmetry method of diagnosing and assessing treatments of certain neuropathologies through analysis of EEG cortical data has been presented [33]. The first step in this analysis of cortical EEG, as illustrated in Figure 6, involves performing a specific binning and mapping procedure and putting the voltages of each surface electrode into three levels motivated by the trion model.

Next, pattern detection algorithms are applied to the spatial array of mapped EEG data [[9],[27],[33]]. (EEG arrays of 128 electrodes are now in use.) Pattern detection determines the number of occurrences of ST patterns, and the numbers of occurrences of all patterns are related to one another by a defined closed set of symmetry relationships (e.g., inversion of the temporal order of pattern elements for each electrode as in Figure 6E or left-right reflection of the patterns on the spatial array of electrodes). A given global (over the array of EEG electrodes) ST pattern and the set of patterns obtained through application of the symmetry relationships comprise a symmetric pattern family. If one of the symmetry operations is performed on all of the members of the pattern family, the individual members transform back into each other, and the family remains unchanged.

A symmetry index is defined [33] whose value (from 0 to 1) indicates the degree to which patterned activity distributes itself across the different symmetrically related patterns of a family. A symmetry index value of 0 corresponds to cortical activity that exhibits a pattern without exhibiting any of its symmetrically related pattern family members (over a given time window). An index value of 1 corresponds to a pattern and all of its symmetrically related family members that occur within some time window, and activity is distributed identically across all of those patterns—each of the patterns occurring the same number of times. The degree of dispersion can be affected by the nature of the patterns themselves, with certain patterns inherently biasing activity towards a low value of the symmetric index as a result of their self-symmetric nature. More specifically, for certain types of patterns, the application of symmetry operations produces the same or self-symmetric pattern. As a result, the possibilities for dispersion of activity between different patterns is reduced or, in certain cases, even eliminated altogether. The persistent excitation of self-symmetric patterns might be a marker of specific pathologies. As a particular example, the extreme case of activity being trapped in a pattern that does not allow (as a result of its self-symmetric nature) the possibility of any dispersion among different symmetrically-related patterns might correspond to an epileptic mode of activity [42].

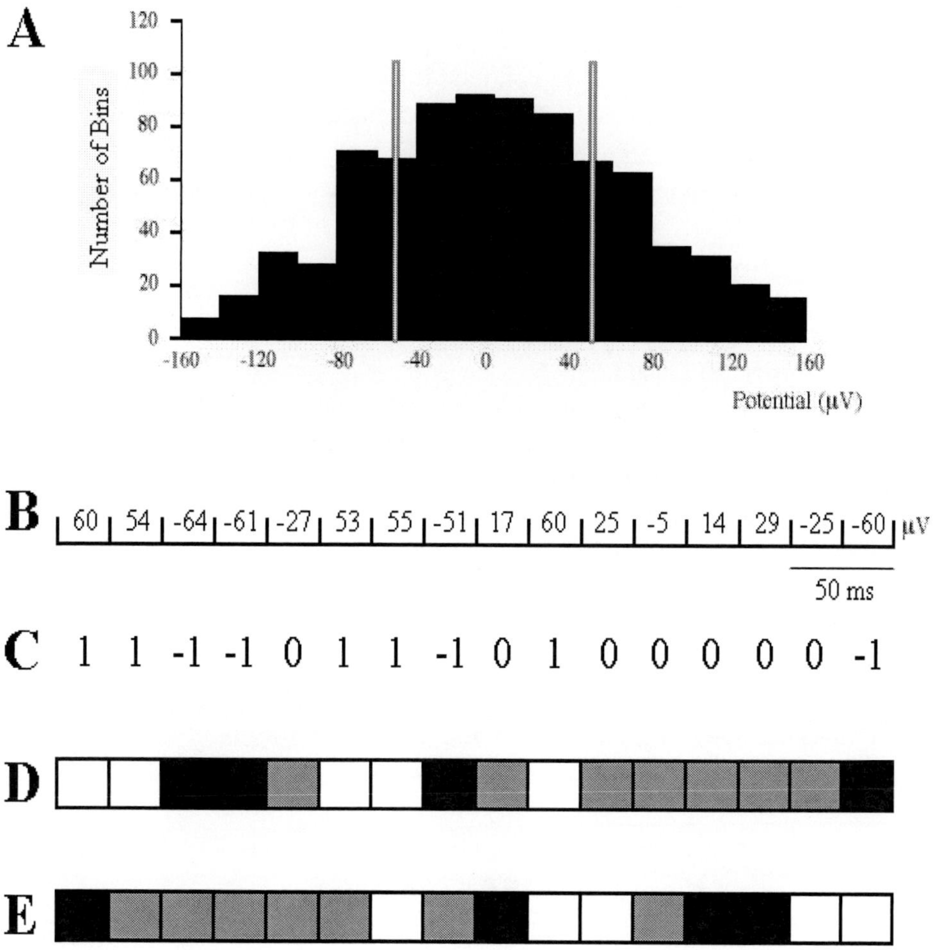

Figure 6. Example of EEG recording for several minutes from a single electrode binned and mapped in three level trion-like temporal patterns. (A) Choosing time bins of size 25 ms, the number of occurrences of the voltages are shown. The average, or 0 level, is determined by going from one standard deviation (σ) below the mean to 1 σ above, as shown by the vertical bars. The above average voltage level 1 corresponds to voltages greater than 1 σ above the mean, and that below level −1 is 1 σ below the mean. (B) A time sequence of voltages. (C) From the mapping in A, the time sequence B is put into the three level form. (D) The sequence in C is put into the gray scale as in the trion model evolutions in Figure 2 with white equal to 1, gray equal to 0, and black equal to −1. (E) The symmetry operator of time reversal acting on the pattern in (D) gives this family-related pattern.

The application of a symmetric pattern analysis towards the activity of the trion model in the sequential and creative regimes (Figure 2A–B) reveals quantitative differences in the symmetry index. In the sequential mode (Figure 2A), the activity evolves through sequences of (symmetrically) unrelated patterns. After an initial homogeneous period, an ST pattern occurs (beginning with the 8th row—the white and black diamond pattern) and continues for 3 cycles. (Allowing a small percentage of fluctuations identifies additional cycles of the pattern.) After this initial pattern a second pattern occurs for some cycles followed by a third pattern. Therefore, all of the activity over this time period consists of multiple cycles of symmetrically unrelated patterns, giving a low symmetry index value in the sequential mode, Figure 2A.

In contrast, a cursory examination of the patterns in the creative mode (Figure 2B) reveals that patterns occur for fewer continuous cycles and that many of the temporally dispersed patterns are related to each other by symmetry operations. For example, the pattern starting at the 14th row of the second column and the pattern occurring near the bottom of the second column are clearly related by a rotational symmetry (the later pattern is identical to the earlier occurring pattern but simply shifted to the right in the representation). Thus, the value of the symmetry index in the creative mode is sizable and clearly different from the sequential mode in these trion model simulations. Note that these insights apply to a single trion cortical column in a limited parameter range and should be taken as a potential guide for evaluating real cortical EEG data.

It is expected that different modes of cognitive activity will correspond to distinct regimes of the symmetry index. Examining the evolution of the symmetry index over time (using different time windows) could identify "switching" between different modes ("normal" function) or indicate that activity is trapped within a particular mode, which might be associated with the particular neuropathologies of schizophrenia or autism, as discussed earlier. Examining the symmetry index in the trion model involving many cortical columns and wide ranges of the parameters should give large insights into these regimes, providing the necessary context for understanding the values and time evolution in real data. This program of interplay of trion model simulations along with analysis of real cortical data gives *a potentially powerful context for understanding and diagnosing normal thought as well as certain neuropathologies, including a means for assessing efficacy of clinical treatment.*

Abbreviations

ST: spatial-temporal; MPs: trion model memory patterns; gMe: generalized Mozart effect.

References

[1] Mountcastle VB. An organizing principle for cerebral function: The unit module and the distributed system. In: Edelman GM, Mountcastle VB. *The Mindful Brain.* Cambridge, MA: MIT Press; 1977:1-50.

[2] Mountcastle VB. The columnar organization of the neocortex. *Brain.* 1997;120:701-722.

[3] Rakic P. Specifications of cerebral cortical areas. *Science*. 1988;241:170-176.

[4] Chenn A, Walsh CA. Regulation of cerebral cortical size by control of cell cycle exit in neural precursors. *Science.* 2002;297:365-369.

[5] Shaw GL, Silverman DJ, Pearson JC. Model of cortical organization embodying a basis for a theory of information processing and memory recall. *Proceedings of the National Academy of Sciences of the United States of America.* 1985;82:2364-2368.

[6] Leng X, Shaw GL. Toward a neural theory of higher brain function using music as a window. *Concepts in Neuroscience.* 1991;2:229-258.

[7] Shenoy KV, Kaufman J, McGrann JV, Shaw GL. Learning by selection in the trion model of cortex. *Cerebral Cortex.* 1993;3:239-248.

[8] McGrann JV, Shaw GL, Shenoy KV, Leng X, Mathews RB. Computation by symmetry operations in a structured model of the brain: recognition of rotational invariance and time reversal. *Physical Review E.* 1994;49:5830-5839.

[9] Shaw GL. *Keeping Mozart in Mind*. 2nd ed. San Diego, CA: Elsevier/Academic Press; 2004.

[10] Sardesai M, Figge C, Bodner M, et al. Reliable short-term memory in the trion model: toward a cortical language and grammar. *Biological Cybernetics.* 2001;84:173-182.

[11] Little WA. The existence of persistent states in the brain. *Mathematical Biosciences.* 1974;19:101-120.

[12] Little WA, Shaw GL. Analytic study of the storage capacity of a neural network. *Mathematical Biosciences.* 1978;39:281-290.

[13] Fisher ME, Selke W. Infinitely many commensurate phases in a simple Ising model. *Physical Review Letters.* 1980;44:1502-1505.

[14] Hebb DO. *Organization of Behavior*. New York, NY: Wiley; 1949.

[15] Rauscher FH, Shaw GL, Ky KN. Music and spatial task performance. *Nature.* 1993;365:611.

[16] Rauscher FH, Shaw GL, Ky KN. Listening to Mozart enhances spatial-temporal reasoning towards a neurophysiological basis. *Neuroscience Letters.* 1995;185:44-47.

[17] Johnson JK, Cotman C, Tasaki CS, Shaw GL. Enhancement in spatial-temporal reasoning after a Mozart listening condition in Alzheimer's disease. *Neurological Research.* 1998;20:61-72.

[18] Johnson JK, Shaw GL, Vuong M, Vuong S, Cotman CW. Short-term improvement on a visual-spatial task after music listening in Alzheimer's disease: a group study. *Activities, Adaptation & Aging.* 2002;26:37-50.

[19] Hughes JR, Daaboul Y, Fino JJ, Shaw GL. The "Mozart effect" on epileptiform activity. *Clinical EEG (Electroencephalography).* 1998;29:101-119.

[20] Hughes JR, Fino JJ, Melyn MA. Is there a chronic change of the "Mozart effect" on epileptiform activity? A case study. *Clinical EEG (Electroencephalography).* 1999;30:44-45.

[21] Rauscher FH, Robinson KD, Jens JJ. Improved maze learning through early music exposure in rats. *Neurological Research.* 1998;20:427-432.

[22] Aoun P, Jones T, Bodner M, Shaw GL. Long-term enhancement of maze learning in mice via generalized Mozart effect. Poster presented at: Society for Neuroscience 33rd annual meeting; New Orleans, LA; 2003.
[23] Sarnthein J, von Stein A, Rappelsberger P, Petsche H, Rauscher FH, Shaw GL. Persistent patterns of brain activity: an EEG coherence study of the positive effect of music on spatial-temporal reasoning. *Neurological Research.* 1997;19:107-116.
[24] Bodner M, Muftuler LT, Nalcioglu O, Shaw GL. fMRI study relevant to the Mozart effect: brain areas involved in spatial-temporal reasoning. *Neurological Research.* 2001;23:683-690.
[25] Muftuler LT, Bodner M, Shaw GL, Nalcioglu O. fMRI study on cortical activation correlates of listening to Mozart and of spatial-temporal processing. Poster presented at: Society for Neuroscience 33rd annual meeting; New Orleans, LA; 2003.
[26] Brothers L, Shaw GL, Wright EL. Durations of extended mental rehearsal are remarkably reproducible in higher level human performance. *Neurological Research.* 1993;15:413-416.
[27] Bodner M, Zhou Y-D, Shaw GL, Fuster JM. Symmetric temporal patterns in cortical spike trains during performance of a short-term memory task. *Neurological Research.* 1997;19:509-514.
[28] Rauscher FH, Shaw GL, Levine LJ, Wright EL, Dennis WR, Newcomb R. Music training causes long-term enhancement of preschool children's reasoning. *Neurological Research.* 1997;19:2-8.
[29] Graziano AB, Peterson M, Shaw GL. Enhanced learning of proportional math through music training and spatial-temporal training. *Neurological Research.* 1999;21:139-152.
[30] Peterson MR, Balzarini D, Bodner M, et al. Innate spatial-temporal reasoning and the identification of genius. *Neurological Research.* 2004;26:2-8.
[31] Bodner M, Derr C, Leng X, et al. The music-math connection. *Early Childhood Connections.* 2002;8:9-16.
[32] Shaw G, Bodner M, Patera J. Innate brain language and grammar: Implications for human language and music. In: Srinivasan SK, Vihayakumar A, eds. *Stochastic Point Processes*. New Delhi, India: Narosa Publishing; 2003:287-305.
[33] Bodner M, Shaw GL, Gabriel R, Johnson JK, Murias M, Swanson J. Detecting symmetric patterns in EEG data: a new method of analysis. *Clinical EEG (Electroencephalography).* 1999;30:143-150.
[34] Chomsky N. *Reflections on Language*. New York, NY: William Morrow; 1975.
[35] Pinker S. *The Language Instinct*. New York, NY: William Morrow; 1994.
[36] Hutsler JJ, Gazzaniga MS. The organization of human language cortex: special adaptation or common cortical design. *The Neuroscientist.* 1997;3:61-72.
[37] Ramus F, Hauser MD, Miller C, Morris D, Mehler J. Language discrimination by human newborns and by cotton-top tamarin monkeys. *Science.* 2000;288:349-351.
[38] Watson S, Wong L, Yee M, Bodner M, Shaw GL. Effective music training for children with autism. *Early Childhood Connections.* 2003;9:27-32.
[39] Smith AD, Olson RJ, Justice JB. Quantitative microdialysis of dopamine in the striatum: effect of circadian variation. *Journal of Neuroscience Methods.* 1992;44:33-41.

[40] McGrann JV, Shaw GL, Silverman DJ, Pearson JC. Higher-temperature phases of a structured neural model of cortex. *Physical Review A.* 1991;43:5678-5682.
[41] Mintz I, Gotow T, Triller A, Korn H. Serotonergic afferents on quantal release at central inhibitory synapses. *Science.* 1989;245:190-192.
[42] Leng X, McGrann JV, Shaw GL. Reversal of epileptic state by patterned electrical stimulation suggested by trion model calculations. *Neurological Research.* 1992;14:57-61.

ACKNOWLEDGEMENTS

It is with great pleasure that we dedicate this chapter to a towering giant in neuroscience, Vernon Mountcastle.

INDEX

A

B

C

D

E

F

G

H

I

J

K

L

M

N

O

P